Calculate with Confidence

Calculate with Confidence

Deborah C. Gray, RN, BSN, MA

Assistant Professor of Nursing

Bronx Community College

Bronx, NY

Contributor

Dorothy Thomas, RN, MSN

Associate Professor of Nursing

St. Louis Community College - Florissant Valley

St. Louis, MO

with 435 illustrations

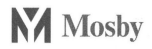

St. Louis Baltimore Boston Chicago London Madrid Philadelphia Sydney Toronto

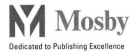
Mosby
Dedicated to Publishing Excellence

Publisher: Alison Miller
Editor-in-Chief: Nancy Coon
Managing Editor: Jeff Burnham
Developmental Editors: Jolynn Gower, Linda Caldwell
Project Manager: Carol Sullivan Wiseman
Production Editor: Shannon Canty
Designer: Betty Schulz
Manufacturing Supervisor: John Babrick
Design and Layout: Ken Wendling
Cover Illustration: Rokusek Design

Printed in the United States of America
Composition by Wordbench
Printing/binding by Von Hoffmann Press

Mosby–Year Book, Inc.
11830 Westline Industrial Drive
St. Louis, MO 63146

Library of Congress Cataloging in Publication Data

Gray, Deborah, RN.
    Calculate with confidence / Deborah Gray ; contributor, Dorothy Thomas.
      p. cm.
    ISBN 0-8016-6961-8
      1. Nursing—Mathematics.   2. Pharmaceutical arithmetic.
  I. Thomas, Dorothy, RN.   II. Title.
      [DNLM: 1. Mathematics—nurses' instruction.   2. Drugs—administration & dosage—nurses' instruction.   QV 748 G778c 1993]
RT68.G43   1993
615'.4—dc20
DNLM/DLC
for Library of Congress   93-36390
                                      CIP

95 96 97   /   9 8 7 6 5 4 3

Preface

Calculate with Confidence is written to meet the needs of the current and potential practitioner of nursing at any level. This book can be utilized for in-service education programs and as a reference for the inactive nurse returning to the work world. This book is suitable for courses of instruction whose content reflects the calculation of dosage and solutions and for any health-care professional whose responsibilities include safe administration of medications and solutions to clients in diverse clinical settings.

Despite the advent of what is called *unit dose* in some institutions, it doesn't completely relinquish health professionals from the responsibility of calculation. A working knowledge in the area of dosage calculation is necessary, regardless of the medication system used in an institution.

Calculate with Confidence offers a simplified approach to the calculation and administration of drug dosages. The book includes theoretical and mathematical concepts related to the administration of medications. An increased need for competency in basic math as a prerequisite to dosage calculation has mandated including a review of basic math skills. A step-by-step approach to dosage calculation by the various routes of administration is included.

Information related to systems of measurements and conversions is discussed. Numerous illustrations including full-color drug labels, syringes, and equipment used in medication administration have been included to enhance learning and application to the clinical setting. Practice problems have been included in each section to test the mastery of content presented. In the area of basic math a pretest and posttest have been included. The pretest will allow students to identify areas that need or do not need review. Shading of syringes has been used to allow for visualization of dosages. Rationale for answers to dosage calculation problems has been included to enhance understanding of principles and answers relating to dosages. Formulas that are simplified and encourage understanding of the dynamics in calculation are presented. Alternative vocabulary has been used in certain areas to enhance the learning of some material presented.

It is my hope that the use of this book will help nurses and potential nurses to calculate dosages accurately and with confidence and ensure administration of medications safely to all clients, which is the primary responsibility of nurses.

Deborah C. Gray

Acknowledgements

I wish to extend sincere gratitude and appreciation to my family, friends and colleagues for their support and encouragement during the time I was compiling this text.

I am indebted to the Nursing Department at Bronx Community College, who listened to me, made pertinent suggestions, helped with validation of content used in this text, and brought me problems from clinical situations, as well as allowing me to use the computerized Assisted Programs in Pharmacology copyrighted by Research Foundation that assisted with development of content, especially on Intravenous Calculations. You told me "I could fly" and your encouragement helped me to "soar like an eagle".

I am sincerely grateful to Professor Marie-Louise Nickerson of the English Department at Bronx Community College who nurtured and encouraged me to consider publication and worked closely with me on a project that resulted in the development of this text for publication. I am grateful to Dr. Gerald S. Lieblich, Chairperson of the Department of Mathematics, who took the time to review and validate content, as well as making pertinent suggestions for the unit on Basic Math. Special thanks to the reviewers; their comments and suggestions were invaluable during the preparation of this text. Thanks to students past and present at Bronx Community College Nursing program that brought some practice problems to my attention.

Thanks to the following companies and hospitals for permission to reproduce records used in the chapters dealing with Medication Records. TDS Health Care Systems Corporation, New York City and Hospitals Corporation, St. Barnabas Hospital (Bronx, NY) and Jack D. Weiler Hospital, a division of Montefiore Medical Center. A special thanks to Norma Dison, Alice J. Smith, Ruth K. Radcliff, Sheila J. Ogden, and Laura K. Hart for use of some illustrations and drug labels from your texts.

I am especially grateful to the staff at Mosby, especially Beverly Copland, Susan Epstein, and Shannon Canty for their support and help in planning, writing, and producing the text. Thanks for all your encouragement, nurturing, and support at times when I felt I wasn't going to complete this project.

To Reginald Morris, thanks for your help and support in making the final drafting of the manuscript for this book a reality.

Finally I wish to thank all of the pharmaceutical companies for permission to reproduce their drug labels in this text.

Dedication

To my family, friends, colleagues, students past and present, but especially with love to my children Cameron, Kimberly, Kanin, and Cory who much of the time had to manage without me while I worked on this book as well as coped with my frustrations. You all light up my life and supported me in whatever I had to do.

To the current practitioner of nursing and future nurses, I hope this book will be valuable in teaching the basic principles of medication administration and ensure safe administration of medications to all clients.

Contents

Unit One   Math Review

Unit Two   Systems of Measurement

Unit Three   Methods of Administration and Calculation

Unit Four   Oral and Parenteral Doseforms, Insulin, and Pediatric Dosage Calculations

Unit Five   Basic I.V., Heparin, and Critical Care Calculations

Unit One

Math Review

This section contains a review of basic math skills that will assist in computation of dosages.

A pretest and a posttest have been included in this section, offering an opportunity for students to evaluate their skills.

Pretest

This test is designed to test your ability in the basic math areas reviewed in Unit I. The test consists of 50 questions that are worth 2 points each. The passing score is 70 or better. If you miss three or more questions in any section, review the chapter relating to the content. Answers are found at the back of the book.

Express the following in Roman numerals.

1. 9 _____

2. 16 _____

3. 23 _____

4. $10\frac{1}{2}$ _____

5. 22 _____

Express the following in Arabic numbers.

6. x̄īss _____

7. x̄īī _____

8. x̄vīīī _____

9. x̄xīv _____

10. v̄ī _____

Reduce the following fractions to lowest terms.

11. $\frac{14}{21}$ _____

12. $\frac{25}{100}$ _____

13. $\frac{2}{150}$ _____

14. $\dfrac{24}{30}$ _____

15. $\dfrac{24}{36}$ _____

Perform the indicated operations; reduce to lowest terms where necessary.

16. $\dfrac{2}{3} \div \dfrac{3}{9} =$ _____

17. $4 \div \dfrac{3}{4} =$ _____

18. $\dfrac{2}{5} + \dfrac{1}{9} =$ _____

19. $7\dfrac{1}{7} - 2\dfrac{5}{6} =$ _____

20. $4\dfrac{2}{3} \times 4 =$ _____

Change the following fractions to decimals; express your answer to the nearest tenth.

21. $\dfrac{6}{7}$ _____

22. $\dfrac{6}{20}$ _____

23. $\dfrac{2}{3}$ _____

24. $\dfrac{7}{8}$ _____

Indicate the largest fraction in each group.

25. $\dfrac{3}{4}, \dfrac{4}{5}, \dfrac{7}{8}$ _____

26. $\dfrac{7}{12}, \dfrac{11}{12}, \dfrac{4}{12}$ _____

Perform the indicated operations with decimals.

27. $20.1 + 67.35 =$ _____

28. 0.008 + 5.0 = _____

29. 4.6 × 8.72 = _____

30. 56.47 − 8.7 = _____

Divide the following decimals; express your answer to the nearest tenth.

31. 7.5 ÷ 0.004 = _____

32. 45 ÷ 1.9 = _____

33. 84.7 ÷ 2.3 = _____

Indicate the larger decimal in each group.

34. 0.674, 0.659 _____

35. 0.375, 0.37, 0.038 _____

36. 0.25, 0.6, 0.175 _____

Solve for x, the unknown value.

37. $8 : 2 = 48 : x$, $x =$ _____

38. $x : 300 = 1 : 150$, $x =$ _____

39. $\dfrac{1}{10} : x = \dfrac{1}{2} : 15$, $x =$ _____

40. $0.4 : 1 = 0.2 : x$, $x =$ _____

Round off to the nearest tenth.

41. 0.43 = _____

42. 0.66 = _____

43. 1.47 = _____

Round off to the nearest hundredth.

44. 0.735 = _____

45. 0.834 = _____

46. 1.227 = _____

Complete the table below, expressing the measures in their equivalents where indicated. Reduce to lowest terms where necessary.

	Percent	Decimal	Ratio	Fraction
47.	6%	_____	_____	_____
48.	35%	_____	_____	_____
49.	_____	_____	_____	5 1/4
50.	_____	0.015	_____	_____

1 Roman Numerals

Objectives

After reviewing this chapter the student will be able to do the following:

1. Change Roman numerals to Arabic numbers
2. Change Arabic numbers to Roman numerals

The Roman numeral system dates back to ancient Roman times and uses letters to designate amounts. Roman numerals are used a great deal, especially in the apothecaries' system of measurement. In the Arabic system numbers, not letters, are used to express amounts. The Arabic system also uses fractions (1/2) and decimals (0.5).

To calculate drug dosages the nurse needs to know both Roman numerals and Arabic numbers. Lower case letters are usually used to express Roman numerals. The Roman numerals that you will see most often in the calculation of dosages are built upon the basic symbols i, v, and x. To prevent errors in interpretation a line is sometimes drawn over the symbol. If this line is used, the lower case "i" is dotted above the line, not below.

Example: two = ii

When the symbol for 1/2 is used in conjunction with Roman numerals, the symbol (ss) is placed at the end.

Example: three and a half = iiiss

The following box shows the common Arabic equivalents for Roman numerals. Review this list before proceeding to the rules pertaining to Roman numerals.

Arabic number	Roman numeral
$\frac{1}{2}$	ss, or $\overline{ss}$
1	i, or $\overline{i}$, I
2	ii, or $\overline{ii}$, II
3	iii, or $\overline{iii}$, III
4	iv, or $\overline{iv}$, IV
5	v, or $\overline{v}$, V
6	vi, or $\overline{vi}$, VI
7	vii, or $\overline{vii}$, VII
8	viii, or $\overline{viii}$, VIII
9	ix, or $\overline{ix}$, IX
10	x, or $\overline{x}$, X
15	xv, or $\overline{xv}$, XV
20	xx, or $\overline{xx}$, XX
30	xxx, or $\overline{xxx}$, XXX

To add, place a Roman numeral that is of lesser value after one of greater value. The numeral of lesser value is then added to the one of greater value. The same numeral is never repeated more than three times.

Example: 25 = $\overline{xxv}$

16 = $\overline{xvi}$

Practice addition, and write the following in Roman numerals:

1. 15   _____

2. 13   _____

3. 30   _____

4. 11   _____

To subtract, place a Roman numeral of lesser value before a numeral of greater value. The numeral of lesser value is then subtracted from the one of greater value.

Example: $\overline{ix}$ = 9

Example: $\overline{xxiv}$ = 24

$\overline{xx}$ = 20, $\overline{iv}$ = 4, v being placed

after $\overline{i}$ is 5 − 1 or 4

10 + 10 and 5 − 1 = 20 + 4 = 24

Practice subtraction on the following problems.

5. 14 _____

6. 29 _____

7. 4 _____

8. 19 _____

Chapter Review

Write the following Arabic numbers as Roman numerals.

1. 6 _____

2. 30 _____

3. $1\frac{1}{2}$ _____

4. 27 _____

5. 12 _____

6. 18 _____

7. 20 _____

8. 3 _____

9. 21 _____

10. 26 _____

Write the following Roman numerals as Arabic numbers.

11. $\overline{\text{viiss}}$ _____

12. $\overline{\text{xix}}$ _____

13. $\overline{\text{xv}}$ _____

14. $\overline{\text{xxx}}$ _____

15. $\overline{\text{ss}}$ _____

16. $\overline{\text{iii}}$ _____

17. $\overline{\text{xxii}}$ _____

18. $\overline{\text{xvi}}$ _____

19. $\overline{\text{v}}$ _____

20. $\overline{\text{xxvii}}$ _____

2 Fractions

Objectives

After reviewing this chapter the student will be able to do the following:

1. Compare the size of fractions
2. Add and subtract fractions
3. Divide and multiply fractions
4. Reduce fractions to lowest terms

Understanding fractions is necessary since the nurse often encounters fractions when dealing with apothecaries' measures in dosage calculation.

A fraction is a part of a whole number. It is a division of a whole into units or parts.

Example: $\frac{1}{2}$ is a whole divided into two parts.

Fractions are composed of two parts: a numerator, which is the top number, and a denominator, which is the bottom number.

$$\frac{\text{Numerator}}{\text{Denominator}} : \frac{\text{how many parts of the whole you are taking}}{\text{how many equal parts the whole is divided into}}$$

Example: In the fraction $\frac{5}{6}$, 5 is the numerator, and 6 is the denominator.

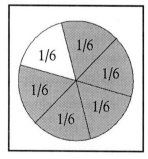

Figure 2.1 Diagram representing fractions of a whole. 5 parts shaded out of 6 parts represents

$$\frac{5}{6} \quad \frac{\text{Numerator}}{\text{Denominator}}$$

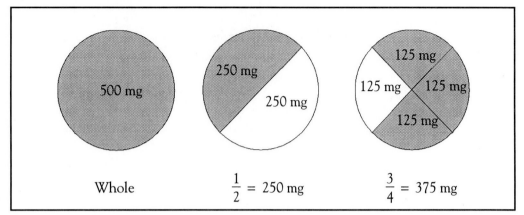

Figure 2.2 Fraction Pie Charts

Types of Fractions

Proper Fraction: Numerator is less than the denominator.

Examples: $\dfrac{1}{8}$, $\dfrac{5}{6}$, $\dfrac{7}{8}$, $\dfrac{1}{150}$

Improper Fraction: Numerator is larger than, or equal to, the denominator.

Examples: $\dfrac{3}{2}$, $\dfrac{7}{5}$, $\dfrac{300}{150}$, $\dfrac{4}{4}$

Mixed Number: Whole number and a fraction.

Examples: $3\dfrac{1}{3}$, $5\dfrac{1}{8}$, $9\dfrac{1}{6}$, $25\dfrac{7}{8}$

Complex Fraction: Numerator, denominator, or both, are fractions.

Examples: $\dfrac{3\frac{1}{2}}{2}$, $\dfrac{\frac{1}{3}}{\frac{1}{2}}$, $\dfrac{2}{1\frac{1}{4}}$, $\dfrac{2}{\frac{1}{150}}$

Whole Numbers: Have an unexpressed denominator of one (1).

Examples: $1 = \dfrac{1}{1}$, $3 = \dfrac{3}{1}$, $6 = \dfrac{6}{1}$, $100 = \dfrac{100}{1}$

An improper fraction can be changed to a mixed number or whole number by dividing the numerator by the denominator.

Examples: $\dfrac{6}{5} = 6 \div 5 = 1\dfrac{1}{5}$, $\dfrac{100}{25} = 100 \div 25 = 4$

A mixed number can be changed to an improper fraction by multiplying the whole number by the denominator, adding it to the numerator, and placing the sum over the denominator.

$$\textbf{Example:} \quad 5\frac{1}{8} = \frac{(5 \times 8) + 1}{8} = \frac{41}{8}$$

Comparing the size of fractions is important in the administration of medications. Here are some basic rules to keep in mind when comparing fractions.

---

1. If the numerators are the same, the fraction with the smaller denominator has the larger value.

   Example 1: $\frac{1}{2}$ is larger than $\frac{1}{3}$

   Example 2: $\frac{1}{150}$ is larger than $\frac{1}{300}$

2. If the denominators are the same, the fraction with the larger numerator has the larger value.

   Example 1: $\frac{3}{4}$ is larger than $\frac{1}{4}$

   Example 2: $\frac{3}{100}$ is larger than $\frac{1}{100}$

Fractions with different denominators can be compared by changing both fractions to fractions with the same denominator. This is done by finding the lowest common denominator (LCD) or the lowest number evenly divisible by the denominators of the fractions being compared.

Example: Which is larger, $\frac{3}{4}$ or $\frac{4}{5}$?

Solution: The lowest common denominator is 20, because it is the smallest number that can be divided by both denominators evenly. Change each fraction to the same terms by dividing the lowest common denominator by the denominator and multiplying that answer by the numerator. The answer obtained from this is the new numerator. The numerators are then placed over the lowest common denominator.

For the fraction $\frac{3}{4}$: $20 \div 4 = 5$; $5 \times 3 = 15$; therefore $\frac{3}{4}$ becomes $\frac{15}{20}$.

For the fraction $\frac{4}{5}$: $20 \div 5 = 4$; $4 \times 4 = 16$; so $\frac{4}{5}$ becomes $\frac{16}{20}$.

Practice Problems

Circle the fraction with the lesser value in each of the following sets.

1. $\dfrac{6}{30}, \dfrac{4}{5}$

2. $\dfrac{5}{4}, \dfrac{6}{8}$

3. $\dfrac{1}{75}, \dfrac{1}{100}, \dfrac{1}{150}$

4. $\dfrac{6}{18}, \dfrac{7}{18}, \dfrac{8}{18}$

5. $\dfrac{4}{5}, \dfrac{7}{5}, \dfrac{3}{5}$

6. $\dfrac{4}{8}, \dfrac{1}{8}, \dfrac{3}{8}$

7. $\dfrac{1}{40}, \dfrac{1}{10}, \dfrac{1}{5}$

8. $\dfrac{1}{300}, \dfrac{1}{200}, \dfrac{1}{175}$

9. $\dfrac{4}{24}, \dfrac{5}{24}, \dfrac{10}{24}$

10. $\dfrac{4}{3}, \dfrac{1}{2}, \dfrac{1}{6}$

Circle the fraction with the higher value in each of the following sets.

11. $\dfrac{6}{8}, \dfrac{5}{9}$

12. $\dfrac{7}{6}, \dfrac{2}{3}$

13. $\dfrac{1}{72}, \dfrac{6}{12}, \dfrac{1}{24}$

14. $\dfrac{1}{10}, \dfrac{1}{6}, \dfrac{1}{8}$

15. $\dfrac{1}{75}, \dfrac{1}{125}, \dfrac{1}{225}$

16. $\dfrac{2}{5}, \dfrac{6}{5}, \dfrac{3}{5}$

17. $\dfrac{1}{8}, \dfrac{4}{6}, \dfrac{1}{4}$ $\dfrac{3}{24}$ $\dfrac{16}{24}$ $\dfrac{6}{24}$

18. $\dfrac{7}{9}, \dfrac{5}{9}, \dfrac{8}{9}$

19. $\dfrac{1}{10}, \dfrac{1}{50}, \dfrac{1}{150}$

20. $\dfrac{2}{15}, \dfrac{1}{15}, \dfrac{6}{15}$

Reducing Fractions

Fractions should always be reduced to their lowest terms.

> To reduce a fraction to its lowest terms, the numerator and denominator are each divided by the largest number by which they are both evenly divisible.

Example 1: Reduce the fraction $\dfrac{6}{20}$.

Solution: Both numerator and denominator are evenly divisible by 2.

$$6 \div 2 = 3 ; \quad 20 \div 2 = 10$$

$$\dfrac{6}{20} = \dfrac{3}{10}$$

Example 2: Reduce the fraction $\dfrac{75}{100}$.

Solution: Both numerator and denominator are evenly divisible by 25.

$$75 \div 25 = 3 ; \quad 100 \div 25 = 4$$

$$\dfrac{75}{100} = \dfrac{3}{4}$$

Practice Problems

Reduce the following fractions to their lowest terms.

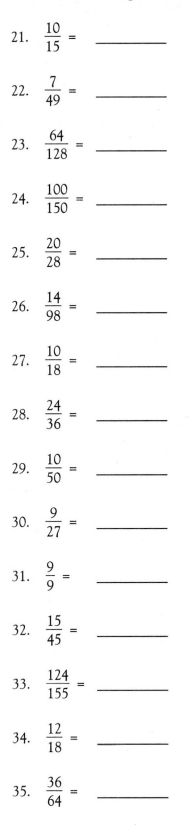

21. $\dfrac{10}{15}$ = _____

22. $\dfrac{7}{49}$ = _____

23. $\dfrac{64}{128}$ = _____

24. $\dfrac{100}{150}$ = _____

25. $\dfrac{20}{28}$ = _____

26. $\dfrac{14}{98}$ = _____

27. $\dfrac{10}{18}$ = _____

28. $\dfrac{24}{36}$ = _____

29. $\dfrac{10}{50}$ = _____

30. $\dfrac{9}{27}$ = _____

31. $\dfrac{9}{9}$ = _____

32. $\dfrac{15}{45}$ = _____

33. $\dfrac{124}{155}$ = _____

34. $\dfrac{12}{18}$ = _____

35. $\dfrac{36}{64}$ = _____

Adding Fractions

> To add fractions with the same denominator, add the numerators, place the sum over the denominator and reduce to lowest terms.

Example 1: $\dfrac{1}{6} + \dfrac{4}{6} = \dfrac{5}{6}$

Example 2: $\dfrac{1}{6} + \dfrac{3}{6} + \dfrac{4}{6} = \dfrac{8}{6}$

$\dfrac{8}{6} = \dfrac{4}{3}$ (See reduction of fractions)

$\dfrac{4}{3} = 1\dfrac{1}{3}$

(Note: In addition to reducing to lowest terms in example 2, the improper fraction was changed to a mixed number.)

> To add fractions with different denominators, change fractions to their equivalent fraction with the least common denominator, add the numerators, write the sum over the common denominator and reduce if necessary.

Example 1: $\dfrac{1}{4} + \dfrac{1}{3}$

Solution: The least common denominator is 12.
Change to equivalent fractions.

$$\dfrac{1}{4} = \dfrac{3}{12}$$

$$+\ \dfrac{1}{3} = \dfrac{4}{12}$$

$$\overline{\qquad\qquad}$$

$$\dfrac{7}{12}$$

Example 2: $\dfrac{1}{2} + 1\dfrac{1}{3} + \dfrac{2}{4}$

Solution: Change the mixed number $1\dfrac{1}{3}$ to $\dfrac{4}{3}$, find the common denominator, change fractions to equivalent fractions, add, and reduce if necessary. The least common denominator is 12.

$$\dfrac{1}{2} = \dfrac{6}{12}$$

$$\dfrac{4}{3} = \dfrac{16}{12}$$

$$+ \quad \dfrac{2}{4} = \dfrac{6}{12}$$

$$\overline{\hspace{3cm}}$$

$$\dfrac{28}{12} = 2\dfrac{4}{12} = 2\dfrac{1}{3}$$

Subtraction of Fractions

To subtract fractions with the same denominator, subtract the numerators, and place this amount over the denominator. Reduce to lowest terms, if necessary.

Example 1: $\dfrac{5}{4} - \dfrac{3}{4} = \dfrac{2}{4} = \dfrac{1}{2}$

Example 2: $2\dfrac{1}{6} - \dfrac{5}{6}$

Solution: Change the mixed number $2\dfrac{1}{6}$ to $\dfrac{13}{6}$.

$$\dfrac{13}{6} - \dfrac{5}{6} = \dfrac{8}{6} = \dfrac{4}{3} = 1\dfrac{1}{3}$$

> To subtract fractions with different denominators, find the lowest common denominator, change to equivalent fractions, subtract the numerators, and place the sum over the common denominator. Reduce to lowest terms, if necessary.

Example 1: $\dfrac{15}{6} - \dfrac{3}{5}$

Solution: The lowest common denominator is 30. Change to equivalent fractions and subtract.

$$\dfrac{15}{6} = \dfrac{75}{30}$$

$$-\ \dfrac{3}{5} = \dfrac{18}{30}$$

$$\dfrac{57}{30} = 1\dfrac{27}{30} = 1\dfrac{9}{10}$$

Example 2: $2\dfrac{1}{5} - \dfrac{4}{3}$

Solution: Change the mixed number $2\dfrac{1}{5}$ to $\dfrac{11}{5}$. Find the lowest common denominator, change to equivalent fractions, subtract, and reduce if necessary. The lowest common denominator is 15.

$$\dfrac{11}{5} = \dfrac{33}{15}$$

$$-\ \dfrac{4}{3} = \dfrac{20}{15}$$

$$\dfrac{13}{15}$$

Multiplying Fractions

> To multiply fractions, multiply the numerators, multiply the denominators, and reduce, if necessary.

Example 1: $\dfrac{3}{4} \times \dfrac{2}{5} = \dfrac{6}{20} = \dfrac{3}{10}$

(Note: If fractions are not in lowest terms, reduction can be done before multiplication.)

Example 2: $6 \times \dfrac{5}{6}$

$$\dfrac{6 \times 5}{6} = \dfrac{30}{6} = 5$$

OR

$$\dfrac{6}{1} \times \dfrac{5}{6} = \dfrac{30}{6} = 5$$

(Note: The whole number 6 is expressed as a fraction here, by placing one (1) as the denominator.)

Example 3: $3\dfrac{1}{3} \times 2\dfrac{1}{2}$

Solution: Change the mixed numbers to improper fractions. Proceed with multiplication.

$$3\dfrac{1}{3} = \dfrac{10}{3} ; \quad 2\dfrac{1}{2} = \dfrac{5}{2}$$

$$\dfrac{10}{3} \times \dfrac{5}{2} = \dfrac{50}{6} = 8\dfrac{2}{6} = 8\dfrac{1}{3}$$

Dividing Fractions

> To divide fractions, invert (turn upside down) the second fraction (divisor), and multiply. Reduce where necessary.

Example 1: $\dfrac{3}{4} \div \dfrac{2}{3}$

Solution: $\dfrac{3}{4} \times \dfrac{3}{2} = \dfrac{9}{8} = 1\dfrac{1}{8}$

Example 2: $1\dfrac{3}{5} \div 2\dfrac{1}{10}$

Solution: Change mixed numbers to improper fractions. Proceed with steps of division.

$$1\dfrac{3}{5} = \dfrac{8}{5}; \ 2\dfrac{1}{10} = \dfrac{21}{10}$$

$$\dfrac{8}{5} \times \dfrac{10}{21} = \dfrac{80}{105} = \dfrac{16}{21}$$

Example 3: $5 \div \dfrac{1}{2}$

Solution: $5 \times \dfrac{2}{1} = \dfrac{10}{1}$

OR

$$\dfrac{5}{1} \times \dfrac{2}{1} = \dfrac{10}{1} = 10$$

(Note: When doing dosage calculations that involve division, the fractions may be

written as follows: $\dfrac{\frac{1}{4}}{\frac{1}{2}}$. In this case $\dfrac{1}{4}$ is the numerator, and $\dfrac{1}{2}$ is the denominator.

Therefore the problem is set up as: $\dfrac{1}{4} \div \dfrac{1}{2}$, which becomes $\dfrac{1}{4} \times \dfrac{2}{1} = \dfrac{2}{4} = \dfrac{1}{2}$.)

Chapter Review

Change the following improper fractions to mixed numbers, and reduce to lowest terms.

1. $\dfrac{10}{8}$ = _____

2. $\dfrac{30}{4}$ = _____

3. $\dfrac{22}{6}$ = _____

4. $\dfrac{11}{4}$ = _____

5. $\dfrac{59}{14}$ = _____

6. $\dfrac{67}{10}$ = _____

7. $\dfrac{9}{2}$ = _____

8. $\dfrac{11}{5}$ = _____

9. $\dfrac{64}{15}$ = _____

10. $\dfrac{100}{13}$ = _____

Change the following mixed numbers to improper fractions.

11. $2\dfrac{1}{2}$ = _____

12. $7\dfrac{3}{8}$ = _____

13. $8\dfrac{3}{5}$ = _____

14. $16\dfrac{1}{4}$ = _____

15. $3\frac{1}{5} =$ _____

16. $2\frac{3}{5} =$ _____

17. $8\frac{4}{10} =$ _____

18. $9\frac{1}{4} =$ _____

19. $12\frac{3}{4} =$ _____

20. $6\frac{5}{7} =$ _____

Add the following fractions and mixed numbers. Reduce to lowest terms.

21. $\frac{2}{5} + \frac{1}{3} + \frac{7}{10} =$ _____

22. $\frac{1}{4} + \frac{1}{6} + \frac{1}{8} =$ _____

23. $20\frac{1}{2} + \frac{1}{4} + \frac{5}{4} =$ _____

24. $\frac{1}{2} + \frac{1}{5} =$ _____

25. $6\frac{1}{4} + \frac{2}{9} + \frac{1}{36} =$ _____

Subtract the following fractions and mixed numbers. Reduce to lowest terms.

26. $\frac{6}{4} - \frac{1}{2} =$ _____

27. $2\frac{1}{4} - 1\frac{1}{2} =$ _____

28. $2\frac{3}{4} - \frac{1}{4} =$ _____

29. $\frac{4}{5} - \frac{1}{6} =$ _____

30. $\dfrac{4}{9} - \dfrac{3}{9} =$ _____

31. $\dfrac{4}{5} - \dfrac{1}{4} =$ _____

32. $\dfrac{4}{6} - \dfrac{3}{8} =$ _____

33. $4\dfrac{1}{6} - 1\dfrac{1}{3} =$ _____

34. $\dfrac{8}{5} - \dfrac{1}{3} =$ _____

35. $\dfrac{4}{7} - \dfrac{1}{3} =$ _____

Multiply the following fractions and mixed numbers. Reduce the answers to lowest terms.

36. $\dfrac{1}{3} \times \dfrac{4}{12} =$ _____

37. $2\dfrac{7}{8} \times 3\dfrac{1}{4} =$ _____

38. $8 \times 1\dfrac{3}{4} =$ _____

39. $15 \times \dfrac{2}{3} =$ _____

40. $36 \times \dfrac{3}{4} =$ _____

41. $\dfrac{5}{4} \times \dfrac{2}{4} =$ _____

42. $\dfrac{2}{5} \times \dfrac{1}{6} =$ _____

43. $\dfrac{3}{10} \times \dfrac{4}{12} =$ _____

44. $\dfrac{1}{9} \times \dfrac{7}{3} =$ _____

45. $\dfrac{10}{25} \times \dfrac{5}{3} =$ _____

Divide the following fractions and mixed numbers. Reduce to lowest terms.

46. $2\dfrac{1}{3} \div 4\dfrac{1}{6} =$ _____

47. $\dfrac{1}{3} \div \dfrac{1}{2} =$ _____

48. $25 \div 12\dfrac{1}{2} =$ _____

49. $\dfrac{7}{8} \div 2\dfrac{1}{4} =$ _____

50. $\dfrac{6}{2} \div \dfrac{3}{4} =$ _____

51. $\dfrac{4}{6} \div \dfrac{1}{2} =$ _____

52. $\dfrac{3}{10} \div \dfrac{5}{25} =$ _____

53. $3 \div \dfrac{2}{5} =$ _____

54. $\dfrac{15}{30} \div 10 =$ _____

55. $\dfrac{8}{3} \div \dfrac{8}{3} =$ _____

3 Decimals

Objectives

After reviewing this chapter the student will be able to do the following:

1. Read and write decimals
2. Compare the size of decimals
3. Change fractions to decimals and decimals to fractions
4. Add, subtract, multiply, and divide decimals
5. Round off decimals to the nearest tenth or hundredth

An understanding of decimals is crucial to the calculation of dosages. Most medications are ordered in metric measures that use decimals.

Example: Digoxin 0.125 mg.

A decimal is a fraction that has a denominator that is a multiple of 10. A decimal fraction is written as a decimal by the use of a decimal point (.). The decimal point is used to indicate place value. Some examples are as follows:

Fraction	Decimal Number
$\dfrac{3}{10}$	0.3
$\dfrac{18}{100}$	0.18
$\dfrac{175}{1000}$	0.175

The decimal point represents the center. Notice that the numbers written to the right of the decimal point are decimal fractions with a denominator of 10, or a multiple of 10, and represent a value that is less than one (1) or part of one (1). Numbers written to the left of the decimal point are whole numbers, or have a value of one (1) or greater.

> The decimal value is determined by its position to the right of the decimal point.

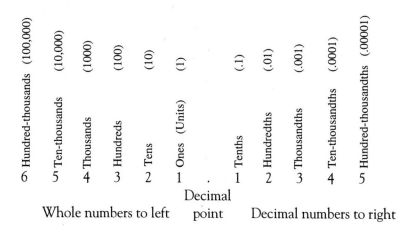

Hundred-thousands (100,000)	Ten-thousands (10,000)	Thousands (1000)	Hundreds (100)	Tens (10)	Ones (Units) (1)		Tenths (.1)	Hundredths (.01)	Thousandths (.001)	Ten-thousandths (.0001)	Hundred-thousandths (.00001)
6	5	4	3	2	1	.	1	2	3	4	5

Decimal

Whole numbers to left   point   Decimal numbers to right

The easiest way to understand decimals is to memorize the place values.

The **first** place to the right of the decimal is tenths.

The **second** place to the right of the decimal is hundredths.

The **third** place to the right of the decimal is thousandths.

The **fourth** place to the right of the decimal is ten-thousandths.

In the calculation of medication dosages it is only necessary to consider three figures after the decimal point (thousandths): e.g., 0.375 mg. It is important to place a zero (0) in front of the decimal point to indicate that it is a fraction, when there is no whole number before it. This will emphasize its value and prevent errors in interpretation.

Reading and Writing Decimals

Once you have an understanding of the place value of decimals, reading and writing them is simple.

To read the decimal numbers read:

(1) The whole number,

(2) the decimal point as "and", and

(3) the decimal fraction.

Example 1: The number 8.3 is read as "eight and three tenths."

Example 2:   The number 0.4 is read as "four tenths."

Example 3:   The decimal 4.06 is read as "four and six hundredths."

Decimals can be read as "point" instead of "and" to indicate a decimal point. When there is only a zero (0) to the left of the decimal, as in example 2, the zero is not read aloud.

To write a decimal number write the following:

(1) The whole number. (If there is no whole number, write zero [0].)

(2) The decimal point to indicate the place value of the rightmost number.

(3) The decimal portion of the number.

Example 1:   Written, seven and five tenths = 7.5

Example 2:   Written, one-hundred-twenty-five thousandths = 0.125

Example 3:   Written, five tenths = 0.5

Practice Problems

Write each of the following numbers in word form:

1.   8.35   _____

2.   11.001 _____

3.   4.57   _____

4.   5.0007 _____

5.   10.5   _____

6.   0.163   _____

Write each of the following in decimal form:

7.   four tenths   _____

8.   eighty-four and seven hundredths   _____

9.   seven hundredths   _____

10.   two and twenty-three hundredths   _____

11.   five hundredths   _____

12.   nine thousandths   _____

Comparing the Value of Decimals

Understanding which decimal is larger or smaller is important in the calculation of dosage problems.

> When decimal numbers contain whole numbers, the whole numbers are compared to determine which is greater.

Example 1:   4.8 is larger than 2.9

Example 2:   11.5 is larger than 7.5

Example 3:   7.37 is larger than 6.94

If the whole numbers being compared are the same, for example 5.6 and 5.2, or if there is no whole number, for example 0.45 and 0.37, then the number in the tenths place determines which decimal is larger.

> If the whole numbers are the same or zero, the decimal with the higher number in the tenths place has the larger value.

Example 1:   0.45 is larger than 0.37

Example 2:   1.75 is larger than 1.25

> If the whole numbers are the same or zero and the numbers in the tenths place are the same, then the decimal with the higher number in the hundredths place has the larger value, and so forth.

Example 1:   0.67 is larger than 0.66

Example 2:   0.17 is larger than 0.14

Note: The addition of zeros at the end of a decimal does not alter its value; they are therefore unnecessary.

Example 1:   0.2 is the same as 0.2000, 0.20

Example 2:   4.4 is the same as 4.40, 4.400

Practice Problems

Circle the decimal with the largest value in the following:

13.   0.5,   0.15,   0.05

14.   2.66,   2.36,   2.87

15.   0.125,   0.375,   0.25

16.   0.175,   0.1,   0.05

17.   7.02,   7.15,   7.35

18.   0.067,   0.087,   0.077

Addition and Subtraction of Decimals

> To add or subtract decimals, place the numbers in columns so that the decimal points are lined up directly under one another, and add or subtract from right to left.

Example 1:   Add 16.4 + 21.8 + 13.2

```
    16.4
    21.8
+   13.2
  _____
    51.4
```

Example 2:   Add 11.2 + 16

```
    11.2
+   16.0        Note the addition of a zero to make the
  _____        columns the same length.
    27.2
```

Example 3:   Subtract 3.78 from 12.84

$$
\begin{array}{r}
12.84 \\
-\ \ 3.78 \\
\hline
9.06
\end{array}
$$

Example 4:   Subtract 0.007 from 0.05

$$
\begin{array}{r}
0.050 \\
-\ 0.007 \\
\hline
0.043
\end{array}
$$
    Note the addition of a zero to make the columns the same length.

Practice Problems

Add the following decimals:

19.   4.7 + 5.3 + 8.4 =   _____

20.   38.52 + 0.029 + 1.90 =   _____

21.   0.7 + 3.25 =   _____

22.   2.2 + 1.67 =   _____

Subtract the following decimals:

23.   3.67 − 0.75 =   _____

24.   64.3 − 21.2 =   _____

25.   0.08 − 0.045 =   _____

26.   6.75 − 0.87 =   _____

Multiplying Decimals

When multiplying decimals be sure the decimal is placed in the correct position in the answer (product).

> To multiply decimals, multiply as with whole numbers. In the answer (product), count off from right to left as many decimal places as there are in the numbers being multiplied.

When there are insufficient numbers in the answer for correct placement of the decimal point, add as many zeros as needed to the left of the answer.

Example 1: 1.35×0.65

$$
\begin{array}{r}
1.35 \\
\times \quad 0.65 \\
\hline
6\,7\,5 \\
8\,1\,0 \\
\hline
8\,7\,7\,5
\end{array}
$$

In this problem 1.35 has two numbers after the decimal, and 0.65 also has two. Therefore you will need to place the decimal point **4** places to the left in the answer (product), and add a zero in front.

Answer: 8775 = 0.8775

Example 2: 0.11×0.33

$$
\begin{array}{r}
0.11 \\
\times \quad 0.33 \\
\hline
3\,3 \\
3\,3 \\
\hline
3\,6\,3
\end{array}
$$

In Example 2, there are four decimal places needed (two numbers after each decimal in 0.11 and 0.33), but there are only three numbers in the product. A zero must be placed to the left of these numbers for correct placement of the decimal point.

Answer: 363 = 0.0363

Multiplication by Decimal Movement

This method may be preferred when doing metric conversions, since it is based upon the decimal system.

> Multiplying by 10, 100, 1000, and so forth can be done by moving the decimal point to the right the same number of places as there are zeros in the number by which you are multiplying.

Example: If multiplying by 10, move the decimal one place to the right; by 100, two places to the right; by 1000, three places to the right, and so forth.

Example 1: $5.2 \times 100 = 520$ (Decimal moved two places to the right.)

Example 2: $1.6 \times 10 = 16$ (Decimal moved one place to the right.)

Practice Problems

Multiply the following decimals.

27. $3.15 \times 0.015 =$ _____

28. $3.65 \times 0.25 =$ _____

29. $9.65 \times 1000 =$ _____

30. $8.9 \times 0.2 =$ _____

31. $14.001 \times 7.2 =$ _____

Division of Decimals

The division of decimals is done in the same manner as dividing whole numbers except for placement of the decimal point. Incorrect placement of the decimal point changes the numerical value and can cause error in calculation.

The parts of a division problem are as follows:

$$\text{Divisor} \overline{\left)\text{Dividend}\right.}^{\text{Quotient}}$$

The number being divided is called the dividend, the number used for the division is the divisor, and the answer is the quotient.

Symbols used to indicate division are as follows:

(1) $\overline{\left)\right.}$

(2) ÷

(3) the horizontal bar with the dividend on the top and the divisor on the bottom.

Example: $\dfrac{27}{9}$

(4) the slanted bar with the dividend to the left and the divisor to the right.

Example: 27 / 9

Dividing a Decimal by a Whole Number

To divide a decimal by a whole number, place the decimal point in the quotient directly above the decimal point in the dividend. Proceed to divide as with whole numbers.

Example:
```
              3 . 5
        5 | 1 7 . 5
        -   1 5
              ‾‾‾‾‾
              2 5
            - 2 5
              ‾‾‾‾‾
                0
```

Dividing a Decimal or a Whole Number by a Decimal

To divide by a decimal, the decimal point in the divisor is moved to the right until the number is a whole number. The decimal point in the dividend is moved the same number of places to the right, and zeros are added as necessary. Proceed to divide as with whole numbers.

Example: Divide 6.96 by 0.3

$$6.96 \div 0.3 = 0.3 \overline{)6.96}$$

Step 1: $3 \overline{)69.6}$ (After moving decimals in the divisor the same number of places as the dividend.)

Step 2:
```
              2 3 . 2
        3 | 6 9 . 6
        -   6
            ‾‾‾
              9
            - 9
              ‾‾‾
                6
              - 6
              ‾‾‾
                0
```

Division by Decimal Movement

> To divide a decimal by 10, 100, or 1000, move the decimal point to the left the same number of places as there are zeros in the divisor.

Example: $0.07 \div 100 = 0.0007$ (The decimal is moved two places to the left)

Rounding Off Decimals

The determination of how many places to carry your division in calculation of dosages is based on the materials being used. Some syringes are marked in tenths, some in hundredths. As you become familiar with the materials used in dosage calculation you will learn how far to carry your division and when to round off. To ensure accuracy, most calculation problems require that you carry your division at least two decimal places (hundredths place) and round off to the nearest tenth.

> To express an answer to the nearest tenth, carry the division to the hundredths place (two places after the decimal). If the number in the hundredths place is 5 or greater, add one to the tenths place. If the number is less than 5, drop the number to the right of the desired decimal place.

Example 1:   Express 4.15 to the nearest tenth.

Answer: 4.2   (The number in the hundredths place is 5, so the number in the tenths place is increased by one. 4.1 becomes 4.2.)

Example 2:   Express 1.24 to the nearest tenth.

Answer: 1.2   (The number in the hundredths place is less than 5, so the number in the tenths place does not change.)

To express an answer to the nearest hundredth, carry the division to the thousandths place (three places after the decimal). If the number in the thousandths place is 5 or greater, add one to the hundredths place. If the number is less than 5, drop the number to the right of the desired decimal place.

Example 1:   Express 0.176 to the nearest hundredth.

Answer: 0.18 (The number in the thousandths place is 6, so the number in the hundredths place is increased by one. 0.17 becomes 0.18.)

Example 2:   Express 0.554 to the nearest hundredth.

Answer: 0.55 (The number in the thousandths place is less than 5, so the number in the hundredths place does not change.)

Practice Problems

Divide the following decimals. Carry division to the hundredths place where necessary.

32. $2 \div 0.5 =$ _____

33. $1.4 \div 1.2 =$ _____

34. $63.8 \div 0.9 =$ _____

35. $39.6 \div 1.3 =$ _____

36. $1.9 \div 3.2 =$ _____

Express the following decimals to the nearest tenth.

37.   3.57   _____

38.   0.95   _____

39.   1.98   _____

Express the following decimals to the nearest hundredth.

40.   3.550   _____

41.   0.607   _____

42.   0.738   _____

Divide the following decimals.

43. $0.005 \div 10$ = _____

44. $0.004 \div 100$ = _____

Multiply the following decimals.

45. 58.4×10 = _____

46. 0.5×1000 = _____

Changing Fractions to Decimals

To change a fraction to a decimal, divide the numerator by the denominator and add zeros as needed. If the numerator doesn't divide evenly into the denominator, carry division three places.

Example 1: $\dfrac{2}{5}$ = $\dfrac{0.4}{5\,\lvert\,2.0}$

Example 2: $\dfrac{3}{8}$ = $\dfrac{0.375}{8\,\lvert\,3.000}$

Changing fractions to decimals can also be a method of comparing fraction size. The fractions being compared are changed to decimals, and the rules relating to comparing decimals are then applied.

Example: Which fraction is larger, $\dfrac{1}{3}$ or $\dfrac{1}{6}$?

Solution: $\dfrac{1}{3}$ = 0.333 as a decimal

$\dfrac{1}{6}$ = 0.166

$\dfrac{1}{3}$ would therefore be the larger fraction.

Changing Decimals to Fractions

To change a decimal to a fraction, simply read the decimal as a fraction and write it as it is read. Reduce if necessary.

Note: See Reading and Writing Decimals.

Example 1:   0.4 is read "four tenths" and

written $\frac{4}{10}$, which $= \frac{2}{5}$ when reduced.

Example 2:   0.65 is read "sixty-five hundredths" and

written $\frac{65}{100}$, which $= \frac{13}{20}$ when reduced.

Practice Problems

Change the following fractions to decimals, and carry the division three places as indicated.

47. $\frac{3}{4}$ _____

48. $\frac{5}{9}$ _____

49. $\frac{1}{2}$ _____

Change the following decimals to fractions, and reduce to lowest terms.

50. 0.75   _____

51. 0.0005   _____

52. 0.04   _____

Points to Remember:

✔ Read them carefully.

✔ Place (0) in front of values when the decimal fraction is not preceded by a whole number to emphasize the number as a fraction and to avoid errors in interpretation.

✔ Add zeros to the right as needed for making decimals of equal spacing for addition and subtraction. These zeros do not change the value.

✔ Double-check work to avoid errors.

Chapter Review

Identify the decimal with the largest value in the following sets.

1. 0.4, 0.44, 0.444

2. 0.8, 0.7, 0.12

3. 1.32, 1.12, 1.5

4. 0.1, 0.05, 0.2

5. 0.725, 0.357, 0.125

Perform the indicated operations.

6. 3.005 + 4.308 + 2.47 = _____

7. 20.3 + 8.57 + 0.03 = _____

8. 5.886 − 3.143 = _____

9. 8.17 − 3.05 = _____

10. 3.8 − 1.3 = _____

Solve the following. Carry division to the hundredths place where necessary.

11. 5.7 ÷ 0.9 = _____

12. 3.75 ÷ 2.5 = _____

13. 1.125 ÷ 0.75 = _____

14. 0.15 × 100 = _____

15. 15 × 2.08 =   _____

16. 472.4 × 0.002 =   _____

Express the following decimals to the nearest tenth.

17. 1.75   _____

18. 0.13   _____

Express the following decimals to the nearest hundredth.

19. 1.427   _____

20. 0.147   _____

Change the following fractions to decimals. Carry division three decimal places as necessary.

21. 8/64   _____

22. 3/50   _____

23. 6 1/2   _____

Change the following decimals to fractions; reduce to lowest terms.

24. 1.01   _____

25. 0.065   _____

4 Ratio and Proportion

Objectives

After reviewing this chapter the student will be able to do the following:

1. Define ratio and proportion
2. Define means and extremes
3. Use ratio and proportion to calculate problems for a missing term (x)

Ratio and proportion is one method for calculating medication dosages. To use this method it is necessary to have an understanding of the concept of ratio and proportion.

Ratios

A ratio is used to indicate a relationship between two numbers. These numbers are separated by a colon (:).

> **Example:** 3 : 4

The colon indicates division, therefore a ratio is a fraction and the numbers or terms of the ratio are the numerator and denominator. The numerator is always to the left of the colon, and the denominator is always to the right of the colon.

> **Example:** 3 : 4   (3 is the numerator, 4 is the denominator,
> and the expression can be written as $\frac{3}{4}$.)

Proportions

A proportion is an equation of two ratios of equal value. The terms of the first ratio have a relationship to the terms of the second ratio. A proportion can be written in any of the following formats:

(1) $3 : 4 = 6 : 8$ (separated with an equal sign)

(2) $3 : 4 :: 6 : 8$ (separated with a double colon)

(3) $\dfrac{3}{4} = \dfrac{6}{8}$ (written as a fraction)

Read as follows: 3 is to 4 equals 6 is to 8; 3 is to 4 as 6 is to 8; or read as a fraction: Three fourths equals six eighths.

Proving that ratios are equal and that the proportion is true can be done mathematically.

Example: $5 : 25 = 10 : 50$

or

$5 : 25 :: 10 : 50$

The terms in a proportion are called the means and extremes. Confusion of these terms can result in an incorrect answer. Let's refer to our example to identify these terms.

The extremes are the outer or end numbers (in the above example 5, 50), and the means are the inner or middle numbers (in the above example 25, 10).

means

Example: $5 : 25 = 10 : 50$

extremes

In a proportion the product of the means equals the product of the extremes.

In other words, the answer obtained when you multiply the means and extremes are equal.

Example: $5 : 25 = 10 : 50$

$25 \times 10 = 50 \times 5$

means   extremes

$250 = 250$

Note: The product of the means, 250, equals the product of the extremes, 250, proving the ratios are equal and the proportion is true.

To verify that the two ratios in a proportion expressed as a fraction are equal and that it is a true proportion, multiply the numerator of each ratio by its opposite denominator. The sum of the products are equal. The numerator of the first fraction and the denominator of the second fraction are the extremes. The numerator of the second fraction and denominator of the first fraction are the means.

Example: 5 : 25 = 10 : 50

$$\frac{5}{25} = \frac{10}{50}$$ (proportion written as a fraction)

$$\frac{5 \text{ (extreme)}}{25 \text{ (mean)}} = \frac{10 \text{ (mean)}}{50 \text{ (extreme)}}$$

Note: When stated as a fraction the proportion is solved by cross multiplication.

$$5 \times 50 = 25 \times 10$$

$$250 = 250$$

Solving For x in Ratio Proportion

Since the product of the means is always equal to the product of the extremes, if three numbers of the two ratios are known the fourth number can be found. In a proportion problem, the unknown quantity is represented by x.

Example: 12 : 9 = 8 : x Steps:

$$12x = 72$$ 1. Multiply the means and extremes.

$$\frac{12x}{12} = \frac{72}{12}$$ 2. Divide both sides of the equation by the number in front of x to obtain the value for x.

$$x = 6$$

Proof: Place the answer obtained for x in the equation, and multiply to be certain that the product of the means equals the product of the extremes.

$$12 : 9 = 8 : 6$$

$$12 \times 6 = 9 \times 8$$

$$72 = 72$$

Solving for x with a proportion in a fraction format can be done by cross multiplication to determine the value of x.

Example: $\dfrac{4}{3} = \dfrac{12}{x}$ Steps

$4x = 36$ 1. Cross multiply to obtain the product of the means and extremes.

$\dfrac{4x}{4} = \dfrac{36}{4}$ 2. Divide by the number in front of x to obtain the value for x.

$x = 9$

Proof: Place the value obtained for x in the equation; the cross products should be equal.

$\dfrac{4}{3} = \dfrac{12}{9}$

$4 \times 9 = 12 \times 3$

$36 = 36$

Solving for x in proportions that involve decimals in the equation can be done by the same process.

Example: $25 : 5 = 1.5 : x$ Steps

$25x = 5 \times 1.5$ 1. Multiply the means and extremes.

$\dfrac{25x}{25} = \dfrac{7.5}{25}$ 2. Divide by the number in front of x to solve for x.

$x = 0.3$

Proof: $25 : 5 = 1.5 : 0.3$

$25 \times 0.3 = 5 \times 1.5$

$7.5 = 7.5$

Proportions with unknowns that also involve fractions may be solved by the same method.

Example: $\frac{1}{5} : 1 = \frac{1}{2} : x$ Steps

$$\frac{1}{5} \times x = \frac{1}{2}$$

1. Multiply the extremes and means.

2. Divide both sides by the number in front

$$x = \frac{1}{2} \div \frac{1}{5}$$

of x. Division of two fractions becomes

multiplication, and the second fraction is

$$x = \frac{1}{2} \times \frac{5}{1}$$

inverted. Multiply numerators and

denominators.

$$x = \frac{5}{2} = 2.5$$

3. Divide the final fraction to solve for x.

Proof: $\frac{1}{5} : 1 = \frac{1}{2} : 2.5$

$$\frac{1}{5} \times 2.5 = 1 \times \frac{1}{2}$$

$$\frac{2.5}{5} = \frac{1}{2}$$

$$0.5 = 0.5 \ (\frac{1}{2} \text{ as a decimal})$$

Note: If the answer is expressed in fraction format for x, it must be reduced to lowest terms. Division should be carried two decimal places when an answer does not work out evenly. When answers do not come out evenly, they may have to be rounded to the nearest tenth to prove the answer correct.

Points to Remember:

✔ Proportions represent two ratios that are equal and have a relationship to each other.

✔ Proportions can be stated using an (=) sign, a double colon (::), or in a fraction format.

✔ Proportions are solved by multiplying the means and extremes.

✔ Ratios are always stated in their lowest terms.

✔ Double-check work.

Chapter Review

Express the following fractions as ratios. Reduce to lowest terms.

1. $\dfrac{2}{3}$ _____

2. $\dfrac{1}{9}$ _____

3. $\dfrac{6}{8}$ _____

4. $\dfrac{1}{5}$ _____

5. $\dfrac{5}{10}$ _____

6. $\dfrac{2}{10}$ _____

Express the following ratios as fractions. Reduce to lowest terms.

7.   3 : 7 _____

8.   4 : 6 _____

9.   1 : 7 _____

10. 8 : 6 _____

11. 3 : 4 _____

Solve for x in the following proportions. Carry division two decimal places as necessary.

12.   20 : 40 = x : 10   _____

13. $\dfrac{1}{4}$: $\dfrac{1}{2}$ = 1 : x _____

14.   0.12 : 0.8 = 0.6 : x _____

15. $\dfrac{1}{250}$: 2 = $\dfrac{1}{150}$: x _____

16. x : 9 = 5 : 10   _____

17. $\dfrac{1}{4} : 1.6 = \dfrac{1}{8} : x$ _____

18. $\dfrac{1}{2} : 2 = \dfrac{1}{3} : x$ _____

19. $125 : 0.4 = 50 : x$ _____

20. $x : 1 = 0.5 : 5$ _____

5 Percentages

Objectives

After reviewing this chapter the student will be able to do the following:

1. Define percent
2. Convert percents to fractions, decimals, and ratios
3. Convert decimals to percents
4. Convert fractions to percents and ratios

Percentages are commonly seen in dosage calculation. Doctors prescribe solutions that are expressed in percentages for external as well as internal use.

> **Example:** Hydrocortisone Cream, Burrow's Solution, and Intravenous Solutions.

In current practice most percentage solutions are prepared by the pharmacy; however there are still some institutions that require nurses to prepare these solutions. Understanding percentages provides the foundation for preparation and calculation of dosages for medications that are ordered in percentages.

The term percent (%) means hundredths. A percentage is the same as a fraction in which the denominator is 100, and the number indicates the part of 100 that is being considered.

> **Example:** $4\% = \dfrac{4}{100}$

The percent symbol may be used with a whole number (15%), a fraction (1/2 %), a mixed number (14 1/2 %), or a decimal (0.6%). Percents therefore can be expressed in different forms without changing the value.

> To change a percent to a fraction, omit the % sign, divide the number by 100, and reduce to lowest terms.

Example 1: $8\% = \dfrac{8}{100}$, reduced is $\dfrac{2}{25}$

Example 2: $\dfrac{1}{4}\% = \dfrac{1}{4} \div \dfrac{100}{1} = \dfrac{1}{4} \times \dfrac{1}{100} = \dfrac{1}{400}$

Practice Problems

Change the following percentages to fractions and reduce to lowest terms.

1. 1% _____

2. 2% _____

3. 50% _____

4. 80% _____

5. 3% _____

> To change a percent to a decimal, drop the percentage symbol, and move the decimal point two places to the left (add zeros as needed).

Example 1:   25% = 0.25

Example 2:   1.4% = 0.014

Note: An alternate method to the above is to drop the % sign, express as a fraction in its lowest terms, and divide the numerator by the denominator to obtain a decimal.

Example: $75\% = \dfrac{3}{4}$ to lowest terms. Divide the numerator of the fraction by the denominator

$$
\begin{array}{r}
0.75 \\
4\overline{)3.00}
\end{array}
$$

Practice Problems

Change the following percents to decimals.

6.   10%   _____

7.   35%   _____

8.   50%   _____

9.   14.2%   _____

10. $\frac{1}{4}$%   _____

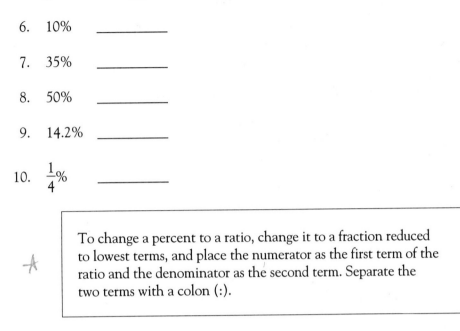

To change a percent to a ratio, change it to a fraction reduced to lowest terms, and place the numerator as the first term of the ratio and the denominator as the second term. Separate the two terms with a colon (:).

Example: 10%   = $\frac{10}{100}$ = $\frac{1}{10}$ = 1 : 10.

Practice Problems

Change the following percents to a ratio. Express in lowest terms:

11.   25%   _____

12.   11%   _____

13.   75%   _____

14.   4.5%   _____

15.   2/5%   _____

Changing Fractions, Decimals, and Ratios to Percentages

To change a fraction to a percent, multiply the fraction by 100, reduce if necessary, and add the symbol for percentage.

Example 1: $\frac{3}{4}$ changed to a percent is

$$\frac{3}{4} \times \frac{100}{1} = \frac{75}{1} = 75$$

Add symbol for percent: 75%

Example 2: $5\frac{1}{2}$: Change to an improper fraction $\frac{11}{2}$

$$\frac{11}{2} \times \frac{100}{1} = \frac{550}{1} = 550$$

Add symbol for percent: 550%

Practice Problems

Change the following fractions to percents.

16. $\frac{2}{5}$ _____

17. $1\frac{1}{4}$ _____

18. $\frac{1}{2}$ _____

19. $\frac{1}{4}$ _____

20. $\frac{7}{10}$ _____

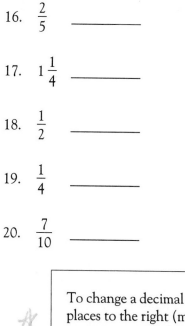

> To change a decimal to a percent, move the decimal point two places to the right (multiply), add zeros if necessary, and add the percentage symbol.

Example 1: Change 0.45 to %

Move the decimal point two places to the right, and add %: The result = 45%

Example 2:   Change 2.35 to %

Move the decimal point two places to the right,
and add %: The result = 235%

Note: A decimal may also be changed to a percent by changing the decimal to a fraction
and following the steps to change a fraction to a percent. If the percentage does not end
in a whole number, express the percentage with the remainder as a fraction, to the nearest whole percent, or to the nearest tenth of a percent.

Example: $0.625 = \dfrac{5}{8} = 62\ 1/2\%,\ 63\%,\ \text{or}\ 62.5\%.$

To change a ratio to percent, change the ratio to a fraction, and
proceed with steps for changing a fraction to percent.

Example: $1 : 4 = \dfrac{1}{4},\ \dfrac{1}{4} \times \dfrac{100}{1} = 25$, add percent symbol

Answer: 25%

Practice Problems

Change the following ratios to percent.

21.   1 : 25   _____

22.   3 : 4   _____

23.   1 : 10   _____

24.   1 : 100   _____

25.   1 : 2   _____

Chapter Review

Express each of the following measures as indicated. Reduce to lowest terms where needed.

	Percent	Ratio	Fraction	Decimal
1.	0.25%	_____	_____	_____
2.	71%	_____	_____	_____
3.	_____	_____	$\dfrac{7}{100}$	_____
4.	_____	1 : 50	_____	_____
5.	_____	_____	_____	0.06
6.	_____	_____	$\dfrac{1}{30}$	_____
7.	_____	_____	$\dfrac{61}{100}$	_____
8.	_____	7 : 1000	_____	_____
9.	5%	_____	_____	_____
10.	2.5%	_____	_____	_____

Post Test

After completing Unit I of this text you should be able to complete this test. The test consists of a total of 50 questions that are worth 2 points each. The passing score is 70 or better. If you miss three or more questions in any section, review the chapter relating to that content.

Express the following in Roman numerals.

1. 5 _____

2. 17 _____

3. 27 _____

4. 29 _____

5. 30 _____

Express the following in Arabic numbers.

6. $\overline{viss}$ _____

7. $\overline{xxiv}$ _____

8. $\overline{xix}$ _____

9. $\overline{xxv}$ _____

10. $\overline{xv}$ _____

Reduce the following fractions to lowest terms.

11. $\frac{8}{6}$ _____

12. $\frac{22}{33}$ _____

13. $\frac{27}{63}$ _____

14. $\frac{10}{15}$ _____

15. $\dfrac{16}{10}$ _____

Perform the indicated operations with fractions; reduce to lowest terms where needed.

16. $\dfrac{5}{6} \div \dfrac{7}{10} =$ _____

17. $5\dfrac{1}{2} \div 4\dfrac{1}{2} =$ _____

18. $6\dfrac{1}{3} \times 4 =$ _____

19. $5\dfrac{1}{5} - 3\dfrac{4}{7} =$ _____

20. $\dfrac{5}{4} + \dfrac{2}{9} =$ _____

Change the following fractions to decimals; express your answer to the nearest tenth.

21. $\dfrac{8}{7}$ _____

22. $\dfrac{1}{8}$ _____

23. $\dfrac{1}{15}$ _____

24. $\dfrac{12}{13}$ _____

Indicate the largest fraction in each group.

25. $\dfrac{1}{2}, \dfrac{2}{3}, \dfrac{5}{9}$

26. $\dfrac{3}{4}, \dfrac{7}{10}, \dfrac{5}{8}$

Perform the indicated operations with decimals.

27. $16.7 + 21.0 =$ _____

28. $0.007 + 17.4 =$ _____

29. $10.57 \times 10 =$ _____

30. $36.8 - 3.86 =$ _____

Divide the following decimals. Express your answer to the nearest tenth.

31. $67.8 \div 0.8 =$ _____

32. $9 \div 0.4 =$ _____

33. $5.01 \div 10 =$ _____

Indicate the largest decimal in each group.

34.   0.850, 0.085

35.   3.002, 0.390, 0.399

36.   0.478, 0.445, 0.493

Solve for x, the unknown value.

37. $10 : 20 = x : 8, \ x =$ _____

38. $500 : x = 200 : 1, \ x =$ _____

39. $0.3 : x = 1.8 : 0.6, \ x =$ _____

40. $\dfrac{1}{4} : x = \dfrac{1}{8} : 2, \ x =$ _____

Round off to the nearest tenth.

41. $0.57 =$ _____

42. $0.99 =$ _____

43. $1.42 =$ _____

Round off to the nearest hundredth.

44. $0.677 =$ _____

45. $0.832 =$ _____

46. $1.222 =$ _____

Complete the table below; express the measures in their equivalents where indicated. Reduce to lowest terms where necessary or round off to nearest hundredth.

	Percent	Decimal	Ratio	Fraction
47.	_____	_____	1 : 10	_____
48.	60%	_____	_____	_____
49.	$66\frac{2}{3}$ %	_____	_____	_____
50.	25%	_____	_____	_____

Unit Two

Systems of Measurement

There are basically three systems of measurement that are used in the computation of medication dosages: metric, apothecaries', and household. To be competent in the administration of medications, it is essential that the nurse be familiar with all three systems and the measures used in the computation of dosages.

1) IF the numeraters are the same, the fraction z the smaller denominator has the larger value.

ex $\frac{1}{2}$ is larger than $\frac{1}{3}$

$\frac{1}{150}$ "   " $\frac{1}{300}$

2) IF the denominators are the same, the fraction z the larger numerator has the larger value.

$\frac{3}{4}$ is larger then $\frac{1}{4}$

IF Denominator's are diff change the Fraction by finding the lowest common Denominator (LCD)

6 Metric System

Objectives

After reviewing this chapter the student will be able to do the following:

1. Express metric measures correctly using rules of the metric system
2. State from memory common equivalents in the metric system that are used for medication administration

The metric system is an international decimal system of weights and measures that was adopted in France in 1795. The metric system is more precise than the apothecaries' or household systems. Apothecaries' and household measures are gradually being replaced with the metric system. More and more in everyday situations we are encountering the use of metric measures. For example, soft drinks come in bottles labeled *liter*; engine sizes are also expressed in liters.

Newborn weights are recorded in grams, and adult weights are expressed in kilograms, as opposed to pounds and ounces. In obstetrics we express fundal height (upper portion of the uterus) in centimeters. Traditional measures are being replaced by metric measures.

Particulars of the Metric System

1. The metric system is based on the decimal system, in which divisions and multiples of ten are used. Therefore a lot of math can be done by decimal movement.

2. There are three basic units of measure used:

   a. gram – the basic unit for weight.
   b. liter – the basic unit for volume.
   c. meter – the basic unit for length.

Dosages are calculated using measurements from the metric system that relate to weight and volume. Meter, which is used for linear (length) measurement, is not used in the calculation of dosages. Linear measurements (meter, centimeter) are commonly used to measure the height of an individual and in determining growth patterns.

3. Common prefixes are used in this system that denote the numerical value of the unit being discussed. Memorization of these prefixes would be helpful.

memorize

Prefix	Numerical Value	Meaning
Kilo	1000	one thousand times
Centi	0.01	hundredth part of
Milli	0.001	thousandth part of
Micro	0.000001	millionth part of

Let's see how using the prefixes can tell us something about a measure by looking at the following example.

> **Example:**   67 milligrams
>
> prefix – milli – measure in thousandths of a unit
> gram – represents a unit of weight
>
> Therefore 67 milligrams = 67 thousandths of a gram.

4. Regardless of the size of the unit, the name of the basic unit is incorporated into the measure. This allows easy recognition of the unit of measure.

> **Example 1:** milliliter – the word liter indicates that you are measuring volume
>
> **Example 2:** kilogram – the word gram indicates that you are measuring weight

5. Abbreviations for units of measure in the metric system are often the first letter of each word. Small letters are used more often than capital letters.

> liter = L (This is the one abbreviation that still uses a capital letter.)

6. When prefixes are used in combination with the basic unit, the first letter of the prefix and the first letter of the unit of measure are written together and expressed in small letters.

> **Example 1:**   milligram – The m is taken from the prefix *milli* and the g from *gram*, the unit of weight.
> Abbreviation = mg
>
> **Example 2:**   microgram – Abbreviated as mcg. Microgram is also written using the symbol (μ) in combination with the letter g from the basic unit *gram*. Using the symbol (μg) should be avoided, and avoid interpreting the abbreviation mcg as mg.
>
> **Example 3:**   milliliter – Abbreviated as mL. Note that when L (liter) is used in combination with a prefix it remains capitalized.

```
Common Metric Abbreviations

gram  =  g
milligram  =  mg
kilogram  =  kg
liter  =  L
milliliter  =  mL
microgram  =  mcg
```

Rules of Metric System

There are rules that are specific to the metric system and are important to remember.

```
1. Arabic numbers are used to express quantities in this system.

2. Parts of a unit or a fraction of a unit are expressed as decimals.

3. The quantity whether in whole numbers or decimals is always
   written before the abbreviation or symbol for a unit of measure.
```

Fractions are not used. Example: 3/4 gram. The fraction 3/4 is incorrect. It must be expressed as a decimal. 0.75 gram is the correct way to express 3/4.

Note: Zeros should always be placed in front of the decimal when the quantity is not a whole number. When the quantity expressed is preceded by a whole number, zeros are not necessary. For example, 2.5 mL is written as 2.5 mL, not 2.50 mL. Addition of unnecessary zeros can lead to errors in reading. 2.50 mL may misread as 250 instead of 2.5 mL.

Example 1:   one thousand milligrams

```
1000        mg
  |          |
quantity   abbreviation for milligram
```

Example 2:   four tenths of a gram

```
0.4         g
  |          |
quantity   abbreviation for gram
```

Units of Measure

Weight: The gram is the basic unit of weight. Some medications are ordered as fractions of grams.

     a. The milligram is smaller than a gram; medications may be ordered in milligrams.
     1000 mg = 1 g

     b. The microgram is smaller than a gram and milligram. The word micro also means tiny or small. Micrograms are tiny parts of a gram.
     1000 mcg = 1 mg. A milligram is one thousand times larger than a microgram. It would take one million micrograms to make one gram.

     c. The kilogram is very large, and is not used for measuring medications. A kilogram is one thousand times larger than the gram.
     1 kg = 1000 g. This measure is frequently used to denote weights of clients upon which medication dosages are based.

Units of Weight to Memorize

1 kilogram (kg) = 1000 grams (g)

1 gram (g) = 1000 milligrams (mg)

1 milligram (mg) = 1000 micrograms (mcg)

Volume:

     a. The liter is the basic unit.

     1000 mL (cc) = 1 L

     b. The milliliter is smaller than a liter. It is abbreviated as mL.

     1 mL = 0.001 L

     c. The cubic centimeter is the amount of space that one milliliter of liquid occupies and is abbreviated as cc.

     1cc = 0.001 L = 1 mL

Cubic centimeter (cc), and milliliter (mL) are considered to be the same and are used interchangeably. (See Figures 6.1 and 6.2 illustrating metric measures.)

13. mL is the same as   _____

14. The prefix kilo- means   _____

15. The prefix milli- means   _____

Using the rules of the metric system, express the following quantities correctly using abbreviations.

16. six tenths of a gram   _____

17. fifty kilograms   _____

18. four tenths of a milligram   _____

19. four hundredths of a liter   _____

20. four and two tenths micrograms _____

21. five thousandths of a gram   _____

22. six hundredths of a gram   _____

23. two and six tenths milliliters _____

24. one hundred milliliters   _____

25. three hundredths of a milliliter _____

7 Apothecaries' and Household Systems

Objectives

After reviewing this chapter the student will be able to do the following:

1. State the common apothecaries' and household equivalents
2. State specific rules that relate to the apothecaries' and household systems
3. Identify symbols and interpret measures in the apothecaries' and household systems

The apothecaries' system is one of the oldest systems of measurement. It was brought to this country from England during the colonial period. In the European countries, the apothecaries' system has been totally replaced by the metric system. This transition in the United States has been a gradual and slow process, with the apothecaries' system still used in dosage calculation.

Doctors order medications in this system that have been in use for many years (morphine, codeine, atropine, aspirin). An example of this would be an order such as "aspirin grains ten." Pharmaceutical companies often label drugs using the apothecaries' system as well as the metric. For example, if we look at a bottle of nitroglycerin tablets we see that while the tablets may be labeled grains 1/150, which is an apothecaries' measure, the label may have 0.4 milligrams in parentheses, which is a metric measure.

Other medications that illustrate the use of both apothecaries' and metric measures include medications such as atropine sulfate, morphine sulfate, and sodium phenobarbital. (See Figure 7.1, illustrating the use of metric and apothecaries' measures on drug labels.) Since the apothecaries' system is still in use, it is necessary for those involved in the administration of medications to be familiar with the basics relating to it.

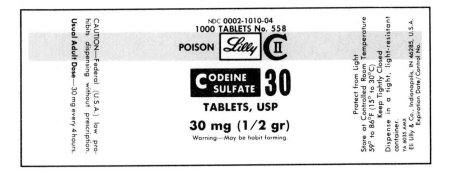

Figure 7.1, A Drug label showing apothecaries' and metric measures. (gr = apothecaries', mg = metric). (From Radcliff R, Ogden S: *Calculation of Drug Dosages,* ed 4, St Louis, 1991, Mosby.)

Figure 7.1, B Drug label showing apothecaries' and metric measures. (gr = apothecaries', mg = metric). (From Radcliff R, Ogden S: *Calculation of Drug Dosages*, ed 4, St Louis, 1991, Mosby.)

Particulars of the Apothecaries' System

1. The measures used in this system are approximates; however, they have become acceptable in the preparation and administration of medications.

2. Roman numerals are often used in this system, as well as Arabic numbers.

3. Fractions are used to express quantities that are less than one, as opposed to the use of decimals in the metric system.

4. The symbol "ss" is used for the fraction 1/2. When used it can be written ss, or s̄s̄.

> **Example:** half of a grain in abbreviated form would be gr ss or gr s̄s̄.

The symbol "ss" can also be used with Roman numerals. When used with Roman numerals, it is placed at the end.

> **Example:** seven and a half grains = gr v̄īīss̄.

5. Unlike the metric system, in the apothecaries' system the abbreviation or symbol for a unit of measure is written before the amount or quantity.

> **Example:** twelve drams. The symbol for dram is (ʒ), or it is abbreviated dr. Therefore twelve drams would be written as ʒ xii, ʒ 12, ʒ x̄īī, dr xii or dr 12.

6. A combination of Arabic numbers and fractions can also be used in this system to express units of measure.

Example: gr 7 1/2

gr   7   1/2
| | |
abbreviation   arabic   fraction

Apothecaries' Units of Measure

The units of measure used for medication administration are few.

Weight: The basic unit for weight is the grain.

a. grain is abbreviated in lower case letters as gr.

b. dram is also a unit of weight, one dram is equal to 60 grains. The symbol for dram is a single-headed (z) with a tail. (ʒ) Dram is abbreviated as dr.

c. Ounce. The symbol for ounce is a double-headed (z) with a tail. (℥) Note: The extra loop on the z differentiates it from a dram. It is important not to confuse the symbols for dram and ounce because of the large difference in measures. A way to avoid confusion is to remember that an ounce is larger than a dram, thus the symbol is bigger. Ounce can be abbreviated as oz.

Volume: The basic unit for volume is the minim.

a. The most current abbreviation for minim is a small case (m). Minims are extremely small (the size of one drop) and are therefore always expressed as whole numbers. A way to remember the size of a minim is to think about the beginning three letters of the word (min), and think of words such as minute and minimal.

b. Volume can also be measured by dram and ounce. To differentiate liquid measures from solid measures, an (f) may be seen before the measure. F = fluid; it is abbreviated with a lower case (f). *(f) is omitted when it is obvious that the measure is a liquid.

Example: f ʒ = fluid dram, f ℥ = fluid ounce.

1 fluid dram = 60 minims. (f ʒ i = m 60).

1 fluid ounce = 8 fluid drams. (f ℥ i = f ʒ viii).

c. The pint and quart are also apothecaries' measures.

Pint is abbreviated as pt. *
1 pint = 16 fluid ounces.
Quart is abbreviated as qt. *
1 quart = 32 fluid ounces or 2 pints.

* Abbreviation used most often.

d. Some apothecaries' measures have equivalents in the metric system that should be memorized:

$$
\begin{aligned}
1\ \text{dram} &= 4\ \text{mL} \\
1\ \text{ounce} &= 30\ \text{mL} \\
1\ \text{pint} &= 500\ \text{mL} \\
1\ \text{quart} &= 1000\ \text{mL}
\end{aligned}
$$

For the purpose of medication administration it is necessary to be familiar with the following units from the apothecaries' system. See Figure 7.2 illustrating apothecaries' fluid measures.

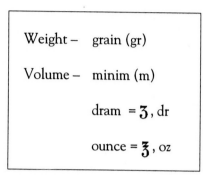

1 dr = 60 gr.

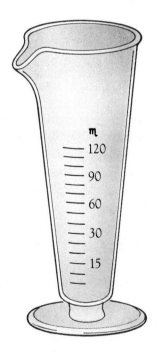

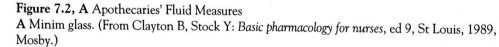

Figure 7.2, A Apothecaries' Fluid Measures
A Minim glass. (From Clayton B, Stock Y: *Basic pharmacology for nurses*, ed 9, St Louis, 1989, Mosby.)

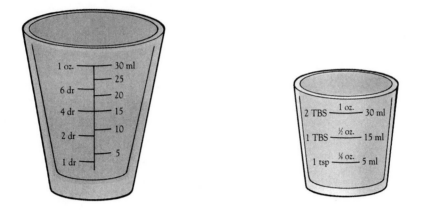

Figure 7.2, B and C Apothecaries' Fluid Measures. **B** Drams, **C** Ounces.

Household System

The household system is still in use for dosages primarily at home, as indicated by the name. The nurse needs to be familiar with household measures since clients freqently use utensils in the home to take prescribed medications. The household system is the least accurate of the three systems of measure. Capacities of utensils such as teaspoon, tablespoon, and cup vary from one house to another; therefore liquid measures are approximate.

Particulars of the Household System

1. Some of the units for liquid measures are the same as those in the apothecaries' system.   **Example:** pint and quart.

2. There are no standard rules for expressing household measures, which accounts for variety in their use.

3. Standard cookbook abbreviations are used in this system.

4. Arabic numbers and fractions are used to express quantities.

5. The basic unit in the household system is the drop (gtt).

Note: Drops should never be used as a measure for medications since the size of drops varies and therefore can be inaccurate. When drops are used as a measure for medications they should be calibrated or used only when associated with a dropper size as in intravenous flow rates.

6. Common household measures and conversions within this system are:
   a. Drop (gtt)
   b. Teaspoon (t, tsp) (60 gtt = 1 tsp)
   c. Tablespoon (T, tbs) (3 tsp = 1 tbs)
   d. Cup (C) (16 tbs = 1 C)
   e. Pint (pt) (2 C = 1 pt)
   f. Quart (qt) (2 pt = 1 qt)

Chapter Review

Using the rules of the apothecaries' system, write the following using the correct abbreviations/symbols.

1. eight and one-half grains   _____

2. three minims   _____

3. five drams   _____

4. eight ounces   _____

5. quart   _____

6. pint   _____

7. one hundred twenty fifth of a grain   _____

8. six and a half fluid drams   _____

9. two fluid ounces   _____

10. five ounces   _____

Complete the following:

11. The volume of one drop equals _____

12. $\text{ʒ}\, i = m$_____

13. $f\,\text{ʒ}\, i = f\,\text{ʒ}$_____

14. $1\ pt = f\,\text{ʒ}$_____

15.   1 qt = f ʒ _____

16.   1 tbs = f ʒ _____

17.   The abbreviation for drop is _____

18.   T is the abbreviation for _____

19.   t is the abbreviation for _____

8 Converting Within and Between Systems

Objectives

After reviewing this chapter the student will be able to do the following:

1. Recall equivalents/conversions from metric, apothecaries', and household systems to convert a given measure
2. Convert a unit of measure to its equivalent within the same system
3. Convert a unit of measure to its equivalent in another system of measure (example: metric to apothecaries', etc.)

Equivalents Among Metric, Apothecaries', and Household Systems

There are some equivalents in one system that have equivalents in another system; however, equivalents are not exact measures, and you will see discrepancies. Several tables have been developed illustrating conversions/equivalents. Sometimes drug companies use equivalents that may be different for a measure. A common discrepancy is with grains, which is an apothecaries' measure. Some tables will indicate 65 mg = gr 1, as opposed to 60 mg = gr 1. Both of these equivalents are correct. However 60 mg = gr 1 is most often used in medication calculations.

Table 8.1 lists some of the equivalents that exist between systems. Memorize these common equivalents!

Household	Apothecaries'	Metric
	m 15, or m 16* =	1 mL (cc)
1 t, 1 tsp =	ʒ i =	4 or 5* mL (cc)
1 T, tbs =	ʒ iv =	15* or 16 mL (cc)
	gr 15 =	1 g (1000 mg)
	gr 1 =	60 mg
	1 oz (ʒ i) =	30 mL
	1 pt (16 oz) =	500 mL (cc)
	1 qt (32 oz) =	1000 mL (cc), 1 L
	2.2 lb =	1 kg (1000 g)

Table 8.1 Equivalents Between Measurement Systems (* equivalent used most often)

Converting

To convert or make a conversion means to change from one form to another. This converting can mean simply changing a measure to its equivalent in the same system. Changing from grams to milligrams illustrates a metric measure changed to another metric measure. When a measurement is converted from one system to another system, this is called converting between systems. For example: conversion of milligrams (metric) to grains (apothecaries'). The measurement obtained when converting between systems is approximate, not exact.

It is important for nurses to be able to make conversions, since all three systems are currently in use. Many times medications may be ordered in a unit of measure that is different from what is available. The nurse therefore must understand the systems of measurement and be able to convert within the same system, as well as from one to another, with accuracy.

Before beginning the actual process of converting there are certain points to remember that can make converting simple.

Points For Converting

1. Memorization of the equivalents/conversions is essential.

2. THINK of memorized equivalents/conversions as essential conversion factors.
   Example: 1000 mg = 1 g is called a conversion factor.

3. Follow basic math principles regardless of the conversion method used.

4. Answers should be expressed applying specific rules that relate to the system to which you are converting.

> **Example:**   The metric system uses decimals; the apothecaries' system uses fractions.

5. Ratio-Proportion is the easiest method to use, and this method can also be used for the calculation of dosages.

Methods of Converting

1. Moving of Decimals: Because the metric system is based on the decimal system, conversions within the metric system can be done easily by movement of the decimals. Conversely, this method could not be applied in the apothecaries' or household systems since decimals are not used in either system. Metric conversions can be done by dividing or multiplying by 1000. Knowledge concerning the size of a unit is important when using this method, since this determines whether division or multiplication is necessary to make the conversion.

   a) To convert a smaller unit to a larger one, divide or move the decimal to the left.

   b) To convert a larger unit to a smaller one, multiply or move the decimal to the right.

Example: 350 mg = _____ g

> After determining that mg is the smaller unit, and you are converting to a larger unit (g), recall the conversion factor that allows you to change milligrams to grams: 1 g = 1000 mg. Therefore 350 is divided by 1000 by moving the decimal three places to the left, indicating 350 mg = 0.35 g.
>
> 3 5 0. = 0.35 g
>
> Note: The final answer is expressed in decimal format. Remember to always place a (0) in front of the decimal point to indicate a value that is less than one.

Example: 0.85 L = _____ cc

> After determining that (L) is the larger unit, and you are converting to a smaller unit (cc), recall the conversion factor that allows you to change Liters to cc.: 1 L = 1000 cc. Therefore 0.85 is multiplied by 1000 by moving the decimal three places to the right, indicating 0.85 L = 850 cc.
>
> 0 . 8 5 0 = 850 cc
>
> Note the addition of a zero here to allow movement of the decimal the correct number of places.

Practice Problems

Convert the following metric measures to the equivalent units indicated.

1. 600 cc = _____ L

2. 0.016 g = _____ mg

3. 4 kg = _____ g

4. 3 mcg = _____ mg

5. 0.3 mg = _____ g

6. 0.01 kg = _____ g

7. 1.9 L = _____ mL

8. 0.5 g = _____ kg

9. 0.07 mg = _____ mcg

10.   650 cc = _____ L

11.   0.04 g = _____ mg

12.   0.12g = _____ kg

13.   180 mg = _____ g

14.   1700 mL = _____ L

15.   15 kg = _____ g

2. Converting by Using Ratio-Proportion: This is one of the easiest ways to make conversions, whether they are within the same system or between systems. The basics on how to state ratio-proportions and how to solve them when looking for one unknown have been presented in Chapter 4. To make conversions using ratio-proportion, a proportion must be set up that expresses a numerical relationship between the two systems. A proportion may be written in a colon format or as a fraction when making conversions. Regardless of the format used there are some basic rules to follow when using this method.

---

1. State the known equivalent first (memorized equivalent).

2. Add the incomplete ratio on the other side of the equal sign, making sure the units of measurement are written in the same sequence.   **Example:**   mg : g = mg : g.

3. Label all terms in the proportion including x. (These labels are ignored when multiplying or dividing.)

4. Solve the problem by using the principles for solving ratio-proportions. (Product of the means equals the product of the extremes.)

5. The final answer for x should be labeled with the appropriate unit of measure or desired unit.

⭐ When using the method of ratio-proportion to make conversions, as with any method used, the known equivalents must be memorized. Stating the proportion in the fraction format may be a way of avoiding confusion with the terms (means and extremes). However, regardless of the format used the terms must correspond to each other in value and have a relationship. Division should always be carried at least two decimal places to ensure accuracy.

Example: 8 mg = _____ g

Solution: State the known equivalent first; add the incompleted ratio, making sure the units are in the same sequence. Label all the terms in the proportion including *x*.

1000 mg : 1 g   =   8 mg : *x* g
(known equivalent)   (unknown)

Read as "1000 mg is to 1 g as 8 mg is to *x* g."

Note: The terms of the proportion are in the same sequence, (mg : g = mg : g) and there is a correspondence in the ratio:

small : large = small : large.

Once the proportion is stated, solve it by multiplying the means (inner terms), and the extremes (outer terms).

Result:

$$\overbrace{1000 \text{ mg} : 1 \text{ g} = 8 \text{ mg} : x \text{ g}}^{\text{means}}$$

extremes

$$1000 \times (x) = 1 \times 8$$

$$\frac{1000x}{1000} = \frac{8}{1000}$$

$$x = \frac{8}{1000}$$

Since the measure you are converting to is metric, the fraction is changed to a decimal by dividing 8 by 1000 to obtain an answer of 0.008 g.

In this example because the measures are metric, perhaps moving the decimal would be the preferred method as opposed to actual division.

An alternate way of stating the problem illustrated in the example on the previous page would be stating it as a fraction and cross multiplying to solve for *x*.

$$\frac{1000 \text{ mg}}{1 \text{ g}} = \frac{8 \text{ mg}}{x \text{ g}}$$

$$\frac{1000 \, x}{1000} = \frac{8}{1000}$$

Note: The known equivalent is stated here as the numerator and denominator of the first fraction and the unknown as the numerator and the denominator of the second fraction.

$$x = 0.008 \text{ g}$$

The remainder of this chapter will show examples of the methods discussed in converting within the same system and between systems.

Converting Within the Same System

Converting within the same system is frequently seen with metric measures; however it can be done using the other systems of measurement, such as one apothecaries' measure being converted to another equivalent within the apothecaries' system. Any one of the methods discussed can be used, but movement of decimals is limited to the metric system. Ratio-proportion can be used for all systems.

Example 1:   (metric)— (metric)

0.6 mg = _____ mcg

Solution: equivalent 1000 mcg = 1mg. (mg is larger than mcg) The answer is obtained by moving the decimals three places to the right (multiply).

Answer: 600 mcg

Alternate: Set up as a proportion following the rules presented, as a fraction, or using the colon.

Example 2:   (apothecaries') — (apothecaries')

f ℨ iv   =   m _____

Solution: m 60   =   f ℨ i

A dram is larger than a minim; the answer is obtained by multiplying 4 by 60.

Answer: m 240

Alternate: Set up as a proportion using the colon format or as a fraction.

Note: Since it may be confusing to write using apothecaries' symbols when stating the proportion, it can be written as follows:

1 fluid dram : 60 minims = 4 fluid dram : *x* minims

OR

$$\frac{1 \text{ fluid dram}}{60 \text{ minims}} = \frac{4 \text{ fluid dram}}{x \text{ minims}}$$

The principles presented relating to solving ratio-proportion problems are used to solve for *x*, when presented in colon format or fraction.

Practice Problems

Convert the following to the equivalent measures indicated.

16.   500 cc = _____ L

17.   4 kg = _____ g

18.   1.4 L = _____ cc

19.   ℨ vi =   ℥ _____

20.   m 120 =   ℨ _____

21.   ℥ ss =   ℨ _____

22.   10 gtt = _____ tsp

23.   60 g = _____ kg

24.   600 mg = _____ g

25.   0.736 mg = _____ mcg

26.   1600 mL = _____ L

27.   15 cc = _____ mL

28.   0.18 g = _____ mg

29.   25 mcg = _____ mg

30.   5.2 g = _____ kg

Converting Between Systems

The methods presented previously can be used to change a measure in one system to its equivalent in another.

Example 1:   (apothecaries')   (metric)

gr 1/100 = _____ mg

Solution: Equivalent gr 1 = 60 mg   (gr is larger than mg).
Multiply 1/100 × 60 to obtain 60/100. Since the final
answer is a metric measure, 60/100 is changed to a
decimal by dividing 100 into 60.

Answer: 0.6 mg

Alternate: Express the conversion in proportion format, and solve for *x*.

gr 1 : 60 mg = gr 1/100 : *x* mg

OR

$$\frac{gr\ 1}{60\ mg} = \frac{gr\ 1/100}{x\ mg}$$

Example 2:   (apothecaries')   (metric)

110 lb   = _____ kg

Solution: Equivalent 1 kg = 2.2 lbs   (lb is smaller than kg)
110 is divided by 2.2.

Answer: 50 kg

Practice Problems

Convert the following to the equivalent measures indicated.

31.   60 lbs = _____ kg

32.   15 mg = gr _____

33.   ʒv = _____ cc

34.   gr v = _____ mg

35.   ʒvii = _____ cc

36.   250 cc = _____ qt

37.   45 mL = _____ tbs

38.   gr 45 = _____ g

39.   gr īss = _____ mg

40.   m 45 = _____ mL

41.   gr 15 = _____ mg

42.   4 qts = _____ mL

43.   72 kg = _____ lbs

44.   gr 1/125 = _____ mg

45.   2.4 L = _____ cc

Points to Remember:

✔ Regardless of the method used for converting, memorizing equivalents is a necessity.

✔ Answers stated in fraction format should be reduced as necessary.

✔ When more than one equivalent is learned for a unit, use the most common equivalent for the measure or use the number that divides equally without a remainder.

✔ Division should be carried out two decimal places to ensure accuracy.

✔ Decimal movement as a method for converting is limited to the metric system; ratio-proportion can be used for all systems of measure.

Chapter Review

Convert the following to the equivalent measures indicated.

1.   0.007 g = _____ mg

2.   1 mg = _____ g

3.   6000 g = _____ kg

4.   5 mL = _____ L

5.   0.45 L = _____ cc

6.   60 mL = ℥ _____

7. gr 1/300 = _____ mg

8. 1 mg = gr _____

9. 12 mL = ℥ _____

10. gr ii = _____ mg

11. 1 1/2 qt = _____ mL

12. 30 mg = gr _____

13. 1.6 L = _____ mL

14. 47 kg = _____ lbs

15. 1 mL = m _____

16. 75 lbs = _____ kg

17. 0.008 g = _____ mg

18. 3 mL = m _____

19. gr 1/2 = _____ mg

20. gr 1/150 = _____ mg

21. 6,172 g = _____ kg

22. 200 mL = _____ tsp

23. 102 lbs = _____ kg

24. 204 g = _____ kg

25. 1.5 L = _____ cc

26. 200 mcg = _____ mg

27. 48.6 L = _____ cc

28. 0.7 L = _____ cc

29. ℥ vss = _____ mL

30. 4 tsp = _____ cc

31. gr iv = _____ mg

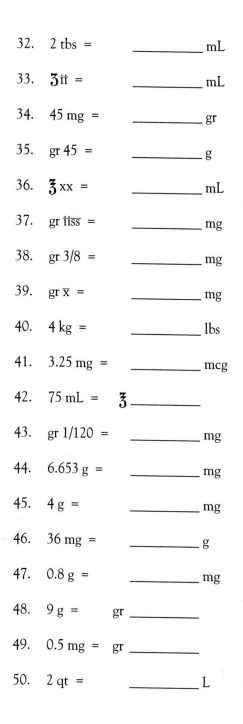

32.   2 tbs = _____ mL

33.   ℥ ii = _____ mL

34.   45 mg = _____ gr

35.   gr 45 = _____ g

36.   ℥ xx = _____ mL

37.   gr iiss = _____ mg

38.   gr 3/8 = _____ mg

39.   gr x̄ = _____ mg

40.   4 kg = _____ lbs

41.   3.25 mg = _____ mcg

42.   75 mL = ℥ _____

43.   gr 1/120 = _____ mg

44.   6.653 g = _____ mg

45.   4 g = _____ mg

46.   36 mg = _____ g

47.   0.8 g = _____ mg

48.   9 g = gr _____

49.   0.5 mg = gr _____

50.   2 qt = _____ L

Unit Three

Methods of Administration and Calculation

The safe and accurate administration of medications to a client is an important and primary responsibility of a nurse. Being able to read and calculate medication orders is necessary for accurate administration.

9 Medication Administration

Objectives

After reviewing this chapter the student will be able to do the following:

1. State the "five rights" of safe medication administration
2. Identify factors that influence medication dosages
3. Identify the common routes for medication administration

Medications are therapeutic measures for a client; however, when administered haphazardly they can cause harmful effects. When a medication error is made it is often caused by multiple factors.

Some causes of medication errors are as follows:

1. The way in which a drug is ordered.
2. Errors in the mathematical calculation of dosages.
3. Incorrect reading of labels on medications.
4. Poor labeling and/or packaging of drugs by the pharmaceutical companies.
5. Lack of knowledge concerning the medication to be administered.
6. Use of improper abbreviations, incorrect expression of drug dosages, or illegible and incorrect preparation of medication records.
7. Failure to properly identify a client before administering medications or failure to listen to a client and double-check when clients raise questions regarding a medication.
8. Failure to educate a client properly about medications they are taking.
9. Administration of medications without any thought.

The reasons for medication errors are not limited to those listed and not limited to nursing errors alone. The best solution for medication errors is prevention. One way to prevent medication errors is for personnel involved in the administration of medications to perform the task properly.

The administration of medications is more than just giving the medication ordered or merely giving it because it is what the doctor ordered. The doctor orders the medication, but the nurse should know the action, uses, side effects, expected response, and the range of dosage for the medication being administered. Nurses must be accountable when administering medications. This includes preparation and administration.

Medication administration is a process that includes assessment, planning, intervention, evaluation, and teaching clients about safe administration. Failure to think about what you are doing, why you are doing it, and failure to assess a client can result in errors.

Factors That Influence Drug Dosages and Action

There are several factors that influence drug dosages and the way they act. These factors include the following:

1. Route of administration.
2. Time of administration.
3. Age of the client.
4. Nutritional status of the client.
5. Absorption and excretion of the drug.
6. Health status of the client.
7. Sex of the client.

All of the above factors affect how an individual reacts to a medication and the dosage they receive. All of these factors must be considered when medications are prescribed and administered. Due to differences in the actions and the types of drugs, clients also respond in various ways, and therefore dosages must be individualized. No two clients will respond to a medication in the same manner.

Special Considerations for the Elderly

Elderly individuals are constant users of our health-care system and may take a large number of either over the counter or prescribed medications. As with children (see Chapter 19), special considerations should be given to the client who is over 65 years of age. With aging comes the slowing down of the body's functions. Some of the changes that occur that can have a direct effect in terms of medication and their action include the following: decrease in circulation, slower absorption, slower metabolism, and a decrease in excretory functions. These physiological changes can cause unexpected drug reactions and cause the elderly individual to be more sensitive to the effects of many drugs. As a rule the elderly client will require smaller doses of medications, and they should be given further apart to prevent accumulation of drugs and toxicity. With aging there may be visual and hearing problems. Special attention must be given when teaching clients about their medications to avoid errors. Take time and talk to the elderly, listen to what they say, and never assume they don't know how much or what medications they are taking.

The "Five Rights" of Medication Administration

When administering medications to a client the "five rights" of medication administration should serve as guidelines. Failure to achieve any of these "rights" constitutes a medication error. The "five rights" should be checked before administering any medication to avoid errors and ensure client safety.

The **"Five Rights"**

1. The right drug.

2. The right dose.

3. The right client.

4. The right route.

5. The right time.

The right drug – When medications are ordered they should be compared with the order that is written. When administering medications the label on the medication container should be checked against the MAR (medication administration record) or medication ticket. Medications should be checked three times: before pouring it, after pouring, and before replacing the container. With "unit dose" (each drug dose is prepared in the prescribed dose, packaged, labeled, and ready to use) the label should still be checked three times.

The right dose – Always perform and check calculations carefully, without ignoring decimals. Have someone else double-check a dosage that causes concern. In some agencies certain medication dosages are always checked by another nurse (for example, insulin and heparin). After dosages are calculated they should be given using standard measurement devices such as calibrated medicine dropper, cups, etc.

The right client – Always make sure you are administering medications to the right client. Ask for the client's name, and check the client's identification bracelet against the medication administration record. If a client does not have an identification brace-let, obtain one; secure the help of a staff member in establishing proper identification. Never go by room number or last name only.

The right route – Medications should be given by the correct route (for example, orally or by injection). The route of the medication should be stated on the order. Do not assume.

The right time – Drugs should be given at the correct time of day and interval (for example, t.i.d. [three times a day], q6h [every six hours], etc). Judgment should be used as to when medications should be given or not given. If several medications are ordered, set priorities and administer medications that must act at a certain time. For example, insulin should be given at an exact time before meals.

Documentation – Medications should be charted accurately, as soon as they are given on the right client's medication record, under the right date, and next to the right time. If a medication is refused it should be documented as such with a notation on the medication record or in the nurse's notes. Never chart a medication as given before administering it or without documentation as to why it was not given. Follow the policy of the institution when documenting. All documentation should be legible. Correct documentation has also been included in the five rights of medication administration and referred to by some as the sixth right.

Routes of Medication Administration

Medications come in several forms for administration.

1. **Oral** – (p.o.) by mouth (for example, tablets, capsules, and liquid solutions). Some medications are given sublingual (placed under the tongue) or buccal (placed against the cheek).

2. **Parenteral** – administration of medications by a route other than by mouth or gastrointesinal tract. Parenteral includes intravenous (IV), intramuscular (IM), subcutaneous (sc), and intradermal.

3. **Insertion** – placing a drug into a body cavity, where the medication dissolves at body temperature (for example, suppositories).

4. **Instillation** – putting a drug in liquid form into a body cavity. This can also include placing an ointment into a body cavity such as erythromycin eye ointment, which is placed in the conjunctiva of the eye. Instillation-type medications also include nose drops and ear drops.

5. **Inhalation** – administration of a drug into the repiratory tract, such as nebulizers used by clients for asthma. In some institutions these medications are administered to the client by use of special equipment, such as positive pressure breathing equipment or the aerosol mask.

6. **Topical** – medications are applied to the external surface of the skin. These include aerosol powders, liquids, ointments, pastes, and transdermal medications (medications in a patch applied to skin and slowly released and absorbed through the skin. These may be effective for hours or days at a time). Examples include Nitro-Dur and Nitropaste used for chest pain.

Forms of oral medications (tablets, capsules), oral solutions, and routes for parenteral medications will be discussed in more detail in later chapters.

Equipment Used In Dosage Calculation

Equipment used for oral administration includes a 30-milliliter or 1-ounce medication cup made of plastic that is used to measure most liquid medications. The cup has measurements that include all three systems of measure. (See Figure 9.1.)

Souffle Cup – A small paper or plastic cup used for solid forms of medication such as tablets and capsules. (See Figure 9.2.)

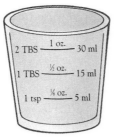

Figure 9.1 Medicine cup.

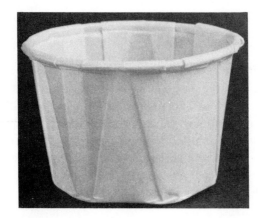

Figure 9.2 Souffle cup. (From Clayton B, Stock Y: *Basic pharmacology for nurses*, ed 10, St Louis, 1993, Mosby.)

Calibrated Dropper – This may be used to administer small amounts of medication to an adult or child. It is usually marked in milliliters or cubic centimeters. The size of the drops varies and depends on the dropper. Since the size of drops varies it is important to remember that drops should not be used as a medication measure unless the dropper is calibrated. Droppers used for the administration of eye, nose, and ear medications are designed for that purpose. Certain medications come with a dropper that is calibrated according to the medication. Examples include children's vitamins and Nystatin oral solutions. (See Figure 9.3 of a calibrated dropper.)

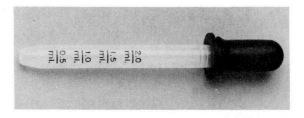

Figure 9.3 Medicine dropper. (From Clayton B, Stock Y: *Basic pharmacology for nurses*, ed 10, St Louis, 1993, Mosby.)

Oral Syringe – This may be used for the administration of liquid medications to adults and children. This type of syringe is designed for the purpose of administering medications orally. No needle is attached. (See Figure 9.4.)

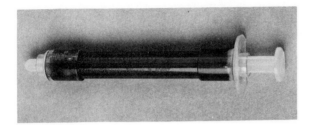

Figure 9.4 Plastic oral syringe. (From Clayton B, Stock Y: *Basic pharmacology for nurses*, ed 10, St Louis, 1993, Mosby.)

Parenteral Syringe – This type of syringe is used for intramuscular, subcutaneous, intradermal, and intravenous drugs. These syringes come in various sizes and are marked in minims and cubic centimeters. Some are marked in units. The specific types of syringes are discussed in more detail in the chapter on parenteral medications. (See Figure 9.5.) The barrel of the syringe holds the medication and has calibrations on it. The needle is attached to the tip. The plunger pushes the medication out. The size of the needle depends on how the medication is given (for example, subcutaneous or intramuscular), the viscosity of the drug, and the size of the client.

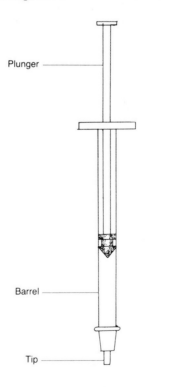

Figure 9.5 Parts of a syringe. (From Clayton B, Stock Y: *Basic pharmacology for nurses*, ed 10, St Louis, 1993, Mosby.)

Chapter Review

1. Name the "five rights" of medication administration

   Right   _drug_

   Right   _dose_

   Right   _Pt_

   Right   _Route_

   Right   _time_

2. Two ways of administering medications to the right client are the following:

   a. ___✓ the Pt ID Bracelet ē M.A.R.___

   b. ___ASK Pt to State their name___

3. A medication label should be read ___3___ times.

4. Medications should be charted ___After___ you have given them.

5. The administration of medications outside the gastrointestinal tract is termed

   ___Parenterce___.

10 Understanding Medication Orders

Objectives

After reviewing this chapter the student will be able to do the following:

1. Identify the components of a medication order
2. Identify the meanings of standard abbreviations used in medication administration
3. Interpret a given medication order

Physicians communicate to the nurse or designated health-care worker which medication or medications to administer to a client by giving a medication order. Medication orders and doctor's orders are used interchangeably. Medication orders can be verbal or written. Verbal orders should only be taken in an emergency situation; however, the verbal order should then be written and signed by the doctor as soon as it is possible to do so. Doctors are usually the only persons allowed to prescribe medications, although in some institutions individuals such as nurse-practitioners, midwives, and physician's assistants may have this privilege as well. In some institutions those persons writing medication orders other than a doctor may require those orders to be countersigned by designated personnel. It is important to be familiar with the specific policies regarding doctor's orders since they vary according to the institution or health-care facility.

The doctor's order indicates the drug plan or medication a doctor has ordered for a client. Before transcribing an order or preparing a dosage, the nurse must be familiar with reading and interpreting an order. A medication order must have certain components and often includes standard abbreviations that the nurse must be able to recall from memory. The abbreviations used in a medication order include units of measure, route, and frequency for the medication ordered. A list of the common abbreviations used in medication administration is found in the following boxes. It is important for you to memorize these abbreviations.

Medication Administration Abbreviations

Abbreviation	Meaning	Abbreviation	Meaning
$\overline{a}$	before	$\overline{p}$	after
$\overline{aa}$, aa	of each	p.c.	after meals
a.c.	before meals	per	through or by
ad.lib.	as desired, freely	per os, p.o.	by or through mouth
b.i.d.	twice a day	p.r.	by rectum
b.i.w.	twice a week	p.r.n.	when necessary/ required
$\overline{c}$	with	q.	every, each
cap, caps	capsule	q.a.m.	every morning
d.c., D/C	discontinue	q.d.	every day
dil.	dilute	q.h.	every hour
DS	double strength	q2h, q4h	every two hours, every four hours
elix.	elixir	qhs, q.h.s.	every night at bedtime
fl, fld.	fluid	q.i.d.	four times a day
gtt	drop	q.n.	every night
h, hr	hour	q.o.d.	every other day
h.s.	hour of sleep, at bedtime	q.s.	a sufficient amount/ as much as needed
I.M.	intramuscular	$\overline{s}$	without
I.V.	intravenous	$\overline{ss}$, ss	one half
IVPB	intravenous piggyback	s.c., S.C., s.q.	subcutaneous
IVSS	intravenous soluset	sl, SL	sublingual
LA	long-acting	sol, soln	solution
LOS	length of stay	s.o.s.	once if necessary
NGT, ng	nasogastric tube	SR	slow-release
n.p.o., NPO	nothing by mouth	stat, STAT	immediately, at once
NS, N/S	normal saline	supp	suppository
o.d.	once a day, every day	susp	suspension
OD	right eye	syp, syr	syrup
o.n.	every night	tab	tablet
os	mouth	t.i.d.	three times a day
OS	left eye	tr., tinct	tincture
OU	both eyes	ung., oint	ointment

Note: Certain abbreviations may be capitalized to indicate different meanings. For example, od in lower case letters means once a day, every day; OD in capital letters pertains to the eye.

Abbreviations/Symbols Used In Medication Administration

Abbreviation/Symbol	Meaning
cc	cubic centimeter
dr, ʒ	dram
g	gram
gr	grain
gtt	drop
kg	kilogram
L	liter
m	minim
mcg	microgram
mEq*	milliequivalent
mg	milligram
mL, ml	milliliter
MU	milliunits
oz, ʒ	ounce
T, tbs	tablespoon
t, tsp	teaspoon
U**	unit

* mEq (milliequivalent) is a drug measure in which electrolytes are measured.

Example: Potassium.

** U (Unit) is a basic quantity in a measurement system that is used to indicate strengths of medications.

Example: Penicillin 50,000 U and Insulin U-100. There is no conversion between units and milliequivalents.

Writing A Medication Order

When a doctor writes a medication order, it is written in a special book for doctor's orders or on a form called the *doctor's order sheet* in the client's chart or hospital record. Doctor's order sheets vary from institution to institution. The order sheet should have the client's name on it. A prescription blank is used to write medication orders for clients who are being discharged from the hospital or are seeing the doctor in an outpatient facility. Nurses frequently have to explain these orders for the client so they have an understanding of the dosages they will be taking.

Components of a Medication Order

When a medication order is written it must contain seven important parts or it is considered invalid or incomplete. The basic parts that a medication order must contain are as follows:

1. The client's full name – This avoids confusion of the client with another, therefore preventing error in administering the wrong medication to the wrong client. Many institutions use a name plate to imprint the client's name and record number on the order sheet. In institutions that use computers, the computer screen will show identifying information for the client, such as age and known drug allergies.

2. Date and time the order was written – This includes the month, day, year, and the time the order was written. This will help in determining the start and stop of the medication order. In many institutions the doctor is required to include the length of time the medication is to be given (Example: 7 days).

Note: A record of the time the order was written is preferred in many institutions, but omission does not invalidate the order.

3. The name of the medication – The medication may be ordered by the generic or brand name. To avoid confusion with another medication, the medication should be written clearly and spelled correctly.

   a) generic name – has to do with the proper name, or chemical compound, and is usually designated in lower case letters.

   b) trade name – refers to the brand name, or the name under which a manufacturer markets the drug. This is usually designated by beginning with a capital letter.

   Example: acetaminophen is the generic name for Tylenol; furosemide is the generic name for Lasix.

4. Dosage of the medication – The amount of the medication as well as the strength should be written clearly to avoid confusion.

   Example: In some institutions when the medication ordered is expressed in units, which is abbreviated (U), the written order is written without abbreviating units to avoid confusion with the (U) being read as a zero (0). When abbreviations for measure are used, only standard abbreviations should be used.

5. Route of administration – This is a very important part of a medication order since medications can be administered by several routes. Never assume that you know which route is appropriate. Standard abbreviations should be used to indicate the route.

Example: p.o. (oral, by mouth).

6. Time and/or frequency of administration – This indicates the times a medication is to be given using standard abbreviations.

Example: q.i.d. (four times a day), STAT (immediately).

The time intervals in which a medication is administered are determined by the institution and most have routine times for administering medications.

Example: t.i.d. (three times a day) may be 9 a.m., 1 p.m., and 5 p.m. or 10 a.m., 2 p.m., and 6 p.m.

Factors such as the purpose of the drug, drug interactions, absorption of the drug, and side effects should be considered when scheduling medication times.

7. Signature of the person writing the order – For a medication order to be legal it must be signed by the doctor. The doctor writing the order must include his or her signature on the order, and it should be legible. In some institutions, depending on the rank of the doctor, an order may have to be co-signed by a senior doctor.

Example: Resident or intern's orders may require the signature of an attending doctor.

In addition to the seven items listed, any special instructions for certain medications need to be clearly written.

Example: Hold if blood pressure is below 100 systolic; administer a half hour before meals.

Medications ordered as needed or whenever necessary (p.r.n.) should indicate the purpose of administration as well.

Example: For chest pain, temperature above 101, or blood pressure greater than 140 systolic and 90 diastolic.

In instances where specific instructions are not stated, nursing judgment must be used to determine whether it is appropriate or not to administer a medication.

For dosage calculations the nurse is usually concerned with components 3 to 6 of a medication order (the drug name, dosage of the drug, route, and time or frequency of administration). This information aids in determining a safe and reasonable dosage for a client.

Interpreting a Medication Order

Medication orders are written in the following order:

1. The name of the drug.

2. The dosage expressed in standard abbreviations or symbols.

3. The route.

4. The frequency.

Example: Colace   100 mg.   p.o.   t.i.d.
↓   ↓   ↓   ↓
name   dosage   route   frequency

This order means the doctor wants the client to recieve 100 milligrams of a stool softener named Colace by mouth three times a day. The use of abbreviations in a medication order is like a form of shorthand; it shortens the amount of writing to give a specific order.

Depending on the policy of the institution the nurse or trained personnel such as the unit secretary (ward clerk) transcribes the medication order to the appropriate MAR or ticket. In facilities where personnel other than the nurse transcribe orders, the nurse still has the responsibility for double-checking and co-signing the order, indicating it has been correctly transcribed.

Transcribing of orders has decreased in institutions where the unit dose is used, resulting in fewer errors. In some institutions that use unit dose, however, more transcribing may be necessary because the MAR may only have the capacity to be used for a 5-day period. Therefore it is necessary to transcribe orders again at the end of the designated time period.

In facilities that use computers, the medication order is placed into the computer, and a printout is generated that lists the currently ordered medications. The use of the computer therefore eliminates the need for transcribing orders. The charting of the medications administered is also done directly into the computer. Computerized charting does not eliminate the responsibility of the nurse to double-check medication orders.

Points to Remember:

✔ A primary responsibility of the nurse is the safe administration of medications to a client.

✔ The seven components of a medication order are as follows:

1. The full name of the client.

2. Date and time the order was written.

3. Name of the medication to be administered.

4. Dosage of the medication.

5. Route of administration.

6. Time or frequency of administration.

7. Signature of the person writing the order.

✔ All medication orders must be legible and use standard abbreviations and/or symbols.

✔ If any of the seven components of a medication order are missing or seem incorrect, don't assume – clarify the order!

Chapter Review

A. List the seven components of a medication order:

1. _____

2. _____

3. _____

4. _____

5. _____

6. _____

7. _____

B. Write the meaning of the following abbreviations:

8. b.i.d. _twice a day_

9. OU _Both Eyes_

10. ad.lib. _as desired_

11. s.c. _Subcutaneous_

12. c̄ _with_

13. a.c. _Before meals_

14. q.i.d. _4 x a day_

15. b.i.w. _twice a week_

16. h.s. _hour of sleep_

17. o.d. _____

18. elix. _Elixer_

19. OS _Left Eye_

20. syr. _Syrup_

21. n.p.o. _Nothing by mouth_

22. sl. _____

C. Give the abbreviations for the following:

23. after meals _p̄ c_

24. three times a day _tid_

25. intramuscular _Im_

26. every eight hours _q8h_

27. suppository _Sup_

28. intravenous _IV_

29. once if necessary _SOS_

30. without _s̄_

31.   immediately   _____ stat _____

32.   right eye   _____ OD _____

33.   ointment   _____ Oint _____

34.   one half   _____ ss _____

35.   milliequivalents   _____ mEq _____

36.   every night at bedtime _____ qhs _____

37.   by rectum   _____ pr _____

D. Interpret the following orders:

38. Methergine 0.2 mg p.o. q4h × 6 doses.   _____

_____

39. Digoxin 0.125 mg p.o. o.d.   _____

_____

40. Regular Humulin Insulin 14 U. s.c. q.d. 7:30 a.m.   _____

_____

41. Demerol 50 mg I.M. and Atropine gr 1/150 I.M. on call to the operating room.

_____

42. Ampicillin 500 mg p.o. stat, and then 250 mg p.o. q.i.d. thereafter.

_____

43. Lasix 40 mg I.M. stat. _____

_____

44. Librium 50 mg p.o. q4h p.r.n. for agitation. _____

_____

45. Potassium Chloride 20 mEq I.V. × 2 Liters. _____

_____

46. Tylenol gr x p.o. q4h p.r.n. for pain. _____

_____

47. Mylicon 80 mg p.o. pc and hs. _____

_____

48. Folic Acid 1 mg p.o. o.d. _____

_____

49. Nembutal 100 mg p.o. h.s. p.r.n. _____

_____

50. Aspirin gr x p.o. q4h p.r.n. for temperature > 101°F. _____

_____

51. Dilantin 100 mg p.o. t.i.d. _____

_____

52. Minipress 2 mg p.o. b.i.d. hold for systolic b/p (blood pressure) < 120. _____

_____

53. Compazine 10 mg. I.M. q4h p.r.n. for nausea and vomiting _____

_____

54. Ampicillin 1 g I.V.P.B. q6h × 4 doses. _____

_____

55. Heparin 5000 U. s.c. q12h. _____

_____

56. Dilantin susp. 200 mg per NGT q a.m. and 300 mg per NGT h.s. _____

_____

57. Benadryl 50 mg p.o. stat. _____

_____

E. Identify the missing part from the following medication orders. Assume the date, time, and signature are included on the orders.

58. Dicloxacillin 250 mg q.i.d.   _Route of administration_

59. Synthroid 0.05 mg p.o.   _Frequency or time of Administration_

60. Nitrofurantoin p.o. q6h × 10 days.   _____

61. 25 mg p.o. q12h, hold if B/P m < 100 systolic. _____

62. Solucortef 100 q6h.   _____

11 Medication Administration Records

Objectives

After reviewing this chapter the student will be able to do the following:

1. Identify the necessary information that must be transcribed to a medication administration record (MAR)
2. Read an MAR and identify medications that are given on a routine basis, including name of the medication, dosage, route of administration, and time of administration
3. Transcribe medication orders to an MAR

The medication record system is the most widely used system for drug administration. The medication record is a way of keeping track of medications that a client has received and is currently receiving. The name of each medication, as well as the dosage, route, and frequency, is written on the client's medication record. A complete schedule is written out of all the administration times for medications that are given on a continuous or routine basis. Each time a dose is given the nurse initials it next to the time. In some institutions separate records are maintained for routine, I.V., p.r.n., and medications administered on a one-time basis, while in others these are kept on the same record in a designated area. The medication record system is the same as the MAR.

For medication records and charting, some institutions use a Kardex, an MAR, or a combination of both. Other institutions use a computerized system in which medication-charting information is entered into the computer, which automatically generates a list of all the medications to be given and the times.

After a doctor's order has been verified, the order is transcribed to the official record used at the institution. As we examine the various medication records presented in this chapter, you will notice that despite the difference in forms, there is essential information that is common to all.

Essential Information on a Medication Record

All of the information that appears on the medication record must be legible and transcribed carefully to avoid a medication error. In addition to client information, the following information is necessary on all medication forms:

1. Dates – This usually includes the date the order was written and the date the medication is to be started (if different from the order date).

2. Medication Information – This includes the drug's full name, the dosage strength, the route, and the frequency. Abbreviations used on the medication record should be standard abbreviations.

3. Time of Administration – This will be based on the desired administration schedule stated on the order, such as "t.i.d." The desired administration time is placed on the medication record and converted to time periods based on the institution's time intervals for scheduled or routine medications. Thus, t.i.d. may mean 9 a.m.–1p.m.–5p.m. at one institution and 10 a.m.–2 p.m.–6 p.m. at another.) Medication times for p.r.n. and one-time doses are recorded at the time they are administered.

4. Initials – Most medication records have a place for the initials of the person transcribing the medication to the MAR and the person administering the medication.

5. Special Instructions – Any special instructions relating to a medication should be indicated on the medication record. For example, "Hold if blood pressure < 100 systolic" or "p.r.n. for pain."

In addition to the above information, some medication records may include space for charting information such as injection site, pulse, and blood pressure if this information is relevant to the medication.

Documentation of Medications Administered

Medication records include an area for documenting medications administered. After administering the medication, the nurse or other qualified personnel must sign their initials next to the time the drug was given. For scheduled medications, a complete schedule is written out, and the person records initials next to each given time. With one-time doses and p.r.n. medication, the time of administration is written and again initialed by the person administering it. The medication form has a place for the full name of each person administering medications, along with the identifying initials. This allows for immediate identification of the person's initials if necessary. When medications are not administered, some records have notations, such as an asterisk (*), that indicate this. The type of notations used will depend on the institution. In addition to the notations made on the medication record, most institutions require documentation in the nurse's notes.

Following are sample forms that are used in medication administration.

Computerized Medication Records

In institutions that use a computerized system, orders are entered directly into the computer by the doctor along with all other essential information relating to the client. The institution generates its own medication record, following a specific format. Figure 11.1 shows a patient care worksheet indicating the medication orders. Figure 11.2 shows the charting of the medications, which is done directly into the computer. The abbreviation GIV next to the medications means that the medications were given. The full name of the nurse administering the medications is listed to the right of the printout. In addition to the printout on an individual, a printout is generated that shows the scheduled medications that are due on the various units. (See Figure 11.3.) Each client's name and room number are also included on the printout.

Unit Dose System

Many institutions have adopted a system of medication administration referred to as *unit dose*. This system has decreased medication preparation time since the medications are prepared in the pharmacy on a daily basis and sent to the unit. The type of medication forms used for this system varies from one institution to another. In some instances this system has decreased the amount of transcription of orders, while in other instances transcription to the medication record is still required. Samples of the type of forms that are used in the unit dose system are illustrated in Figures 11.4 to 11.6.

Figure 11.4 shows a sample of a doctor's order sheet used at an institution that uses unit dose. This form requires the doctor to write the medication order on a form that is in triplicate. The original copy is placed on the MAR. The second copy is sent to the pharmacy, and the last copy remains in the client's chart. This eliminates checking the order in the chart since the original is attached to the MAR. Transcription of the order is therefore not required. Figure 11.5 illustrates placement of the medication order on the medication administration record. Figure 11.6 shows an MAR used at some institutions for p.r.n. medications, one-time dose orders, and intravenous therapy. Note that on the sample medication records shown in Figures 11.5 and 11.6, the charting of medications administered is alongside the actual doctor's order.

In some institutions using unit dose, however, transcription of medication orders to the MAR is required. The doctor's orders are therefore written on a separate order sheet. Figure 11.7 illustrates the transcription of orders to the MAR. Figure 11.8 illustrates the back of the medication record shown in Figure 11.7.

In institutions that do not use unit dose or computers, standard-type medication sheets may be used that require the nurse to transcribe the medications to the MAR from the doctor's order sheet. It is important to notice that regardless of the form used, the data relating to medications are the same. Figure 11.9 shows a standard MAR that might be used.

```
1S   -0882        TDS HEALTHCARE DEMO HOSPITAL
09/12/89  07:37 AM              (QAB$$N)                    PAGE 001
==========================================
BAKER, SAMUEL              M   68
MR#: 10017598       ACCT#: 5029541I            PATIENT CARE SUMMARY
SERV: CARD          1S        106A
MD: PIERCE,BENJAMIN     ADM: 09/11/89
DX: CHF
==========================================
SUMMARY: 09/12 07:00 AM TO 03:30 PM


PATIENT INFORMATION:
     09/11       ADMIT DX:CHF

ALL CURRENT MEDICAL ORDERS:

   NURSING ORDERS:
     09/11  10. ACTIVITY, BEDREST, (BP ).
     09/11  11. POSITION: ELEVATE HD OF BED 30 DEG, (BP ).

   DIET:
     09/11   1. DIET: CARDIAC, SODIUM CONTROLLED: 2000MG (87 MEQ),
                  (BP ).

   SCHEDULED MEDICATIONS:
     09/11   2. LASIX FUROSEMIDE TAB 40MG, #1, PO, Q12H, (09/11/89
                  09AM-..), (BP ).  09
     09/11   3. DIGOXIN TAB 0.25MG, #1, PO, QD, (09/11/89 02PM-..),
                  (BP ).  02
     09/12  13. ARTIFICIAL TEARS ARTIFICIAL TEARS (15ML),, 3 GTTS,
                  BOTH EYES, Q4H, WHILE AWAKE, (09/12/89 09AM-..), (MC )
                  . 09 01
     09/12  15. METAMUCIL PSYLLIUM HYDROPHILIC MUCILLOID PKT (LIME
                  FLAVORED), PO, WITH WATER, BID, (09/12/89 09AM-..),
                  (MC ). 09

   PRN MEDICATIONS:
     09/11   8. DALMANE FLURAZEPAM CAP 15MG, #1, PO, QHS, PRN,
                  (09/11/89 10PM-..), (BP ).
     09/11   9. DALMANE FLURAZEPAM CAP 15MG, #1, PO REP X1, (BP ).

   DRUG INTERACTIONS:
     09/11       DRUG INTERACTION: .
                 KALURETICS INCREASE THE EFFECT OF DIGITALIS.
                 DIGOXIN TAB 0.25MG, #1, PO, QD  (09/11/89 02PM-..)
                 ENTERED FOR: PIERCE,BENJAMIN 09/11/89.
                 FUROSEMIDE TAB 40MG, #1, PO Q12H  (09/11/89 09AM-..)
                 ENTERED FOR: PIERCE,BENJAMIN 09/11/89 SEVERITY: 2
                 HANSTEN 4TH: 277 DRUG INTER. FACTS: 249,253

   LABORATORY:
    # 09/11   6. (IN PROCESS)H&H, TOMORROW, (09/12/89), (BP ).
    # 09/11   7. (IN PROCESS)ELECTROLYTES, TOMORROW, (09/12/89), (BP ).

   RADIOLOGY:
     09/11   4. X-RAY: CHEST, PA & LAT, INDICATION: --CHF, PRECAUTION:
                  OXYGEN, HANDLING: BEDSIDE/PORTABLE, SCHEDULE: STAT,

                           CONTINUED
==========================================
BAKER, SAMUEL              10017598           PATIENT CARE SUMMARY


09/12/89  07:37 AM              (QAB$$N)                    PAGE 002
==========================================
BAKER, SAMUEL              M   68
MR#: 10017598       ACCT#: 5029541I            PATIENT CARE SUMMARY
SERV: CARD          1S        106A
MD: PIERCE,BENJAMIN     ADM: 09/11/89
DX: CHF
==========================================
SUMMARY: 09/12 07:00 AM TO 03:30 PM

                  (BP ).

   ANCILLARY:
     09/11   5. NASAL CANNULA: 2 LPM --CONTINUOUSLY....INDICATION:
                  IMPROVE DISTRIBUTION OF VENTILATION, (BP ).

                           LASTPAGE
```

Figure 11.1 Sample computer printouts relating to medication administration. (Used with permission from TDS-Hospital Information Systems, sample clinical reports, pp. 45-46, 200 Ashford Center North, Atlanta, GA 30338.)

```
MEDICATIONS:
INDERAL, PROPRANOLOL TAB 40MG,
  09/12 09:00AM #1, PO,GIV                              MCKINNEY,PATRICIA
  09/12 05:00PM #1, PO,GIV                              MCKINNEY,PATRICIA
DIGOXIN TAB 0.25MG,
  09/12 09:00AM #1, PO,GIV                              MCKINNEY,PATRICIA
LASIX, FUROSEMIDE TAB 20MG,
  09/12 09:00AM #1, PO,GIV                              MCKINNEY,PATRICIA
  09/12 09:00PM #1, PO,GIV                              MCKINNEY,PATRICIA
```

Figure 11.2 Sample computer printout relating to medication administration. (Used with permission from TDS-Hospital Information Systems, sample clinical reports, p. 48, 200 Ashford Center North, Atlanta, GA 30338.)

```
1S   -0829        TDS HEALTHCARE DEMO HOSPITAL
             09:00 AM SCHEDULED MEDICATIONS DUE 1S    A  09/12/89
                                           ISSUED 06:28 AM 09/12/89


100P   SANDERS, JOHN                                          GIV NGIV

INDERAL PROPRANOLOL TAB 40MG, #1, PO, Q8H, (09/11/89 09AM-..)
, (MC ).                                                      --- ---

LASIX FUROSEMIDE TAB 20MG, #1, PO, BID, (09/12/89 09AM-..),
(MC ).                                                        --- ---

DIGOXIN TAB 0.25MG, #1, PO, DAILY AT, 9AM, STARTING TODAY,
(09/12/89 09AM-..), (MC ).                                    --- ---


101P   JOHNSON, ANDY                                          GIV NGIV

PROCARDIA NIFEDIPINE CAP 10MG, #1, PO, Q8H, (09/11/89 05PM-
..), (MC ).                                                   --- ---


103B   EDGAR, SHARON                                          GIV NGIV

PREDNISONE TAB 5MG, #1, PO, DAILY, X4DAY, (09/12/89 09AM-
09/15/89 09AM), (PN ).                                        --- ---


106A   BAKER, SAMUEL                                          GIV NGIV

LASIX FUROSEMIDE TAB 40MG, #1, PO, Q12H, (09/11/89 09AM-..),
(BP ).                                                        --- ---

ARTIFICIAL TEARS ARTIFICIAL TEARS (15ML),, 3 GTTS, BOTH EYES,
Q4H, WHILE AWAKE, (09/12/89 09AM-..), (MC ).                  --- ---

METAMUCIL PSYLLIUM HYDROPHILIC MUCILLOID PKT (LIME FLAVORED),
PO, WITH WATER, BID, (09/12/89 09AM-..), (MC ).               --- ---


106B   DIXON, PAUL                                            GIV NGIV

KEFZOL CEFAZOLIN IVPB 1GM,  D5W 50ML, ADMINISTER OVER 20 MIN,
Q8H, X21DOSES, (09/12/89 09AM-09/19/89 01AM), (MC ).          --- ---

GENTAMICIN INJ IVPB 80MG, D5W 100ML, ADMINISTER OVER 60 MIN,
Q12, X14DOSES, (09/12/89 09AM-09/18/89 09PM), (MC ).          --- ---


110A   MATTHEWS, ELIZABET                                     GIV NGIV

HEPARIN BEEF LUNG (10000U/ML) INJ 5000U SC, Q8H, (09/11/89
09AM-..), (BHA).                                              --- ---




1S   -0892        TDS HEALTHCARE DEMO HOSPITAL
             05:00 PM UNREPORTED SCHEDULED MEDS 1S    A  09/11/89
                                           ISSUED 08:09 AM 09/12/89


100P   SANDERS, JOHN                                          GIV NGIV

INDERAL PROPRANOLOL TAB 40MG, #1, PO, Q8H, (09/11/89 09AM-..)
, (MC ).                                                      --- ---


101P   JOHNSON, ANDY                                          GIV NGIV

PROCARDIA NIFEDIPINE CAP 10MG, #1, PO, Q8H, (09/11/89 05PM-
..), (MC ).                                                   --- ---


110A   MATTHEWS, ELIZABET                                     GIV NGIV

HEPARIN BEEF LUNG (10000U/ML) INJ 5000U SC, Q8H, (09/11/89
09AM-..), (BHA).                                              --- ---
```

Figure 11.3 Printout of medications for unit. (Used with permission from TDS-Hospital Information Systems, sample clinical reports, pp. 31-32, 200 Ashford Center North, Atlanta, GA 30338.)

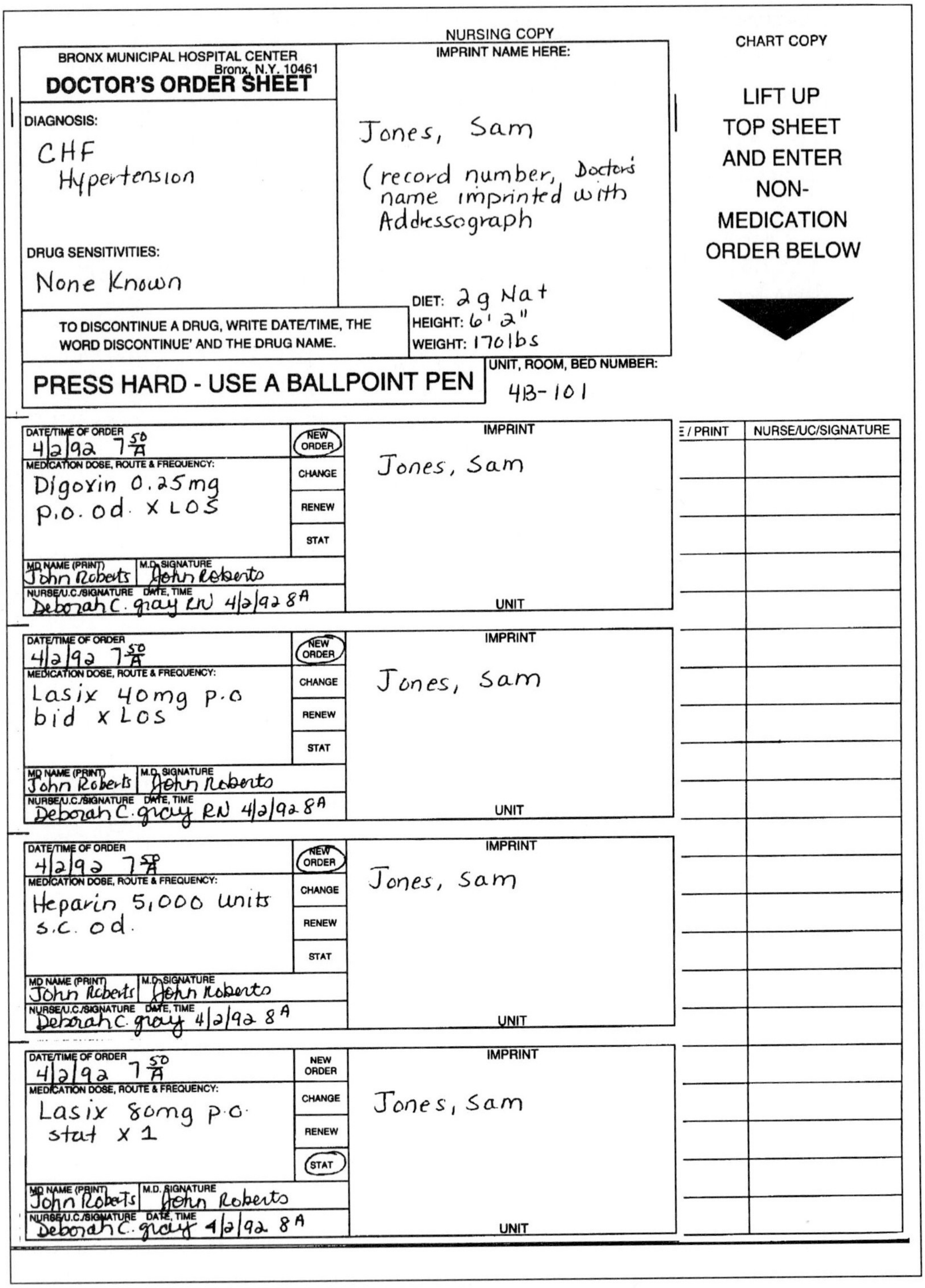

Figure 11.4 Sample of doctor's order sheet. (Used with permission from Bronx Municipal Hospital Center, Bronx, New York.)

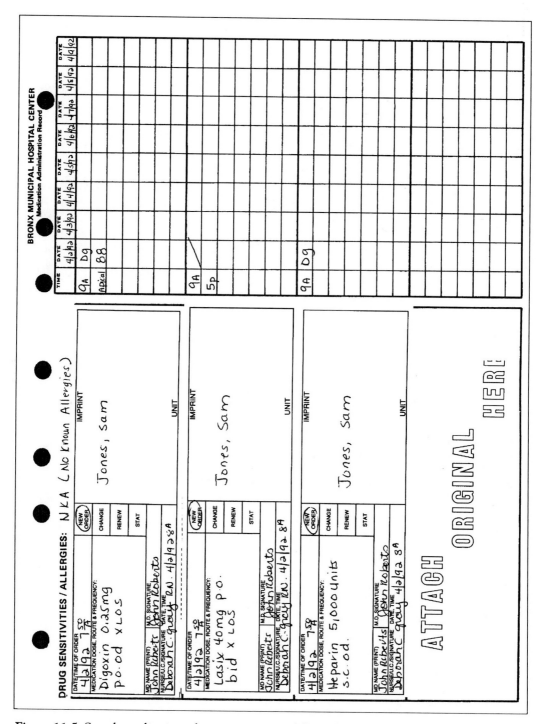

Figure 11.5 Sample medication administration record (MAR). (Used with permission from Bronx Municipal Hospital Center, Bronx, New York.)

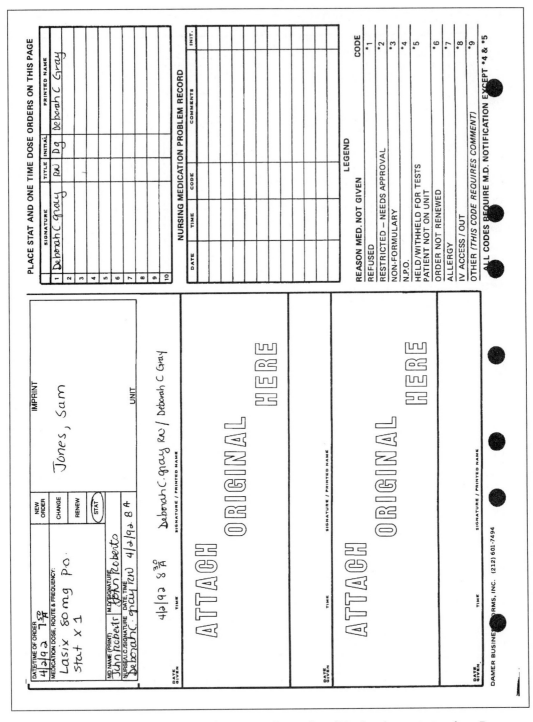

Figure 11.6 Sample MAR for stat and one-time dose orders. (Used with permission from Bronx Municipal Hospital Center, Bronx, New York.)

ST. BARNABAS HOSPITAL

BRONX, NY • DEPARTMENT OF NURSING

MEDICATION ADMINISTRATION RECORD

DIAGNOSES
Bi-polar Disorder

Addressograph with
Patient Identification

ALLERGIC TO: Aspirin   DATE 5/7/92

USE RED ASTERISK (*) TO INDICATE DOSES NOT GIVEN-EXPLAIN IN NURSES NOTES

PAGE _1_ OF _1_

ORDER DATE / EXP. DATE	STANDING MEDICATIONS / MED-DOSE-FREQ-ROUTE	DATE / HOUR	5/7 INIT	5/8 INIT	5/9 INIT	5/10 INIT	5/11 INIT	5/12 INIT	5/13 INIT	5/14 INIT	5/15 INIT
Dg R.N. INIT. 5/7/92 6/7/92	Thorazine 200mg p.o. t.i.d.	9a 1P 5P	Dg								
Dg R.N. INIT. 5/7/92 6/7/92	Dilantin 100mg p.o. bid	9A 5P	Dg								
Dg R.N. INIT. 5/7/92 6/7/92	Ensure 1 can p.o. t.i.d.	9A 1P 5P	Dg								
Dg R.N. INIT. 5/7/92 6/7/92	Benadryl 25mg p.o. H.S	9p	Dg								
R.N.											

PHR-002

INJECTION CODES: RT = RIGHT THIGH   RA = RIGHT ARM   LU = LEFT UPPER GLUTEAL   ↑ RAB = UPPER RIGHT ABDOMEN   ↑ LAB = UPPER LEFT ABDOMEN
LT = LEFT THIGH   LA = LEFT ARM   RU = RIGHT UPPER GLUTEAL   ↓ RAB = LOWER RIGHT ABDOMEN   ↓ LAB = LOWER LEFT ABDOMEN

Figure 11.7 Transcription of medication orders to MAR. (Used with permission from St. Barnabas Hospital, Bronx, New York.)

SINGLE-STAT-PREOP ORDERS

ORDER DATE	NURSE INIT	MED-DOSE-ROUTE	TO BE GIVEN				ORDER DATE	NURSE INIT.	MED-DOSE-ROUTE	TO BE GIVEN		
			DATE	TIME	NURSE INIT				DATE	TIME	NURSE INIT.

P.R.N. MEDICATION

ORDER DATE /EXP DATE	REORD DATE /EXP DATE	MED-DOSE-FREQ-ROUTE		DOSES GIVEN
Dg 5/7/92		Tylenol 650mg p.o. q4h prn for headache	DATE 5/8 TIME 5p SITE PO INIT. Dg	
REORD 6/7/92				

INITIAL IDENTIFICATION

	INITIAL	PRINT NAME, TITLE		INITIAL	PRINT NAME, TITLE		INITIAL	PRINT NAME, TITLE
1	Dg	Deborah C. Gray RN	5			9		
2			6			10		
3			7			11		
4			8			12		

Figure 11.8 Back of medication record in Figure 11.7. (Used with permission from St. Barnabas Hospital, Bronx, New York.)

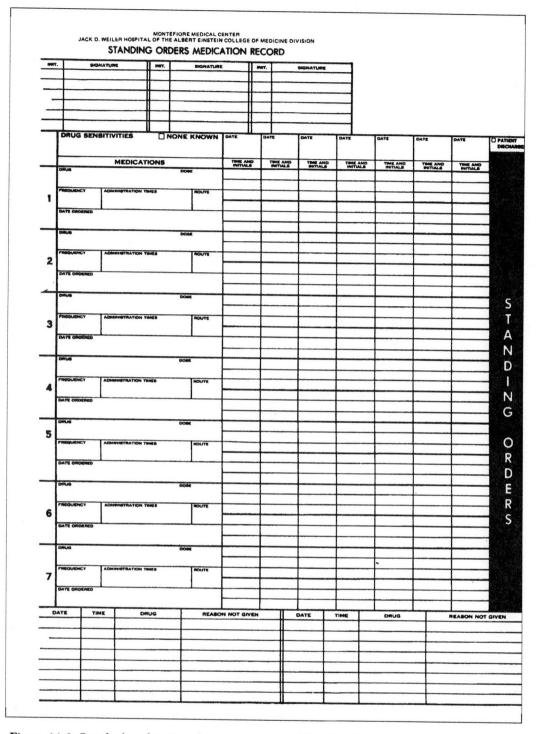

Figure 11.9 Standard medication administration record (MAR). (Used with permission from Montefiore Medical Center, Jack D. Weiler Hospital of the Albert Einstein College of Medicine Division, Bronx, NY.)

Points to Remember:

✔ The system used for medication administration plays a role in determining the type of medication record used and whether transcription of orders is necessary.

✔ Regardless of the type of medication record used at an institution, the nurse should know the data that is essential for the medication record and understand the importance of determining accuracy and clarity of medication orders.

✔ Persons transcribing orders should transcribe them in ink and write legibly to avoid medication errors. All essential notations or instructions should be clearly written on the medication record.

✔ Documentation of medications administered should be done accurately and only by the person administering them.

Practice Exercise

Using the medication administration record on the next page (Figure 11.10), list the medication, dosage, route, and time for the medications given by DG (Deborah C. Gray) on 4/6/92 and 4/8/92.

Practice Exercise

Transcribe the following orders to the practice medication sheets provided. When you have completed this, place your initials in the appropriate space on the medication form. Use the forms provided labeled Standing Orders (Figure 11.11) and STAT/PRN (Figure 11.12). Use the times indicated and the date 4/9/92.

1. Potassium Chloride 20 mEq p.o. od × LOS (9A)

2. Digoxin 0.125 mg p.o. od × LOS (9A)

3. Lasix 30 mg p.o. bid × LOS (9A and 5P)

4. Aldomet 500 mg p.o. b.i.d. × LOS (9A and 5P)

5. Percocet 2 tabs p.o. q 3-4h p.r.n. for pain × 2 days. Chart that you administered it on 4/9/92 at 2 p.m.

6. Tylenol 650 mg p.o. q4h p.r.n. temp > 38.2° C × LOS

Note: The abbreviation LOS = length of stay. When not written as part of the order, it is implied unless stated otherwise.

Check your medication sheet against the medication sheet in the answers section.

MONTEFIORE MEDICAL CENTER
JACK D. WEILER HOSPITAL OF THE ALBERT EINSTEIN COLLEGE OF MEDICINE DIVISION
STANDING ORDERS MEDICATION RECORD

INIT.	SIGNATURE	INIT.	SIGNATURE	INIT.	SIGNATURE
Dg	Deborah C gray				
mB	mary Brown				
AS.	ann Smith				

Addressograph with
Patient Identification

DRUG SENSITIVITIES □ NONE KNOWN		DATE 4/6/92	DATE 4/7/92	DATE 4/8/92	DATE 4/9/92	DATE 4/10/92	DATE 4/11/92	DATE 4/12/92	□ PATIENT DISCHARGE
PCN, Sulfa									
MEDICATIONS		TIME AND INITIALS	TIME AND INITIALS	TIME AND INITIALS	TIME AND INITIALS	TIME AND INITIALS	TIME AND INITIALS	TIME AND INITIALS	
1 DRUG Digoxin DOSE 0.25mg		9A MB ap 76	9A AS ap 72	9A Dg ap 88					
FREQUENCY OD ADMINISTRATION TIMES 9A ROUTE PO.									S
DATE ORDERED 4/6/92									T
2 DRUG Lasix DOSE 20mg		9A mB 5P mB	9A AS 5P AS	9A Dg 5P Dg					A
FREQUENCY bid ADMINISTRATION TIMES 9A -5P ROUTE P.O.									N
DATE ORDERED 4/6/92									D
3 DRUG Procardia DOSE 10mg		9A mB 1P mB 5P Dg	9A AS 1P AS 5P mB	9A Dg 1P Dg 5P Dg					I
FREQUENCY tid ADMINISTRATION TIMES 9A -1P -5P ROUTE SI									N
DATE ORDERED 4/6/92									G
4 DRUG Colace DOSE 100 mg		9A mB 5P mB	9A AS 5P AS	9A Dg 5P Dg					
FREQUENCY bid ADMINISTRATION TIMES 9A -5P ROUTE PO									O
DATE ORDERED 4/6/92									R
5 DRUG Heparin DOSE 5,000 U		9A mB	9A AS	9A Dg					D
FREQUENCY od ADMINISTRATION TIMES 9A ROUTE S.C.									E
DATE ORDERED 4/6/92									R
6 DRUG DOSE									S
FREQUENCY ADMINISTRATION TIMES ROUTE									
DATE ORDERED									
7 DRUG DOSE									
FREQUENCY ADMINISTRATION TIMES ROUTE									
DATE ORDERED									

DATE	TIME	DRUG	REASON NOT GIVEN	DATE	TIME	DRUG	REASON NOT GIVEN

Figure 11.10 Medication administration record for practice questions. (Used with permission from Montefiore Medical Center, Jack D. Weiler Hospital of the Albert Einstein College of Medicine Division, Bronx, NY.)

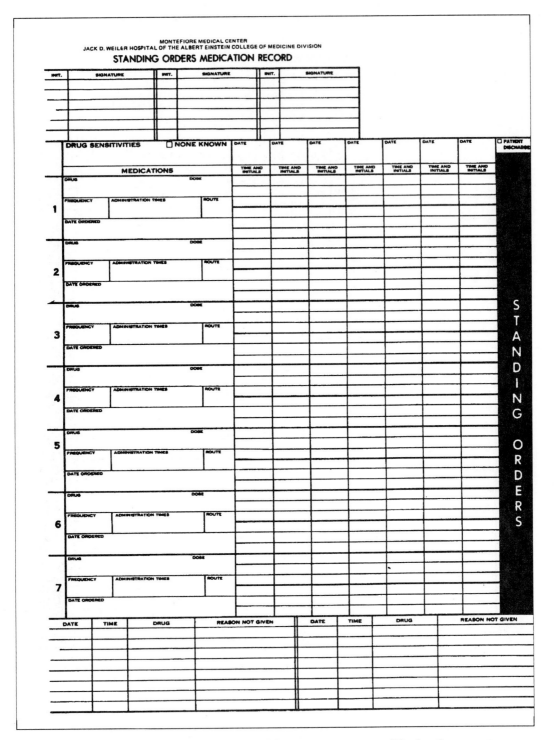

Figure 11.11 Medication administration record for practice questions. (Used with permission from Montefiore Medical Center, Jack D. Weiler Hospital of the Albert Einstein College of Medicine Division, Bronx, NY.)

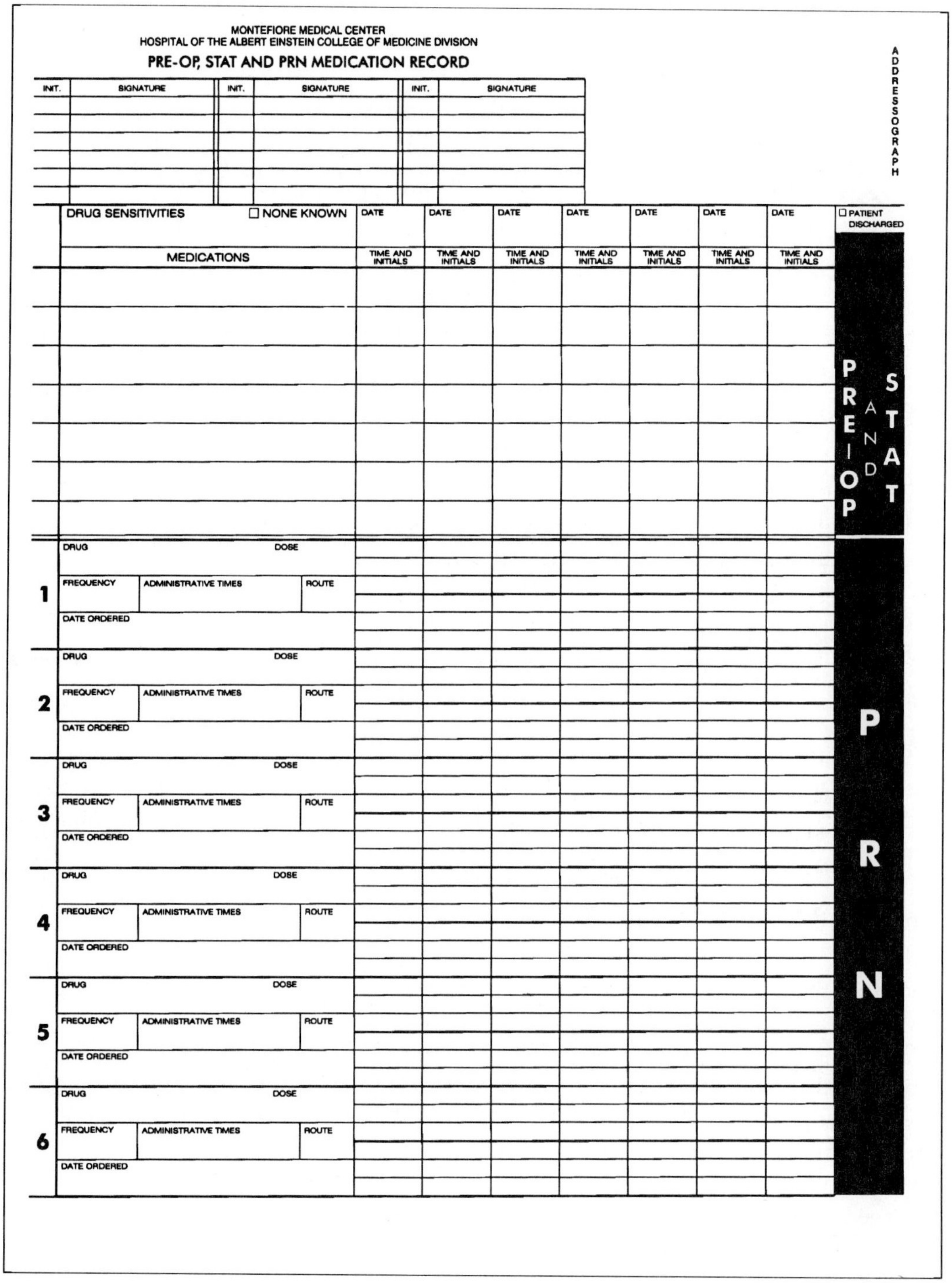

MONTEFIORE MEDICAL CENTER
HOSPITAL OF THE ALBERT EINSTEIN COLLEGE OF MEDICINE DIVISION
PRE-OP, STAT AND PRN MEDICATION RECORD

ADDRESSOGRAPH

INIT.	SIGNATURE	INIT.	SIGNATURE	INIT.	SIGNATURE

DRUG SENSITIVITIES ☐ NONE KNOWN	DATE	DATE	DATE	DATE	DATE	DATE	DATE	☐ PATIENT DISCHARGED
MEDICATIONS	TIME AND INITIALS	TIME AND INITIALS	TIME AND INITIALS	TIME AND INITIALS	TIME AND INITIALS	TIME AND INITIALS	TIME AND INITIALS	PRE-OP AND STAT
1 DRUG / DOSE / FREQUENCY / ADMINISTRATIVE TIMES / ROUTE / DATE ORDERED								PRN
2 DRUG / DOSE / FREQUENCY / ADMINISTRATIVE TIMES / ROUTE / DATE ORDERED								
3 DRUG / DOSE / FREQUENCY / ADMINISTRATIVE TIMES / ROUTE / DATE ORDERED								
4 DRUG / DOSE / FREQUENCY / ADMINISTRATIVE TIMES / ROUTE / DATE ORDERED								
5 DRUG / DOSE / FREQUENCY / ADMINISTRATIVE TIMES / ROUTE / DATE ORDERED								
6 DRUG / DOSE / FREQUENCY / ADMINISTRATIVE TIMES / ROUTE / DATE ORDERED								

Figure 11.12 Medication administration record for practice questions. (Used with permission from Montefiore Medical Center, Jack D. Weiler Hospital of the Albert Einstein College of Medicine Division, Bronx, NY.)

12 Reading Medication Labels

Objectives

After reviewing this chapter the student will be able to do the following:

1. Identify the trade and generic names of medications
2. Identify the dosage strength of medications
3. Identify the form in which the medication is supplied
4. Identify the total volume of the medication container where indicated
5. Identify directions for mixing or preparing a drug where necessary

To administer medications safely to a client, nurses must be able to read and interpret the information on a medication label. Medication labels indicate the dosage contained in the package. It is important to read the label carefully and recognize essential information.

Reading Medication Labels

The nurse should be able to recognize the following information on a medication label:

1. Generic name – This is a name given by the manufacturer that first develops the medication. Medications have only one generic name. Doctors are ordering medications more often by the generic name, so nurses need to know the generic name as well as the trade name. Pharmacists in many institutions are dispensing medications by generic name to decrease costs. Sometimes only the generic name may appear on a medication label or package.

2. Trade name – This is also referred to as the brand name. It is important to remember that a drug may be marketed under different trade names by different manufacturers.

3. Dosage strength – This refers to the weight of the medication per unit of measure (the weight per tablet, capsule, milliliter, etc.). In solutions, the medication may be stated as 80 mg/2 mL.

Example: 50 mg per tablet.

4. Form – This specifies the type of preparation in the container or package.

Example: tablets, capsules. For solutions it may indicate milliliters (mL) or cubic centimeters (cc).

5. Route of administration – This will tell how the medication is to be administered.

Example: orally, injectable, intravenous.

6. Total volume – On solutions or oral liquids the total volume of the vial or ampule is stated.

Example: 30 mL may be total volume on a medication label, but it contains 2 mg per mL. It's important to recognize the difference between amount per mL and the total volume to avoid confusion and errors.

7. Directions for mixing or reconstituting a medication – When medications come in a powdered form the directions for how to mix or reconstitute them and with what solution are found on the label.

Medication labels also contain information such as the expiration date, storage information, lot numbers, the name of the drug manufacturer, and a National Drug Code Number (NDC number). Some medication labels will be more detailed than others; however recognition of pertinent information on a medication label is an absolute requirement before calculation and administration.

Let's examine some medication labels for pertinent information.

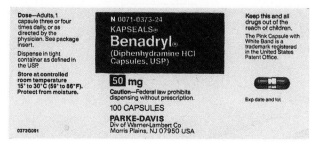

1. On the label note:

a) Benadryl is the brand name.

b) Diphenhydramine HCl is the generic name.

c) The drug form is capsule.

d) The dosage strength is 50 mg per capsule.

e) The drug manufacturer is Parke-Davis.

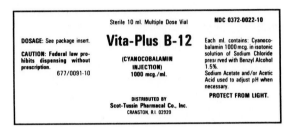

2. On this label:

a) Vita-Plus B-12 is the trade name.

b) Cyanocobalamin is the generic name.

c) Injection is the drug form or route.

d) 10 mL is the total volume of the vial.

e) 1000 mcg per mL is the dosage strength.

f) Protect from light are the directions for storage.

g) Scot-Tussin Pharmacal Co., Inc. is the drug manufacturer.

h) 0372-0022-10 is the NDC (National Drug Code Number).

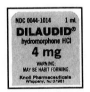

3. On this label:

a) Dilaudid is the trade name.

b) Hydromorphone HCl is the generic name.

c) 1 mL is the total volume of the ampule.

d) 4 mg per mL is the dosage strength.

e) 0044-1014 is the NDC (National Code Number).

f) Knoll Pharmaceuticals is the drug manufacturer.

g) May be habit forming is the warning.

NDC 0002-1444-01
VIAL No. 657

℞ *Lilly*

VANCOCIN® HCl
sterile vancomycin
hydrochloride, usp

Intra Venous
Equiv. to
500 mg
Vancomycin

FOR INTRAVENOUS USE
IMPORTANT—Read literature
for precautions and directions
before use.
Usual Adult Dose—2 g daily.
Dilute with 10 mL of Sterile
Water for Injection.
After Dilution—Refrigerate.
Prior to Reconstitution: Store at
59° to 86°F.
MUST BE FURTHER DILUTED
BEFORE USE—SEE LITERATURE
Lyophilized
YD 2651 AMX Mfd. by
Eli Lilly Industries, Inc.
Carolina, Puerto Rico 00630, a subsidiary of
Eli Lilly & Co., Indianapolis, IN, U.S.A.

4. On this label:

a) Vancocin HCl is the trade name.

b) Vancomycin hydrochloride is the generic name.

c) Dilute with 10 mL of sterile water for injection are the directions for mixing.

d) 500 mg/10 mL is the dosage strength (50 mg/mL).

e) Injection is the form. It specifies intravenous use.

f) After dilution refrigerate are the directions after reconstitution.

g) Eli Lilly Industries, Inc. is the drug manufacturer.

In this chapter a sample of medication labels is presented to assist you in the recognition of essential information on a drug label. It is important to note that some drugs may not give or indicate their strength. A common one is the multivitamin, which is usually ordered by a number of tablets. For example: "Multivitamin tablet one p.o. everyday."

In hospitals that use unit dose, the medications will come to the unit in individually wrapped packets that are labeled. The label includes the generic or trade name or sometimes both. The strength is indicated on the medication label. The nurse must read the label on unit-dose packages and note that sometimes even with this method calculation may be necessary. The pharmacy usually provides the unit with a 24-hour supply of medications that are available on units in multi-dose containers.

Example: Aspirin.

Most hospital units have a combination of unit dose and multi-dose. Figure 12.1 shows examples of unit-dose packaging.

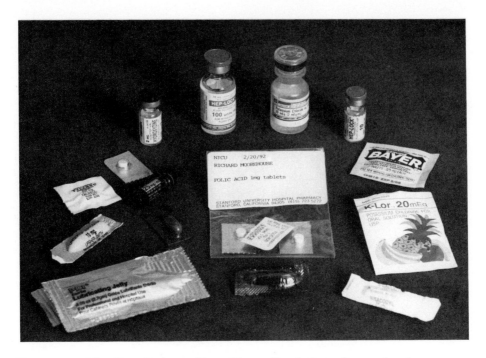

Figure 12.1 Unit Dose Packages (From Clayton/Stock: *Basic pharmacology for nurses,* ed 10, St Louis, 1993, Mosby.)

Points to Remember:

✔ Read medication labels 3 times.

✔ Read directions for mixing when indicated, and check expiration dates.

✔ Read labels carefully and don't confuse medication names; they are often deceptively similar. When in doubt check appropriate resources such as a reference book or the hospital pharmacist.

Chapter Review

NDC 0663-4310-71

250 Capsules

Minipress®

prazosin hydrochloride

1 mg †

CAUTION: Federal law prohibits dispensing without prescription.

6505-01-039-6320

RECOMMENDED STORAGE
STORE BELOW 86° F (30° C)
Dispense in tight, light resistant containers (USP).
†Each capsule contains prazosin hydrochloride equivalent to 1 mg of prazosin.
Manufactured by
Pfizer Pharmaceuticals, Inc., Barceloneta, P.R. 00617

4444

READ ACCOMPANYING
PROFESSIONAL INFORMATION
DOSAGE: See accompanying prescribing information.
IMPORTANT: This closure is not child-resistant.
U.S. Pat. No. 3,511,836

Pfizer Distributed by LABORATORIES DIVISION
New York, N.Y. 10017

1. Generic name _____ Drug form _____

   Trade name _____ Dosage strength _____

2 ml
LANOXIN®
(DIGOXIN)
INJECTION
500 µg (0.5 mg)
in 2 ml
(250 µg [0.25 mg] per ml)
DILUTION NOT REQUIRED
PROPYLENE GLYCOL 40%
ALCOHOL 10%
Store at 15°-30°C (59°-86°F).
Protect from light.

54281

FOR I.V. OR I.M. USE
BURROUGHS WELLCOME CO.
Research Triangle Park, NC 27709

LOT   EXP.

2. Generic name _____ Dosage strength _____

   Trade name _____ Drug form _____

   Total volume _____

USUAL ADULT DOSAGE:
See accompanying circular.
This is a bulk package and not intended for dispensing.
CAUTION: Federal (USA) law prohibits dispensing without prescription.

100 | No. 7592   7273206

MSD

NDC 0006-0020-68
100 TABLETS

Decadron®
(Dexamethasone, MSD)

0.25 mg

MERCK SHARP & DOHME
DIVISION OF MERCK & CO., INC.
WEST POINT PA 19486 USA

Lot   Exp.

3. Generic name _____ Drug form _____

   Trade name _____ Dosage strength _____

SCHERING

20 ml Multiple Dose Vial   Sterile
For use in preparation of large volume parenterals

Garamycin® Injectable

brand of gentamicin sulfate injection, USP

40 mg/ml
20 ml = 800 mg

For Parenteral Administration
Caution: Federal law prohibits dispensing without prescription.
Schering Pharmaceutical Corporation (PR), Manati, Puerto Rico 00701
An Affiliate of Schering Corporation, Kenilworth, N.J. 07033

11788815 Rev. 1/81

Usual Adult Dose: See package insert.
Each ml of aqueous solution contains:
gentamicin sulfate, USP equivalent to
40 mg gentamicin, 1.8 mg methylparaben
and 0.2 mg propylparaben as preservatives, 3.2 mg sodium bisulfite, and
0.1 mg edetate disodium.
Store between 2° and 30°C (36° and 86°F).
GARAMYCIN Injectable should not be
physically premixed with other drugs.

Read accompanying directions carefully.
Control No.
Exp. Date.

4. Generic name   _____   Dosage strength   _____

   Trade name   _____   Drug form   _____

   Total volume _____   Instructions _____

NDC 0002-1060-02
100 TABLETS No. 1703

℞   *Lilly*   POISON

CRYSTODIGIN®

DIGITOXIN TABLETS
USP

0.1 mg

CAUTION—Federal (U.S.A.) law
prohibits dispensing without
prescription.
Keep Tightly Closed
Store at 59° to 86°F
WW 2160 AMX
ELI LILLY AND COMPANY
Indianapolis, IN 46285, U.S.A.
Exp. Date/Control No.

Usual Maintenance Dose—
0.05 to 0.3 mg a day.
Each Tablet Contains: Crystalline Digitoxin, 0.1 mg
See accompanying literature.
Indiscriminate use may be
dangerous.
Dispense in a tight, light-
resistant container.

5. Generic name   _____   Drug form   _____

   Trade name   _____   Dosage strength _____

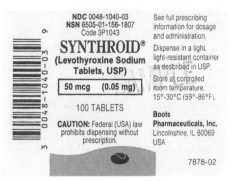

6. Generic name _____ Drug form _____

Trade name _____ Dosage strength _____

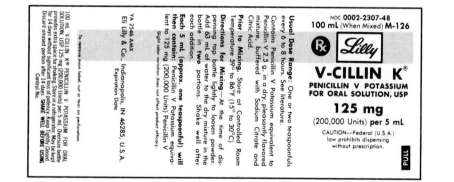

7. Generic name _____ Dosage strength _____

Trade name _____ Directions for storage _____

Total volume _____

LyphoMed®
POTASSIUM CHLORIDE
INJECTION, USP
(2 mEq/mL)

40 mEq

20 mL
Single Dose Vial

N 0469-6520-15 Sterile. Nonpyrogenic. 965-20

MUST BE DILUTED PRIOR TO IV ADMINISTRATION

Each mL contains: Potassium Chloride 149 mg;
Water for Injection q.s. pH adjusted with HCl or
KOH if necessary. 4000 mOsmol/L.

Usual Dose: See Package Insert.

LyphoMed, Inc., Rosemont, IL 60018   B-87

8. Generic name   _____   Drug form   _____

   Trade name   _____   Dosage strength   _____

An aid in the treatment of temporary constipation.
Keep this and all medication out of the reach of children.
Warning: As with any drug, if you are pregnant or nursing a baby, seek the advice of a health professional before using this product.
Caution: If cramping pain occurs, discontinue the medication.
Manufactured by R.P. Scherer
Clearwater, Florida 33518
Expressly for:
HOECHST-ROUSSEL Pharmaceuticals Inc.
Somerville, New Jersey 08876
REG TM HOECHST AG
60210-2/85

NDC 0039-0002-10
Surfak®
docusate calcium USP
STOOL SOFTENER

Seal Under Cap
Printed Hoechst-Roussel

100 CAPSULES
50 MG EACH

Each capsule contains 50 mg docusate calcium USP and the following inactive ingredients: alcohol USP up to 1.3% (w/w), corn oil NF, FD&C Red #3, FD&C Red #40, gelatin NF, glycerin USP, parabens NF, sorbitol NF, soybean oil USP and other ingredients.
Usual Dosage: Adults—two or three capsules daily; children 6 to 12 and adults with minimal needs — one to three capsules daily. Continue for several days or until bowel movements are normal. For children under 6 consult a physician. Preserve in a tight container. Store at controlled room temperature (59° 86°F) in a dry place.

9. Generic name   _____   Drug form   _____

   Trade name   _____   Dosage strength   _____

Sterile
Streptomycin Sulfate, USP
Equivalent to 5.0 g of Streptomycin Base

5.0 g
FOR INTRAMUSCULAR USE ONLY

CAUTION: Federal law prohibits dispensing without prescription.

ROERIG Pfizer
A division of Pfizer Inc. N.Y., N.Y. 10017

RECOMMENDED STORAGE
IN DRY FORM
STORE BELOW 86° F (30° C)
MADE IN U.S.A.
Sterile reconstituted solutions should be protected from light and may be stored at room temperature for four weeks without significant loss of potency.

Usual Daily Dosage
Adults: Varies with infection— consult package insert.
Adult average single injection:
0.5 to 1.0 g

mg/ml of Solution
400 mg/ml

ml Diluent added
9.0 ml

The dry powder is dissolved by adding Water for Injection, USP or Sodium Chloride Injection, USP in an amount to yield the desired concentration.

PATIENT

ROOM NO.

DATE DILUTED

10. Generic name   _____

    Trade name   _____

    Form   _____

    Directions for mixing   _____

    Dosage strength after reconstitution   _____

    Storage instructions   _____

13 Calculation of Dosages Using Ratio-Proportion

Objectives

After reviewing this chapter the student will be able to do the following:

1. State a ratio-proportion to solve a given dosage calculation problem
2. Solve simple calculation problems using the ratio-proportion method

---

There are several methods used for calculating dosages. The most common methods are ratio-proportion or use of a formula. After presentation of the various methods, students can choose the method that they find easiest to use. First let's discuss calculating using ratio-proportion. If necessary review Chapter 4 on ratio-proportion.

Use of Ratio-Proportion in Dosage Calculation

Ratio-proportion is useful and easy to use in dosage calculation, because frequently it is necessary to find one unknown quantity.

For example, suppose you had a medication with a dosage strength of 50 milligrams in 1 milliliter, and the doctor orders a dosage of 25 milligrams. A ratio-proportion could be used to solve this. 50 mg : 1mL is the known ratio, and x would be used to represent the unknown mL that would contain 25 milligrams. Therefore to set this problem up in a ratio-proportion the known ratio (50 mg : 1 mL) would be stated first, then the unknown ratio (25mg : x mL). The known ratio is what you have available, or the information on the drug label.

An important thing to remember is when stating the ratios, the units of measure should be stated in the same sequence (In the example, mg : mL = mg : mL).

Example 1:   50 mg : 1 mL = 25 mg : x mL
             (known)   (unknown)

Solution: To solve for x the principles presented in Chapter 4 on ratio-proportion are used.

50 mg : 1 mL = 25 mg : x mL

$50\,x$ = product of extremes

25 = product of means

$50\,x$ = 25 is the equation

$$\frac{50x}{50} = \frac{25}{50}$$ (divide both sides by 50, the number in front of x)

x = 0.5 mL

Note: As shown in Chapter 4 on ratio-proportion, this proportion could also be stated in fraction format.

Important Points When Calculating Dosages Using Ratio-Proportion

1. Make sure that everything is in the same unit and system of measure before calculating. If not a conversion will be necessary before calculating the dosage. Conversions can be made by changing what's ordered to the units in which the medication is available or by changing what's available to the units in which the medication is ordered. Try to be consistent as to how you make conversions. It is usual to convert what is ordered to the same unit and system of measure you have available.

2. Before calculating the dose make an estimate of what the approximate and reasonable answer would be.

3. Set up the proportion labeling all of the terms in the proportion. This includes x. State the known ratio first (what's available or on the drug label).

4. Make sure the terms of the ratios are stated in the same sequence.

5. Label the value you obtain for x. For example: mL, tabs, etc.

Let's look at some more problems using ratio-proportion to solve them.

Example 2:   The doctor orders 40 mg p.o. of a drug.
Available: 20 mg tablets.

Solution: 20 mg : 1 tab = 40 mg : x tab
  (known)   (unknown)

$$\frac{20x}{20} = \frac{40}{20}$$

x = 2 tabs

Note: When setting up the ratios both followed the sequence in stating the terms.
For example,   mg : tab = mg : tab.

This proportion could also be stated as a fraction and solved by cross multiplication.

Known   Unknown

$$\frac{20 \text{ mg}}{1 \text{ tab}} = \frac{40 \text{ mg}}{x \text{ tab}}$$

Here the known is stated as the first fraction and the unknown as the second.

Example 3:   Doctor's order: 1 g p.o. of an antibiotic.

Available: 500 mg capsules. How many capsules will you give?

Solution: Notice the dosage ordered is a different unit from what is available.
Proceed first by changing the units of measure so they are the same.
As shown in Chapter 8, ratio-proportion can be used for conversion.

After making the conversion, set up the problem and calculate the
dosage to be given. In this example the conversion required is
within the same system (metric).

In this example the g would be converted to mg by using the
equivalent 1000 mg = 1 g. After making the conversion of
1 g to 1000 mg, the ratio would be stated as follows:

500 mg : 1 caps = 1000 mg : x caps
  (known)   (unknown)

x = 2 caps

An alternate method of solving might be to convert mg to g. In doing this 500 mg would be converted to g using the same equivalent 1000 mg = 1 g. However decimals are common when measures are changed from smaller to larger in the metric system. 500 mg = 0.5 g. Even though converting the mg to g would net the same final answer, conversions that net decimals are frequently the source of calculation errors. Therefore if possible avoid conversions that require their use. As a rule, it is best to convert to the measure stated on the drug label. Doing this consistently can prevent confusion. As with the other examples this proportion could be stated as a fraction as well.

For the purpose of learning to calculate dosages using ratio-proportion, emphasis was placed in this chapter on the mathematics of the answer. Determining whether an answer is logical will come in the discussion of calculation of dosages by the various routes in later chapters.

Points to Remember:

✔ When stating the ratios the known ratio is stated first. The known ratio is what is available, on hand, or the information obtained from the drug label.

✔ The unknown ratio is stated second. The unknown ratio is the dose desired, or what the doctor has ordered.

✔ The terms of the ratio in a proportion must be written in the same sequence of measurement.

✔ Label all terms of the ratios in the proportion including (x).

✔ When conversion of units is required it is usually easier to convert to the unit of measure on the drug label, or what the medication is available in.

✔ Estimate the answer.

✔ Label all answers obtained.

✔ A proportion may be stated in horizontal fashion or as a fraction.

✔ Double check all work.

✔ Be consistent in how ratios are stated and conversions are done.

Practice Problems

Answer the following problems by indicating less than 1 tablet or more than 1 tablet:

1. A client is to receive gr 1/300 of a drug. The tablets available are gr 1/150. How many tablets do you need?

2. A client is to receive gr 1/15 of a drug. The tablets available are gr 1/30. How many tablets do you need?

3. A client is to receive gr 1/8 of a drug. The tablets available are gr 1/4. How many tablets do you need?

4. A client is to receive gr 1/2 of a drug. The tablets available are gr 1/4. How many tablets do you need?

5. A client is to receive gr 1/6 of a drug. The tablets available are gr 1/8. How many tablets do you need?

Solve the following problems using ratio-proportion calculations. Express your answer to the nearest tenth.

6. The doctor orders 7.5 mg p.o. of a drug. Available are tablets labeled 5 mg.

7. The doctor orders gr 1/4 p.o. of a drug. Available are tablets labeled 15 mg.

8. The doctor orders gr iss p.o. of a drug. Available are capsules labeled 100 mg.

9. The doctor orders 0.25 mg I.M. of a drug. Available 0.5 mg per cc.

10. The doctor orders gr 1/4 I.M. of a drug. Available gr 3/4 per cc.

11. The doctor orders Potassium Chloride 20 mEq I.V. Available Potassium Chloride 40 mEq per 10 cc.

12. The doctor orders 5000 U. s.c. of a drug. Available 10,000 U. per cc.

13. The doctor orders 50 mg I.M. of a drug. Available 80 mg per 2 cc.

14. The doctor orders 0.5 g p.o. of an antibiotic. Available capsules labeled 250 mg.

15. The doctor orders 400 mg p.o. of a liquid medication. Available 125 mg per 5cc.

Chapter Review

Part I
Directions: Read the medication label provided, and calculate the tablets or capsules necessary to provide the dosage ordered.

1. Doctor's order: gr 1/4 p.o. of Phenobarbital t.i.d.

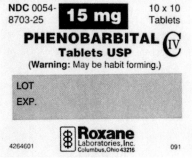

2. Doctor's order: Ampicillin 0.25 g p.o. q.i.d

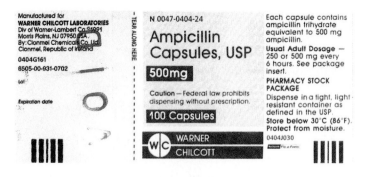

3. Doctor's order: Ampicillin 1 g p.o. q6h

4. Doctor's order: Phenobarbital 60 mg p.o. h.s.

5. Doctor's order: Baclofen 20 mg p.o. t.i.d

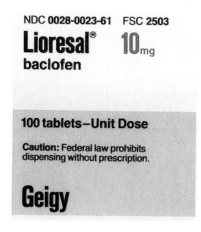

6. Doctor's order: Isosorbide Dinitrate 20 mg p.o. t.i.d.

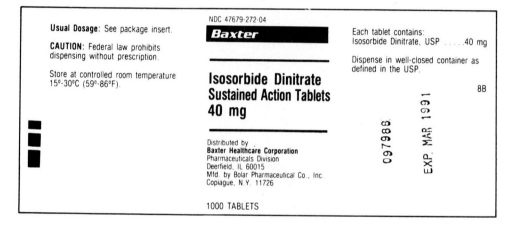

7. Doctor's order: Dexamethasone 4 mg p.o. q6h

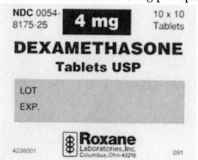

8. Doctor's order: Diabinese 250 mg p.o. q.d.

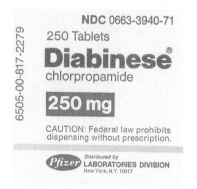

9. Doctor's order Digoxin 125 mcg p.o. q.d.

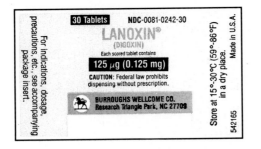

10. Doctor's order: Synthroid 0.05 mg p.o. q.d.

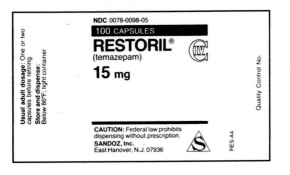

11. Doctor's order: Restoril 30 mg p.o h.s. p.r.n.

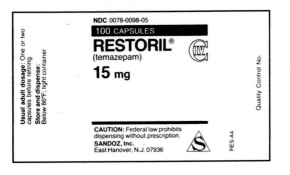

12. Doctor's order: Phenobarbital gr i p.o. h.s.

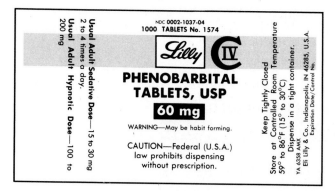

13. Doctor's order: Macrodantin 100 mg p.o. t.i.d.

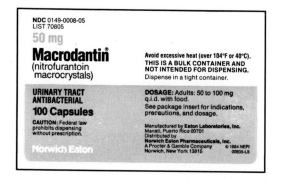

14. Doctor's order: Keflex 0.5 g p.o. q.i.d.

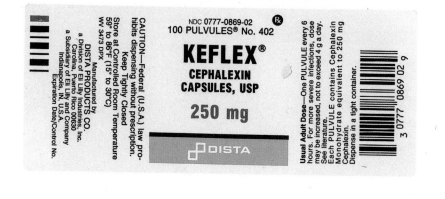

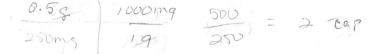

Part II

Directions: Read the medication labels provided, and calculate the volume necessary to provide the dosage ordered. Express your answer as a decimal fraction to the nearest tenth where indicated.

15. Doctor's order: Dilantin 100 mg via gastrostomy tube t.i.d.

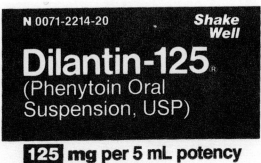

N 0071-2214-20   **Shake Well**

Dilantin-125®
(Phenytoin Oral Suspension, USP)

125 mg per 5 mL potency

Important—Another strength available; verify unspecified prescriptions.

Caution—Federal law prohibits dispensing without prescription.

8 fl oz (237 mL)

PARKE-DAVIS
Div of Warner-Lambert Co/ Morris Plains, NJ 07950 USA   2214G013

Shake well before using.
Each 5 mL contains phenytoin, 125 mg with a maximum alcohol content not greater than 0.6 percent.

Usual Dose—Adults, 1 teaspoonful three times daily; Children, see package insert.

See package insert for complete prescribing information.

Store below 30° C (86° F). Protect from freezing.

Keep this and all drugs out of the reach of children.

Exp date and lot

6505-00-890-1110

16. Doctor's order: Benadryl 50 mg p.o. h.s.

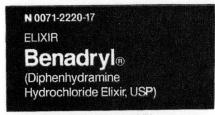

N 0071-2220-17

ELIXIR

Benadryl®
(Diphenhydramine Hydrochloride Elixir, USP)

Caution—Federal law prohibits dispensing without prescription.

4 FLUIDOUNCES

PARKE-DAVIS
Div of Warner-Lambert Co
Morris Plains, NJ 07950 USA

Elixir P-D 2220 for prescription dispensing only.

Contains—12.5 mg diphenhydramine hydrochloride in each 5 mL. Alcohol, 14%.

Dose—Adults, 2 to 4 teaspoonfuls; children over 20 lb, 1 to 2 teaspoonfuls; three or four times daily.

See package insert.

Keep this and all drugs out of the reach of children.

Store below 30°C (86°F). Protect from freezing and light.

Exp date and lot

2220G102

17. Doctor's order: Gentamicin 50 mg I.M. q8h

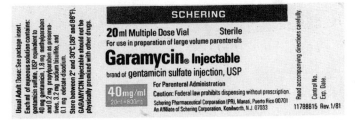

Usual Adult Dose: See package insert.
Each ml of aqueous solution contains: gentamicin sulfate, USP equivalent to 40 mg gentamicin, 1.8 mg methylparaben and 0.2 mg propylparaben as preservatives, 3.2 mg sodium bisulfite, and 0.1 mg edetate disodium.
Store between 2° and 30°C (36° and 86°F).
GARAMYCIN Injectable should not be physically premixed with other drugs.

SCHERING

20 ml Multiple Dose Vial   Sterile
For use in preparation of large volume parenterals

Garamycin® Injectable
brand of gentamicin sulfate injection, USP

40 mg/ml
20ml ÷ 830mg

For Parenteral Administration
Caution: Federal law prohibits dispensing without prescription.
Schering Pharmaceutical Corporation (PR), Manati, Puerto Rico 00701
An Affiliate of Schering Corporation, Kenilworth, N.J. 07033   11788815 Rev. 1/81

Read accompanying directions carefully.

Control No.
Exp. Date.

18. Doctor's order: Vibramycin 100 mg p.o. q12h

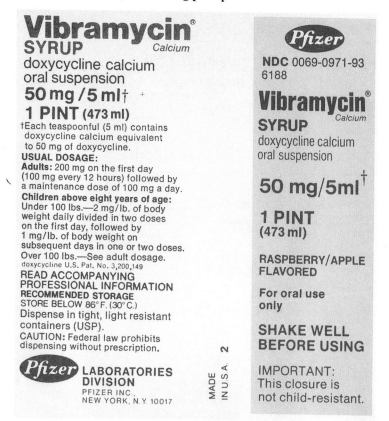

19. Doctor's order: Meperidine Hydrochloride 50 mg I.M. q4h p.r.n. for pain

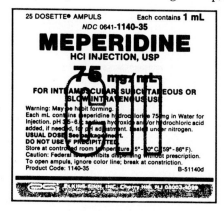

20. Doctor's order: Gentamicin 90 mg I.V. q8h.

2.25 ml

2.3 ml

2.25
40⟌9000
   80
   100
    80
   200

40 mg : 1 ml = 90 mg : x ml

$$\frac{40x}{40} = \frac{90}{40}$$

21. Doctor's order: Morphine gr 1/4 s.c. q4h p.r.n.

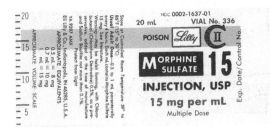

22. Doctor's order: Vitamin B₁₂ 1000 mcg I.M. once monthly.

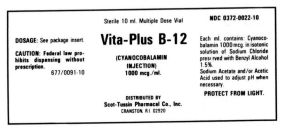

23. Doctor's order: Morphine 10 mg s.c. stat. Express answer in hundredths.

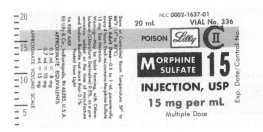

24. Doctor's order: Kaon-Cl 20 mEq p.o. o.d.

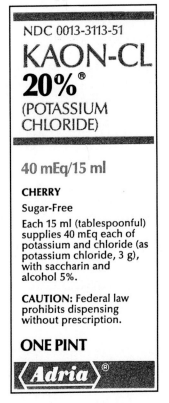

25. Doctor's order: Nystatin Oral Suspension 100,000 U. swish and swallow q6h

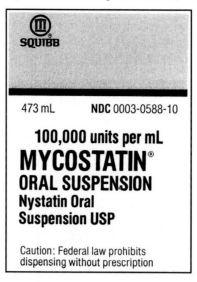

26. Doctor's order: Heparin 5000 U. s.c. o.d.

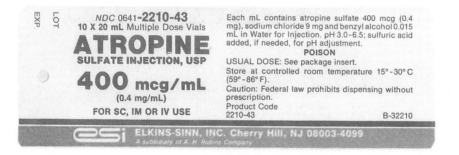

27. Doctor's order: Atropine 0.2 mg s.c. stat

28. Doctor's order: Amoxicillin 500 mg p.o. q6h x 7 days.

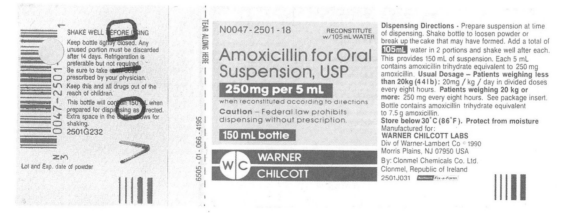

29. Doctor's order: Heparin 7500 U. s.c. o.d. Express answer in hundredths.

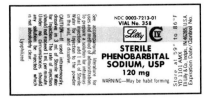

30. Doctor's order: Solumedrol 70 mg I.V. o.d.

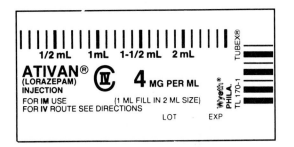

31. Doctor's order: Ativan 2 mg I.M. q4h p.r.n. agitation

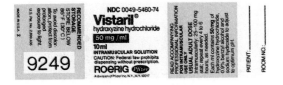

32. Doctor's order: Vistaril 25 mg I.M. on call to OR.

33. Doctor's order: Phenobarbital gr iss I.M. stat.

34. Doctor's order: Aminophylline 100 mg I.V. q6h

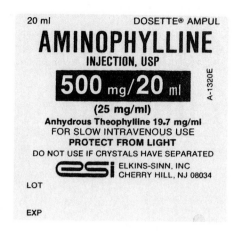

14 Dosage Calculation Using the Formula Method

Objectives

After reviewing this chapter the student will be able to do the follwoing:

1. Identify the information from a calculation problem to place into the formula given
2. Solve problems using the stated formula

This chapter shows how to use a formula for dosage calculation. Using the formula method requires substituting information from the problem into the formula. The formula presented can be used when calculating dosages in the same system or after converting when the dosage desired and the dosage on hand are in different systems.

$$\text{Formula:} \quad \frac{D}{H} \times Q = X$$

Meaning of Initials in Formula:

D = represents the dosage desired, or what the doctor has ordered including the weights. Example: 5 mg, 1/2 gr, 1 g, etc.

H = represents the dosage strength that is available, what is on hand, or the weight of the drug on the label, including the weights. Example: 25 mg, 1 gr, 10 g, etc.

Q = quantity, or the unit of measure that contains the dose that is available. When solving problems that involve solid forms of medication (tabs, caps), the Q is always 1 and can therefore be eliminated from the equation. When solving problems for medications in solution the amount for Q varies and must always be included.

X = represents the unknown, the dosage you are looking for. The dosage you are going to administer. How many mL, tab, etc. you will give.

Steps For Use of the Formula

1. Memorize the formula.

2. Place the information from the problem into the formula in the correct position.

3. Make sure all measures are in the same units and system of measure or a conversion must be done before calculating the dosage.

4. Think logically, and consider what a reasonable amount would be to administer.

5. Calculate your answer.

6. Label all answers. For example tabs, caps, mL, etc.

Now we will look at sample problems illustrating the use of the formula method of calculation.

Example 1:   The doctor orders 0.375 mg p.o. of a drug.
The tablets available are 0.25 mg.

Solution Using Formula:

The dosage 0.375 mg is desired, the dosage strength available is 0.25 mg per tablet.

Note: Since this problem involves a solid form of medication (tablets) where the Q is always 1, the Q could be eliminated from the formula without changing the value.

No conversion is necessary. What is desired is in the same system and unit of measure as what you have on hand. The desired (D) is 0.375 mg. You have available or on hand (H) 0.25 mg per (Q) 1 tablet. The label on x is tablet. Notice the label that is on x is always in the same form as you have on hand.

Therefore it would be set up in formula as follows:

$$\frac{(D)\ 0.375\ mg}{(H)\ 0.25\ mg} \times (Q)\ 1\ tab = x\ (tab)$$

$$\frac{0.375\ mg}{0.25\ mg} \times 1 = x$$

$$\frac{0.375}{0.25} = x$$

$x = 1.5$ tabs, or 1 1/2 tabs. (0.375 mg is larger than 0.25 mg, therefore you would need more than 1 tablet to administer 0.375 mg.)

Note: Although 1.5 tabs is the same as 1 1/2 tabs, in terms of administration it would be best to state as 1 1/2 tabs.

Example 2: The doctor orders 7000 U. s.c. of a drug. The drug is available 10,000 U. in 2 mL.

Solution: $\dfrac{\text{(D) } 7000\ \text{U.}}{\text{(H) } 10{,}000\text{U.}} \times$ (Q) 2 mL = x (mL)

$$\dfrac{7000}{10{,}000} \times 2 = x$$

$$\dfrac{14{,}000}{10{,}000} = 1.4 = x$$

x = 1.4 mL (7000 U. × 2 is more than 10,000 U., therefore it would take more than 1 mL to administer the dose.)

Note: Since this problem involves medication in liquid form the Q must be included.

Example 3: The doctor orders gr 1/2 p.o. Available are tablets labeled 15 mg.

Note: What is desired and what is available must be in the same units and system of measure. Remember it is usual to convert what is desired to what is available. Therefore change gr to mg; this will also eliminate the fraction and decrease the chance of error in calculation.

Rule: Whenever the desired amount and the dosage on hand are in different units or systems of measure you do the following:

1. Choose the approximate equivalent.

2. Convert what is ordered to the same units or system of measure as what is available or on hand by using one of the methods presented in the chapter on converting.

3. Use the formula $\dfrac{D}{H} \times Q = X$ to calculate the dosage to administer.

Solution: Convert gr 1/2 to mg. The equivalent to use is 60 mg = gr 1. Therefore gr 1/2 = 30 mg.

Now that you have everything in the same system and units of measure, use the formula to calculate the dosage to be administered.

$$\frac{\text{(D) 30 mg}}{\text{(H) 15 mg}} \times \text{(Q) 1 tab} = x \text{ (tab)}$$

$$\frac{30}{15} = x$$

x = 2 tabs. (30 mg is a larger dose than 15 mg, therefore it would take more than 1 tablet to administer the desired dose.)

Example 4: The doctor orders gr 1/6 of a drug. The drug is available gr 1/2 per mL.

Solution: $\dfrac{\text{(D) gr } \dfrac{1}{6}}{\text{(H) gr } \dfrac{1}{2}} \times \text{(Q) 1 mL} = x \text{ (mL)}$

$$\frac{1}{6} \div \frac{1}{2} = \frac{1}{6} \times \frac{2}{1} = \frac{2}{6} = \frac{1}{3}$$

$$\frac{1}{3} = x$$

x = 0.33 = 0.3 mL, 0.3 cc. (1/2 is a larger dose than 1/6, therefore it would take less than a cc to administer the required dose.

Points to Remember:

✔ The formula $\dfrac{\text{D}}{\text{H}} \times \text{Q} = \text{X}$ can be used to calculate the dose to be administered.

✔ The Q is always 1 for solid forms of medications (tab, caps) but varies for medications in solution.

✔ Before calculating the dosage to be given the dosage desired must be in the same units and system of measure as the dosage available or a conversion is necessary.

✔ Double-check all of your math, and think logically about the answer obtained.

✔ Label all answers obtained.

Chapter Review

Calculate the following problems using the formula presented in this chapter.

1. Doctor orders gr 1/150 p.o. Available tablets labeled gr 1/300.

2. Doctor orders 0.75 g p.o. Available capsules labeled 250 mg.

3. Doctor orders 90 mg p.o. Available tablets labeled 60 mg.

4. Doctor orders 7.5 mg p.o. Available tablets labeled 2.5 mg.

5. Doctor orders 0.05 mg p.o. Available tablets labeled 25 mcg.

Calculate the following problems in mL; express your answer to the nearest tenth.

6. Doctor orders 40 mg I.M. Available 80 mg per 2 mL.

7. Doctor orders 4500 U. s.c. Available 5000 U. per mL.

8. Doctor orders gr 1/200 I.M. Available 0.3 mg per mL.

9. Doctor orders 0.75 mg I.M. Available 0.25 mg per mL.

10. Doctor orders gr 1/6 s.c. Available 15 mg per mL.

Read the medication label provided, and calculate the dosage ordered.

11. Doctor's order: Phenobarbital gr ss p.o. t.i.d.

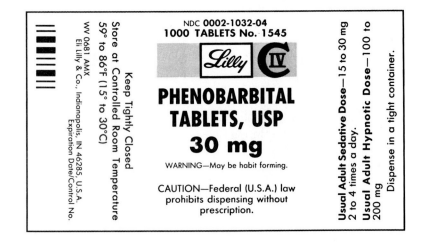

12. Doctor's order: Gantrisin 500 mg p.o. q.i.d.

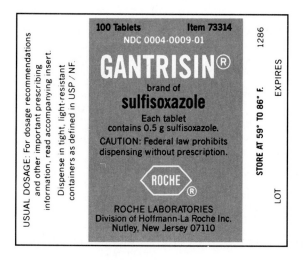

13. Doctor's order: Indocin 50 mg p.o. t.i.d.

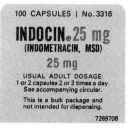

14. Doctor's order: Hydrochlorothiazide 50 mg p.o. b.i.d.

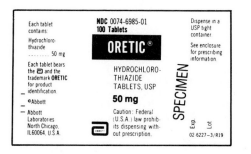

15. Aspirin gr x p.o. q4h p.r.n. for pain.

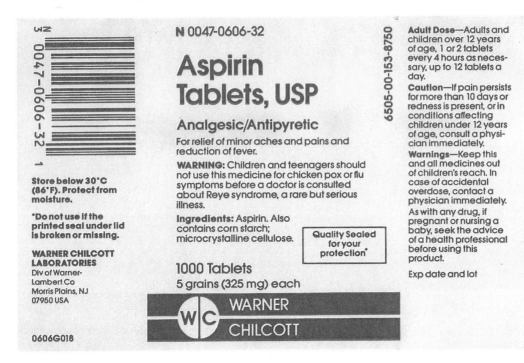

16. Doctor's order: Digoxin 0.375 mg p.o. o.d.

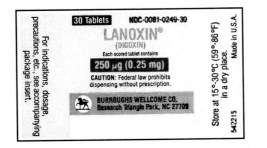

17. Doctor's order: Keflex 0.25 g p.o. q6h.

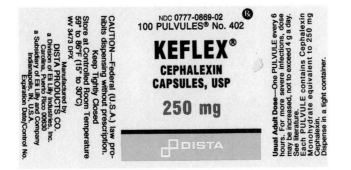

18. Doctor's order: Seconal 100 mg p.o. h.s.

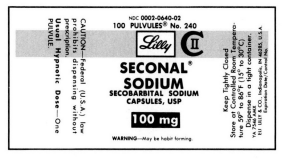

19. Minipress 2 mg p.o. b.i.d. X 2 days.

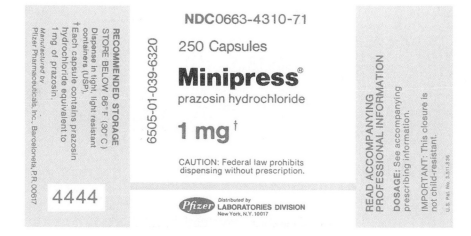

20. Crystodigin 0.2 mg p.o. o.d.

21. Codeine gr 3/4 p.o. q4h p.r.n. for pain.

22. Doctor's order: Cephradine 0.5 g p.o. q6h.

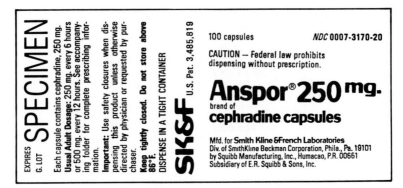

23. Cogentin 0.5 mg p.o. h.s.

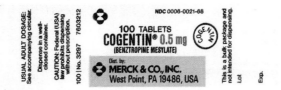

24. Doctor's order: Thorazine 75 mg p.o. b.i.d.

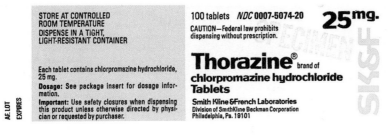

25. Dilantin 60 mg p.o. b.i.d.

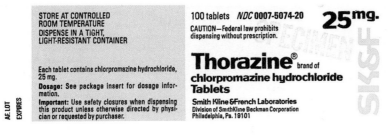

26. Doctor's order: Meperidine Hydrochloride 50 mg I.M. q4h p.r.n. for pain.

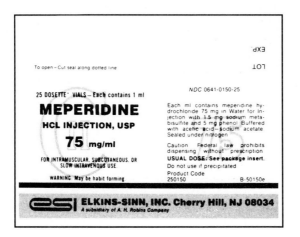

27. Doctor's order: Solu-Medrol 60 mg I.V. o.d.

28. Amikacin 90 mg I.M. q12h.

29. Doctor's order: Amoxicillin 300 mg p.o. q8h.

30. Doctor's order: V-cillin K 300,000 U. p.o. b.i.d.

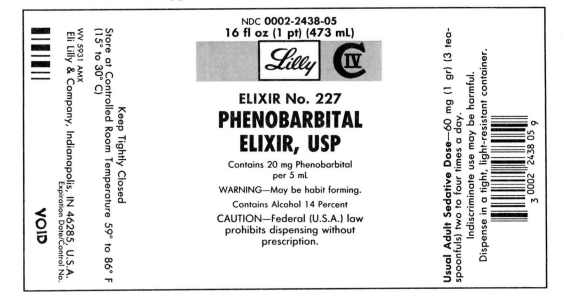

NDC 0002-2307-48
100 mL (When Mixed) M-126

℞ Lilly

V-CILLIN K®
PENICILLIN V POTASSIUM
FOR ORAL SOLUTION, USP

125 mg
(200,000 Units) per 5 mL

CAUTION—Federal (U.S.A.)
law prohibits dispensing
without prescription.

PULL

Usual Dose Range: One or two teaspoonfuls
every 6 to 8 hours. See literature.
Contains Penicillin V Potassium equivalent to
Penicillin V 2.5 g. in a dry, pleasantly flavored
mixture, buffered with Sodium Citrate and
Citric Acid.

Prior to Mixing, Store at Controlled Room
Temperature 59° to 86°F (15° to 30°C).

Directions for Mixing—At the time of dispensing tap bottle lightly to loosen powder.
Add 63 ml of water to the dry mixture in the
bottle in **two** portions. Shake well after
each addition.

Each 5 mL (approx. one teaspoonful) will
then contain: Penicillin V Potassium equivalent to 125 mg (200,000 Units) Penicillin V.

Slight color variation does not affect product efficacy.

YA 2546 AMX
Eli Lilly & Co.,
Indianapolis, IN 46285, U.S.A.
Expiration Date

To remove main label, cut or tear on perforation.

100 mL V-CILLIN K® PENICILLIN V POTASSIUM FOR ORAL
SOLUTION, USP 125 mg (200,000 Units) per 5 mL. Oversize bottle
provides extra space for shaking. Store in a refrigerator. May be kept
for 14 days without significant loss of potency. Keep tightly closed.
Discard unused portion after 14 days. SHAKE WELL BEFORE USING.
Control No.

31. Phenobarbital Elixir 45 mg p.o. b.i.d.

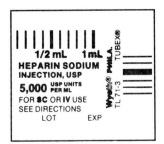

NDC 0002-2438-05
16 fl oz (1 pt) (473 mL)

Lilly ℂ IV

ELIXIR No. 227
PHENOBARBITAL
ELIXIR, USP

Contains 20 mg Phenobarbital
per 5 mL

WARNING—May be habit forming.

Contains Alcohol 14 Percent

CAUTION—Federal (U.S.A.) law
prohibits dispensing without
prescription.

Keep Tightly Closed

Store at Controlled Room Temperature 59° to 86° F
(15° to 30° C)

WV 5931 AMX
Eli Lilly & Company, Indianapolis, IN 46285, U.S.A.
Expiration Date/Control No.

VOID

Usual Adult Sedative Dose—60 mg (1 gr) (3 tea-
spoonfuls) two to four times a day.
Indiscriminate use may be harmful.
Dispense in a tight, light-resistant container.

3 0002 2438 05 9

32. Doctor's order: Heparin 3000 U. s.c. b.i.d.

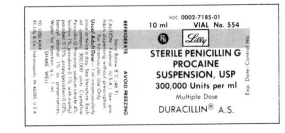

1/2 mL   1 mL
HEPARIN SODIUM
INJECTION, USP
5,000 USP UNITS PER ML
FOR **SC** OR **IV** USE
SEE DIRECTIONS
LOT   EXP

TUBEX® Wyeth® PHILA.   L71-3

33. Doctor's order: Procaine Penicillin 600,000 U. I.M. q12h

NDC 0002-7185-01
10 ml   VIAL No. 554

℞ Lilly

STERILE PENICILLIN G
PROCAINE
SUSPENSION, USP
300,000 Units per ml
Multiple Dose

DURACILLIN® A.S.

REFRIGERATE   AVOID FREEZING

Store Below 8°C (46°F).
CAUTION—Federal (U.S.A.) law pro-
hibits dispensing without prescription.
For Intramuscular Use Only

Usual Adult Dose—1 ml intramuscularly
once or twice a day. See literature. Each
ml contains: 300,000 units Crystalline
Penicillin G Procaine sodium citrate 4%,
lecithin 1%, povidone 0.1% with methylparaben 0.15%, propylparaben 0.02%,
benzyl alcohol 1% as preservatives,
Water for Injection, q.s. 1 ml.
SHAKE WELL

YD 1050 AMX
Eli Lilly & Co.
Indianapolis, IN 46285, U.S.A.

Exp. Date/Control No.

34. Doctor's order: Gentamicin 70 mg I.V. q8h.

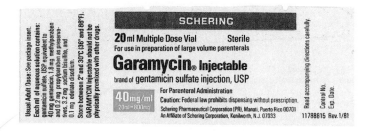

35. Doctor's order: Add Potassium Chloride 20 mEq to each I.V. bag.

POTASSIUM CHLORIDE
INJECTION, USP
2mEq/mL

FOR IV USE AFTER DILUTION

20mL MULTIPLE DOSE VIAL

AMERICAN REGENT
LABORATORIES, INC.
SUBSIDIARY OF
LUITPOLD PHARMACEUTICALS, INC.
SHIRLEY, NY 11967

NDC 0517-2120-01
Each mL contains Potassium Chloride 149mg(2mEq), Methylparaben 0.05%, Propylparaben 0.005%, Water for Injection q.s. pH adjusted with Hydrochloric Acid. 4mOsmol/mL

Sterile, nonpyrogenic

CAUTION: Federal Law (USA) Prohibits Dispensing Without Prescription.

WARNING: USE ONLY IF SOLUTION IS CLEAR

Directions for use:
8/86   See Insert

36. Doctor's order: Depo-Medrol 60 mg I.M. q. Monday X 2 weeks.

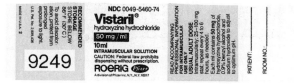

37. Doctor's order: Vistaril 100 mg I.M. stat.

NDC 0049-5460-74
Vistaril®
hydroxyzine hydrochloride
50 mg / mL
10mL
INTRAMUSCULAR SOLUTION
CAUTION: Federal law prohibits dispensing without prescription.
ROERIG Pfizer
A division of Pfizer Inc, N.Y., N.Y. 10017

9249

38. Morphine sulfate 6 mg s.c. q4h p.r.n. for pain

LIGHT SENSITIVE: Keep covered
in this box until ready to use.
To open—Cut seal along dotted line

25 DOSETTE VIALS—Each contains 1 ml

NDC 0641-0180-25

MORPHINE
SULFATE INJECTION, USP
10 mg/ml
FOR SUBCUTANEOUS, INTRAMUSCULAR
OR SLOW INTRAVENOUS USE
NOT FOR EPIDURAL OR INTRATHECAL USE
WARNING: May be habit forming
PROTECT FROM LIGHT
DO NOT USE IF PRECIPITATED
CAUTION: Federal   law   prohibits   dispensing
without prescription.

EXP
LOT

Each ml contains morphine sulfate 10
mg. sodium dihydrogen phosphate 10
mg. disodium hydrogen phosphate
2 8 mg. sodium formaldehyde
sulfoxylate 3 mg and phenol 2 5 mg in
Water for Injection. Sulfuric acid used
to adjust pH to 2 5 - 6 0. Sealed under
nitrogen
USUAL DOSE: See package insert for
complete prescribing information.
NOTE: Slight discoloration will not
alter efficacy. Discard if markedly
discolored.
Product Code 0180-25   B-50180d

ESI   ELKINS-SINN, INC. Cherry Hill, NJ 08034
A subsidiary of A. H. Robins Company

39. Atropine 0.3 mg I.M. stat.

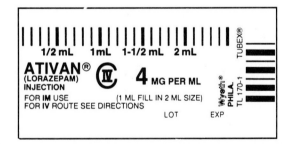

NDC 0002-1675-01
20 mL   VIAL No. 419
℞
POISON   *Lilly*

ATROPINE
SULFATE
INJECTION, USP
**0.4 mg
per mL**
CAUTION—Federal (U.S.A.) law
prohibits dispensing without
prescription.

40. Doctor's order: Stadol 1 mg I.M. q4h p.r.n. for pain.

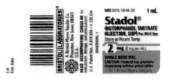

NDC 0015-5846-20   1 mL

Stadol
BUTORPHANOL TARTRATE
INJECTION, USP) For IM/IV Use
Store at Room Temp.

2 mg (2 mg per mL)

SINGLE DOSE VIAL
CAUTION: Federal law prohibits
dispensing without prescription.
©1977, Bristol-Myers Company

BRISTOL LABORATORIES

41. Doctor's order: Ativan 1 mg I.M. stat.

| | | | | | | | | | | | | | | | | | | | | | | |

1/2 mL   1 mL   1-1/2 mL   2 mL   TUBEX®

ATIVAN®   **IV**   **4** MG PER ML
(LORAZEPAM)
INJECTION
FOR **IM** USE   (1 ML FILL IN 2 ML SIZE)
FOR **IV** ROUTE SEE DIRECTIONS
                          LOT   EXP

Wyeth® PHILA.
TL 170-1

42. Doctor's order: Kanamycin 250 mg I.M. q6h.

NDC 0015-3502-20
EQUIVALENT TO
500 mg KANAMYCIN per 2 mL
KANTREX®
Kanamycin Sulfate
Injection, USP
FOR IM OR IV USE
CAUTION: Federal law prohibits
dispensing without prescription.

43. Doctor's order: Robinul 0.4 mg I.M. stat on call to OR.

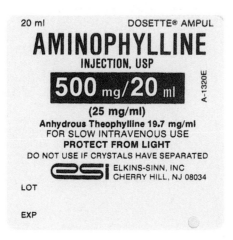

44. Doctor's order: Aminophylline 80 mg I.V. q6h.

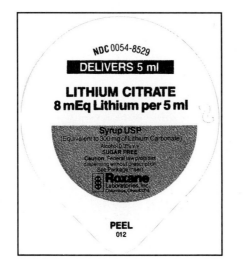

45. Doctor's order: Lithium Citrate oral solution 300 mg t.i.d.

Unit Four

Oral and Parenteral Doseforms, Insulin, and Pediatric Dosage Calculations

Oral medications are the easiest, most economical, and most frequently used medications, but sometimes parenteral (non-gastrointestinal tract) dosage routes are necessary. Both oral and parenteral drugs can be administered in liquid or powder form. In addition to oral and parenteral doseforms, this unit examines the varying types of insulin, as well as pediatric dosage calculations.

15 Calculation of Oral Medications

Objectives

After reviewing this chapter the student will be able to do the following:

1. Identify the forms of oral medication
2. Identify the terms on the medication label to be used in calculation of dosages
3. Calculate dosages for oral and liquid medications using ratio-proportion or the formula method
4. Apply principles learned concerning tablet and liquid preparations to obtain a rational answer

---

The easiest, most economical, and most frequently used method of medication administration is the oral route (p.o. or by mouth). Drugs for oral administration are available in solid forms like tablets and capsules or as liquid preparations. To calculate dosages appropriately the nurse needs to understand the principles that apply to administration of medications by this route.

Forms of Solid Medications

1. Tablets – Tablets are preparations of powdered drugs that have been molded into various sizes and shapes. Tablets come in a variety of dosages that can be expressed in apothecary or metric measures, for example milligrams (mg) and grains (gr) (Figure 15.1).

There are different types of tablets.

a) Scored tablets – These are tablets that are designed to administer a dose that is less than what is available in a single tablet. In other words scored tablets have indentations or markings that allow you to break the tablet into halves or quarters. Only scored tablets may be broken. Examples of scored tablets are Digoxin and Capoten (Figure 15.2).

b) Enteric coated tablets – These are tablets with a special coating that protects the tablet from the effects of gastric secretions and prevents it from dissolving in the stomach.

They are dissolved and absorbed in the intestines. The enteric coating also prevents the drug from becoming a source of irritation to the gastric mucosa, therefore preventing gastrointestinal upset. Examples include enteric coated Aspirin and iron tablets such as Ferrous Gluconate. Enteric coated tablets should never be crushed, since crushing them would destroy the special coating on them and defeat its purpose (Figure 15.3).

c) Sublingual tablets – These tablets are designed to be placed under the tongue where they dissolve in saliva and the medication is absorbed. Sublingual tablets should never be swallowed because this will prevent them from achieving their desired effect. Nitroglycerine, which is used for the relief of acute chest pain, is usually administered sublingually.

In addition to the types of tablets mentioned there are "timed release" tablets available. Medication from these tablets is released over a period of time, at specific time intervals.

2. Capsules – A capsule is a form of medication that contains a powder, liquid, or oil enclosed in a hard or soft gelatin. Capsules come in a variety of colors, sizes, and dosages. Some capsules have special shapes and colorings to identify which company produced them. Capsules and tablets are also available as "timed release" and work over a period of time. Capsules are not dividable and cannot be crushed. Capsules should only be administered as a whole. Examples of medications that come in capsule form are Ampicillin, Tetracycline, Colace, and Lanoxicap (Figure 15.4).

Although there are other forms of solid preparations for oral administration, such as lozenges and troches, tablets and capsules are the most frequent forms of solids encountered by the nurse that require calculation.

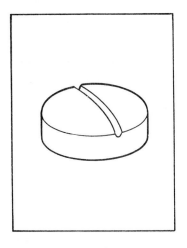

Figure 15.1 Tablet Scored in 1/2 (From Clayton/Stock: *Basic pharmacology for nurses,* ed 10, St Louis, 1993, Mosby.)

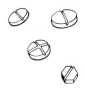

Figure 15.2 Various tablets (From Smith: *Dosages and solutions calculations,* St Louis, 1989, Mosby.)

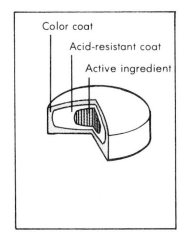

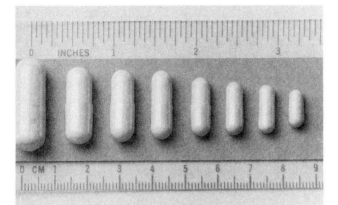

Figure 15.3 Enteric coated tablet (From Clayton/Stock: *Basic pharmacology for nurses*, ed 10, St Louis, 1993, Mosby.)

Figure 15.4 Various sizes and numbers of gelatin capsules (From Clayton/Stock: *Basic pharmacology for nurses*, ed 10, St Louis, 1993, Mosby.)

Calculating Dosages Involving Tablets and Capsules

When administering medications you will have to calculate the number of tablets or capsules needed to administer the dosage ordered. Remembering some important points when calculating dosages that involve tablets and capsules can assist you in determining whether what you have calculated is sensible, accurate, and can safely be administered.

Points to Remember:

✔ Converting drug measures from one system to another and one unit to another to determine the dosage to be administered can result in discrepancies depending on the conversion factor used.
Example: Aspirin may indicate on the label 5 grains (325 mg). This is based on the equivalency that 65 mg = gr 1. On the other hand, another label on Aspirin may indicate 5 grains (300 mg). Here the equivalent 60 mg = gr 1 was used. Both of the equivalents are correct. Remember equivalents are not exact. Use the common equivalents when making conversions, for example 60 mg = gr 1.

✔ When the precise number of tablets or capsules is determined and you find that administering the amount calculated is unrealistic or impossible, always use the following rule to avoid an error in administration: No more than 10% variation should exist between the dosage ordered and the dosage administered. For example, you may determine a client should receive 0.9 tablet or 0.9 capsule. Administration of such an amount accurately would be impossible. Following the stated rule, if you determined that 0.9 tablet or 0.9 capsule should be given, you could safely administer 1 tablet or 1 capsule.

✔ Capsules are not scored and are not dividable. They are administered in whole amounts only. If a client has difficulty swallowing a capsule, check to see if a liquid preparation of the same drug is available. Never crush, open, or empty the contents of a timed release capsule into a liquid or food; this may cause release of all the medication at once.

✔ Tablets and capsules may be available in different strengths for administration, and you may have a choice when giving a dosage. For example, 75 mg of a drug may be ordered. When you check what is available, it may be in tablet or capsule form as 10, 25, and 50 mg respectively. In deciding the best combination of tablets or capsules to give the nurse should always choose the strength that would allow the least number of tablets or capsules to be administered without breaking a tablet. In the example given the best combination to use to administer 75 mg would be 1 of the 50 mg tablets or capsules and 1 of the 25 mg tablets or capsules.

✔ The maximum number of tablets or capsules given to a client to achieve a certain dosage is usually 3. Any more than this is unusual and may indicate an error in the interpretation of the order or in calculation.

✔ When using the formula or ratio-proportion method to calculate tablet and capsule problems, remember each tablet and capsule contains a certain weight of the drug. The weight indicated on a label is per tablet or per capsule. This is particularly important when reading a medication label on bottles or single packages such as unit dose.

✔ In calculating oral dosages you may encounter measures other than apothecary or metric measures. For example electrolytes such as Potassium will indicate the number of milliequivalents (mEq) per tablet. Units (U.) is another measure you may see for oral antibiotics or vitamins. For example a Vitamin E capsule will indicate 400 U. per capsule. Units and milli-equivalents are measurements that are specific to the drug they are being used for. There is no conversion that exists between these and apothecary or metric measures.

Remembering the points mentioned will be helpful when we start to calculate dosages. Any of the methods presented in Chapters 13 and 14 can be used to determine the dosage to be administered.

To compute dosages accurately it is necessary to review a few pointers as a refresher that were presented in previous chapters.

Reminders:

1. Read the problem carefully and identify:
   a) Known factors in the problem.
   b) Unknown factors in the problem.
   c) Eliminate unnecessary information that is not relevant.

2. Make sure that what is ordered and what is available is in the same system of measurement and units or a conversion will be necessary. When a conversion is necessary, it is usual to convert what the doctor has ordered into what you have available or is indicated on the drug label. You can however convert the measures the drug is available into the same units and system of measure as the dosage ordered. The choice is usually based upon whichever is easier to solve. Make conversions consistently one way to avoid confusion. Conversions can be made using any of the methods presented in Chapter 8. If necessary go back and review that chapter.

3. Consider what would be a reasonable answer based on what you are ordered to give.

4. Set the problem up using ratio-proportion or the formula method:

$$\frac{D}{H} \times Q = x$$

5. Label the final answer (tablet, capsule).

Let's look at some sample problems calculating the number of tablets or capsules to administer.

Example 1:   Doctor's Order: Digoxin 0.375 mg p.o. o.d.
Available: Scored tablets labeled 0.25 mg.

1. No conversion is necessary, the units are the same and in the same system of measure.
   Order: 0.375 mg.
   Available: 0.25 mg.

2. Think: Tablets are scored. 0.375 mg is larger than 0.25 mg, therefore you will need more than 1 tablet to administer the correct dosage.

3. Solve using ratio-proportion or the formula method.

Solution Using Ratio-Proportion Method:

$$0.25 \text{ mg} : 1 \text{ tab} = 0.375 \text{ mg} : x \text{ tab}$$

(Known)   (Unknown)
(what's available)   (what's ordered)

$$0.25\, x = 0.375$$

$$x = \frac{0.375}{0.25}$$

$x = 1.5$ tabs or 1 1/2 tabs. (It is best to state as 1 1/2 tabs for administration purposes.)

Note: You can administer 1 1/2 tabs because the tablets are scored. The above ratio-proportion could have been written as a fraction as well. (If necessary review the chapter on Ratio-Proportion.)

Solution Using the Formula Method:

$$\frac{D}{H} = \frac{0.375 \text{ mg}}{0.25 \text{ mg}} = 1\frac{1}{2} \text{ tablets}$$

Example 2:   Doctor's Order: Ampicillin 0.5 g p.o. q6h.
Available: Capsules labeled 250 mg per capsule.

1. Note: A conversion is necessary. The ordered dose and the available dose are in the same system of measurement (metric), but the units are different (g and mg). Before calculating the dosage to be administered, the ordered dose and the available dose must be in the same units.
Order: 0.5 g.
Available: 250 mg capsules.

2. After making the necessary conversion, think, what is a reasonable amount to administer?

3. Calculate the dosage to be administered using ratio-proportion or the formula method.

4. Label your final answer (tablets, capsule).

Problem Set-up:

1. Convert g to mg. Equivalent: 1000 mg = 1 g.

$$1000 \text{ mg} : 1 \text{ g} = x \text{ mg} : 0.5 \text{ g}$$

$$x = 1000 \times 0.5$$

$x = 500$ mg

0.5 g therefore is equal to 500 mg. Converting the g to mg eliminated a decimal, which is often the source of calculation errors. Converting mg to g would necessitate a decimal.
Whenever possible, conversions that result in a decimal should be avoided to decrease the chance of error in calculating. Remember a ratio-proportion could also be stated as a fraction. If necessary, review the chapter on ratio-proportion. Since the measures are metric in this problem, (g, mg) the other method that could have been used was to move the decimal the desired number of places (0.5g = 500 mg).

2. After making the conversion you are now ready to calculate the dosage to be given using ratio-proportion or the formula method. In this problem we will use the answer obtained from converting what was ordered to what's available (0.5 g = 500 mg).

Solution Using Ratio Proportion:

250 mg : 1 cap = 500 mg : x caps

$250 x = 500$

$$x = \frac{500}{250}$$

$x = 2$ caps.

Note: 2 capsules is a logical answer. Capsules are administered in whole amounts; they are not dividable. Using the conversion obtained from converting mg to g in this problem would also net a final answer of 2 caps.

Solution Using the Formula:

$$\frac{D}{H} = \frac{500 \text{ mg}}{250 \text{ mg}} = 2 \text{ capsules}$$

Example 3:   Doctor's Order: Nitroglycerine gr 1/150 sublingual p.r.n. for chest pain.
Available: Sublingual tablets labeled 0.4 mg.

Problem Set-up:

1. Conversion is required.
   Doctor's order: gr 1/150
   Available: 0.4 mg.

Equivalent 60 mg = gr 1. Convert what is ordered to the same system and units of what is available (gr is apothecary, mg is metric).

$$60 \text{ mg} : \text{gr } 1 = x \text{ mg} : \text{gr } \frac{1}{150}$$

$$x = 60 \times \frac{1}{150}$$

$$x = \frac{60}{150}$$

$$x = 0.4 \text{ mg.}$$

Note: In this problem it was easier to change gr to mg. gr 1/150 is equal to 0.4 mg.

2. Think – It's obvious after making conversion that you will give 1 tablet.

3. Solve to obtain the desired dose.

Solution Using Ratio-Proportion:

$$0.4 \text{ mg} : 1 \text{ tab} = 0.4 \text{ mg} = x \text{ tab}$$

$$0.4 \, x = 0.4$$

$$x = \frac{0.4}{0.4}$$

$$x = 1 \text{ tab.}$$

Solution Using Formula:

$$\frac{D}{H} = \frac{0.4}{0.4} = 1 \text{ tab}$$

Note: This involved the division of decimals. Remember the rule for dividing decimals. If necessary review the chapter on decimals.

Alternate Method of Doing Example 3:

An alternate way of doing the problem in Example #3 would be to eliminate the decimal and therefore convert 0.4 mg to gr. In doing this more mathematical steps are involved. The same equivalent would be used.

$$60 \text{ mg} : \text{gr } 1 = 0.4 \text{ mg} : x \text{ gr.}$$

$$60 x = 0.4$$

$$x = \frac{0.4}{60}$$

Remember: Apothecary measures are expressed using fractions. Therefore 0.4 must be divided by 60. To divide 0.4 by 60, the decimal point in the numerator is eliminated by moving the decimal one place to the right to make it 4. For every place the decimal is moved to make it a whole number, a zero is added to the denominator, therefore it would be as follows:

$$\frac{0.4}{60} = \frac{4}{600}$$

$$\frac{4}{600} = \frac{1}{150}$$

Converting this way will net the same answer when calculating the dosage to be given.

Alternate Solution Using Ratio-Proportion:

$$\text{gr } \frac{1}{150} : 1 \text{ tab} = \text{gr } \frac{1}{150} : x \text{ tab}$$

$$\frac{1}{150} x = \frac{1}{150}$$

$$x = \frac{1}{150} \div \frac{1}{150}$$

$$x = \frac{1}{150} \times \frac{150}{1}$$

$$x = \frac{150}{150}$$

$$x = 1 \text{ tab.}$$

Alternate Solution Using Formula:

$$\frac{D}{H} = \frac{\text{gr } \dfrac{1}{150}}{\text{gr } \dfrac{1}{150}} = 1 \text{ tab}$$

Example 4:   Doctor's Order: Nembutal gr 1 1/2 p.o. h.s. p.r.n.
Available: Capsules labeled 100 mg.

Problem Set-up:

1. Convert gr 1 1/2 to mg.

$$60 \text{ mg} : \text{gr } 1 = x \text{ mg} : \text{gr } 1 \text{ 1/2}$$

gr 1 1/2 can be written as 3/2.

$$60 \text{ mg} : \text{gr } 1 = x \text{ mg} : \text{gr } 3/2$$

$$x = 60 \times \frac{3}{2} = \frac{180}{2}$$

$$x = 90 \text{ mg}$$

2. Solve for the dosage to be administered.

Solution Using Ratio-Proportion:

$$100 \text{ mg} : 1 \text{ cap} = 90 \text{ mg} : x \text{ caps.}$$

$$100 x = 90$$

$$x = \frac{90}{100}$$

$$x = 0.9 \text{ caps.}$$

$$x = 1 \text{ cap.}$$

Note: Capsules are not dividable. 0.9 is closer to 1 capsule; it is safe to administer 1 capsule. 1 capsule falls within the 10% variation allowed between the dosage ordered and the dosage given.

Solution Using Formulas:

As already discussed alternate equivalents may be used to achieve the same answer in terms of the dosage to be administered. Using for example 65 mg = gr 1, if this equivalent was used to convert gr 1 1/2 to mg the answer for the conversion would be 97.5 mg.

Therefore in calculating the dose to administer the answer would have been 0.975 capsules precisely. This would still require that 1 capsule be administered. Remember there is a 10% margin because of approximate equivalents. Another alternative to the conversion for this problem may have been to think 1000 mg = 1 g. Therefore since gr 15 = 1 g, 100 mg could be converted to gr as follows:

$$1000 \text{ mg} : \text{gr } 15 = 100 \text{ mg} : x \text{ gr}$$

$$1000 \, x = 1500$$

$$x = \frac{1500}{1000}$$

$$x = \text{gr } 1\ 1/2$$

Converting in this manner will give the same answer of 1 capsule as illustrated using the ratio-proportion method to calculate the dosage to be given.

$$\text{gr } 1\ 1/2 : 1 \text{ cap} = \text{gr } 1\ 1/2 : x \text{ caps}$$

gr 1 1/2 can be changed to an improper fraction for the purpose of calculating.

$$\text{gr } 3/2 : 1 \text{ cap} = \text{gr } 3/2 : x \text{ caps}$$

$$\frac{3}{2}x = \frac{3}{2}$$

$$x = \frac{3}{2} \div \frac{3}{2}$$

$$x = \frac{3}{2} \times \frac{2}{3}$$

$$x = \frac{6}{6}$$

$$x = 1 \text{ cap.}$$

Example 5:   Doctor's Order: Thorazine 100 mg p.o. t.i.d.
Available: Tablets labeled 25 mg and 50 mg.

1. No conversion is necessary.

2. Think: 100 mg is larger than 25 or 50 mg. Therefore more than 1 tablet would be needed to administer the dosage. The client should always be given the strength of tablets or capsules that would require the least number to be taken.

3. In this problem, selection of the 50 mg tablets would require the client to receive 2 tablets, while using 25 mg tablets would require 4 tablets to be administered.

Solution Using Ratio-Proportion:

$$50 \text{ mg} : 1 \text{ tab} = 100 \text{ mg} : x \text{ tab}$$

$$50\,x = 100$$

$$x = 2 \text{ tabs (50 mg each)}.$$

Solution Using Formulas:

$$\frac{D}{H} = \frac{100 \text{ mg}}{50 \text{ mg}} = 2 \text{ tabs of 50 mg each}$$

Note: In Example #5 not only is the number of tablets specified but the strength of tablets chosen is specified as well.

Variation of Tablet and Capsule Problems

To decide how many tablets or capsules are needed frequently requires knowing the dosage and the frequency.

Example 1: Doctor's Order: Valium 10 mg p.o. q.i.d.
How many 5-mg tablets would be needed for 7 days?

Solution: To obtain 10 mg the client requires 2 5-mg tablets each time. Therefore 8 5-mg tablets are necessary to administer the dose q.i.d. (four times a day).

(number of days ordered for)
↓
$$8 \times 7 = 56$$
↑
(# of tabs needed per day)

Answer: Total number of tablets needed would be 56 tablets for 7 days.

Determining the Dosage to be Given Each Time

Example 2: A client is to receive 1g p.o. daily of a drug. The drug should be given in four equally divided doses. How many mg should the client receive each time the medication is administered?

Solution: $$\frac{\text{Total daily allowance}}{\text{\# of doses per day}} = \text{dosage amount to be administered}$$

Answer: $$\frac{1 \text{ g (1000 mg)}}{4} = 250 \text{ mg}.$$

Points to Remember:

✔ The maximum number of tablets and capsules to administer to achieve a desired dose is usually 3.

✔ Before calculating a dose make sure that the dosage ordered and what's available is in the same system of measurement and units. When a conversion is required, it is usually best to convert the dosage ordered to what's available.

✔ No more than a 10% variation should exist between the dosage ordered and the dosage administered.

✔ Regardless of the method used to calculate a dosage, it is important to develop the ability to think about what is a reasonable amount.

Practice Problems

Directions: Calculate the correct number of tablets or capsules to be administered in the following problems. Use any of the methods presented to calculate the dosage. Remember to label your answers.

1. Doctor's Order: Synthroid 0.025 mg p.o. o.d.
    Available: Scored tablets labeled 50 mcg.

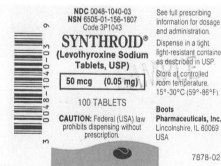

2. Doctor's Order: Capoten 6.25 mg p.o. b.i.d.
    Available: Tablets scored in fourths labeled 25 mg.

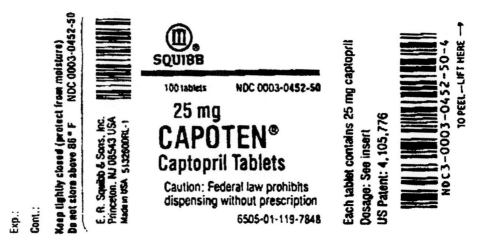

3. Doctor's Order: Ethambutol 1.2 g p.o. o.d.

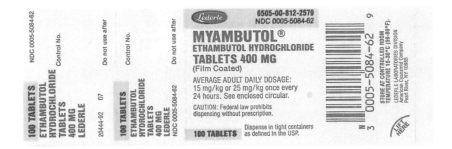

4. Doctor's Order: Coumadin 7.5 mg p.o. h.s.
    Available: Scored tablets labeled 5 mg and 2.5 mg.
    What would be the appropriate strength tablet to use?

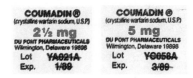

5. Doctor's Order: Lanoxin 0.125 mg p.o. o.d.
    Available: Scored tablets labeled 125 mcg and 500 mcg.
    (a) What would be the appropriate strength tablet to use?
    (b) What will you prepare to administer?

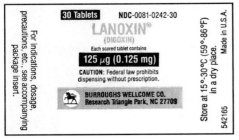
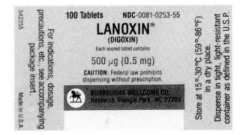

6. Doctor's Order: Ampicillin 1 g p.o. q6h.
    Available: Capsules labeled 500 mg and 250 mg.
    (a) Which strength of capsules would be appropriate to use?
    (b) How many capsules are needed for one dose?
    (c) What is the total number of capsules needed if the medication is ordered for
         7 days?

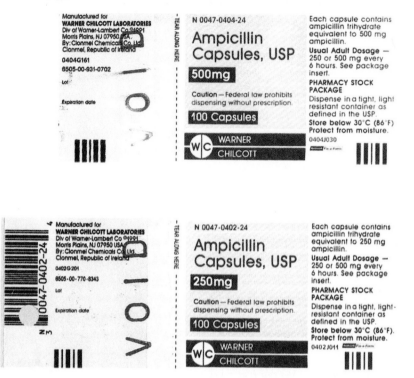

7. Doctor's Order: Reglan 10 mg p.o. t.i.d. 1/2 hr a.c.
    Available: Tablets labeled 5 mg.

8. Doctor's Order: Baclofen 15 mg p.o. t.i.d. x 3 days.
    Available: Scored tablets labeled 10 mg.
    (a) How many tablets are needed for one dose?
    (b) What is the total number of mg the client will receive in 3 days?

9.   Doctor's Order: Synthroid 0.075 mg p.o. q.d.
      Available: Scored tablets labeled 50 mcg.

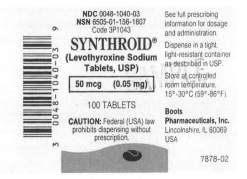

10.   Doctor's Order: Calcium Carbonate 1.3 g p.o. o.d.
      Available: Tablets labeled 650 mg.

11.   Doctor's Order: Dilantin 90 mg p.o. t.i.d.
      Available: Capsules labeled 30 mg.

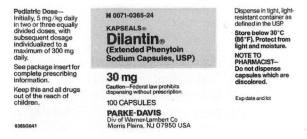

12.   Doctor's Order: Tegretol 200 mg p.o. t.i.d.
      How many tablets will you administer for each dose?

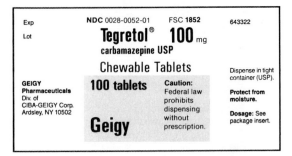

13. Doctor's Order: Dicloxacillin 1 g p.o. as an initial dose and 0.5 g p.o. q6h thereafter.
     Available: Capsules labeled 500 mg per capsule.
     (a) How many capsules will you need for the initial dose?
     (b) How many capsules are needed for each subsequent dose?

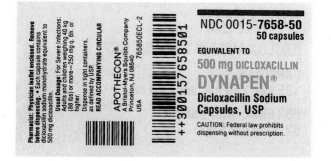

14. Doctor's Order: Aldomet 250 mg p.o. b.i.d.
     How many tablets will you administer for each dose?

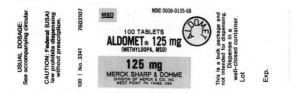

15. Doctor's Order: Phenobarbital gr iss p.o. h.s.
     (a) Which strength of tablets would be the best to administer?
     (b) How many tablets of which strength will you prepare to administer?

16.   Doctor's Order: Decadron 3 mg p.o. b.i.d. x 2 days
Which would be the best strength to administer?

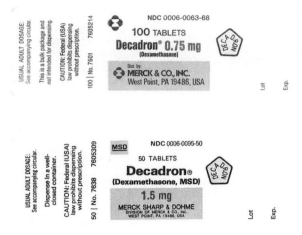

17.   Doctor's Order: Thorazine 100 mg p.o. t.i.d.
How many tablets are needed for 3 days?

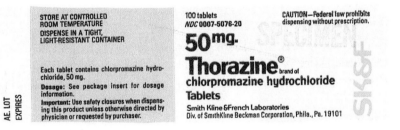

18.   Doctor's Order: Verapamil 120 mg. p.o. t.i.d. Hold for systolic blood pressure < 100,
Heart rate < 55.
Available: Scored tablets labeled 80 mg and 40 mg.
(a) Which would be the best strength tablets to use?
(b) How many of which strength tablet will you administer?

19. Doctor's Order: Acetaminophen gr x p.o. q4h p.r.n. for a temp > 101° F.
    Available: Tablets labeled 325 mg.

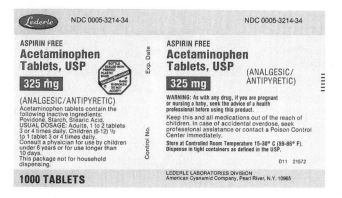

20. Doctor's Order: Cogentin 1 mg p.o. t.i.d.
    Available: Tablets labeled 0.5 mg.

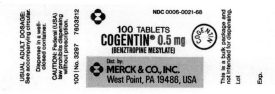

21. Doctor's Order: Prazosin Hydrochloride 3 mg. p.o. b.i.d.
    Available: Capsules labeled 1 mg.

NDC0663-4310-71

250 Capsules

Minipress®

prazosin hydrochloride

1 mg †

CAUTION: Federal law prohibits
dispensing without prescription.

Pfizer Distributed by
LABORATORIES DIVISION
New York, N.Y. 10017

6505-01-039-6320

4444

RECOMMENDED STORAGE
STORE BELOW 86° F (30° C)
Dispense in tight, light resistant
containers (USP).
† Each capsule contains prazosin
hydrochloride equivalent to
1 mg of prazosin.

Manufactured by
Pfizer Pharmaceuticals, Inc., Barceloneta, P.R. 0617

READ ACCOMPANYING
PROFESSIONAL INFORMATION

DOSAGE: See accompanying
prescribing information.

IMPORTANT: This closure is
not child-resistant.

U.S. Pat. No. 3,511,836

22. Doctor's Order: Nitroglycerine gr 1/150 SL. p.r.n.
    Available: Tablets labeled 0.4 mg.

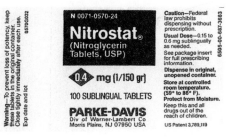

23.   Doctor's Order: Dexamethasone 6 mg p.o. o.d.
       Available: Tablets (scored) labeled 0.5 mg, 4 mg, and 6 mg.
       How many of which strength tablets will you give?

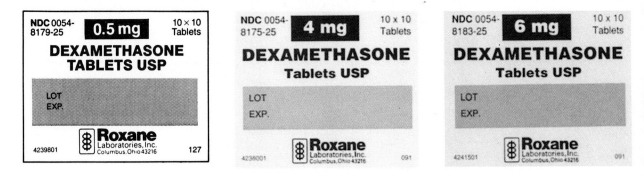

24.   Doctor's Order: Pyridium 0.2 g p.o. q8h.

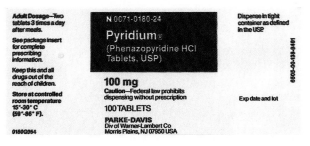

25.   Doctor's Order: Lasix 60 mg p.o. stat.
       Available: Scored tablets labeled 40 mg.

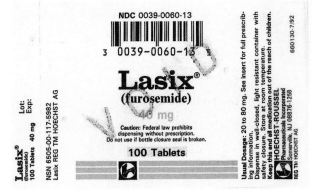

26.   Doctor's Order: Glyburide 2.5 mg p.o. o.d.
       Available: Scored tablets labeled 5 mg.
       How many tablets will you administer for each dose?

27.   Doctor's Order: Tagamet 400 mg p.o. b.i.d.
       Available: Tablets labeled 200 mg.
       How many tablets will you administer for each dose?

28.   Doctor's Order: Indocin 150 mg p.o. b.i.d.
       Available: Indocin sustained release capsules.
       How many capsules will you administer for each dose?

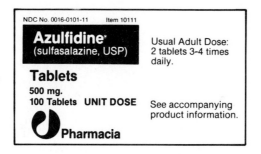

29.   Doctor's Order: Sulfasalazine 1.0 g p.o. q6h.
       Available: Tablets labeled 500 mg.
       How many tabs will you administer for each dose?

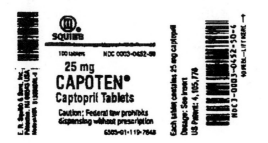

30.   Doctor's Order: Capoten 12.5 mg p.o. b.i.d.
       Available: Scored tablets (quarters) labeled 25 mg.
       How many tabs will you administer for each dose?

31.   Doctor's Order: Synthroid 100 mcg p.o. o.d.
      Available: Tablets labeled 75 mcg and 25 mcg.
      How many tablets of which strength will you use to administer the dose?

NDC 0048-1020-03
Code 3P1023

SYNTHROID®
(Levothyroxine Sodium
Tablets, USP)

25 mcg   (0.025 mg)

100 TABLETS

CAUTION: Federal (USA) law
prohibits dispensing without
prescription.

See full prescribing
information for dosage
and administration.

Dispense in a tight,
light-resistant container
as described in USP.

Store at controlled
room temperature,
15°-30°C (59°-86°F).

Boots
Pharmaceuticals, Inc.
Lincolnshire, IL 60069
USA

7882-01

NDC 0048-1050-03
Code 3P1053

SYNTHROID®
(Levothyroxine Sodium
Tablets, USP)

75 mcg   (0.075 mg)

100 TABLETS

CAUTION: Federal (USA) law
prohibits dispensing without
prescription.

See full prescribing
information for dosage
and administration.

Dispense in a tight,
light-resistant container
as described in USP.

Store at controlled
room temperature,
15°-30°C (59°-86°F).

Boots
Pharmaceuticals, Inc.
Lincolnshire, IL 60069
USA

7880-01

Calculating Oral Liquids

Medications are also available in liquid form for oral administration. Liquid medications are desirable to use for clients who have dysphagia (difficulty swallowing) or who are receiving medications by tubes such as nasogastric (tube in nose to stomach), gastrostomy (tube placed directly into stomach), or jejunostomy (tube directly into intestines). Liquid medications are also desired for use in young children and infants. When medications are ordered that cannot be crushed for administration, the availability of the medication in liquid form should be investigated. Medications in liquid form contain a specific amount or weight of a drug in a given amount of solution that is indicated on the label. Liquid medications are prepared in different forms.

The different forms of oral liquids are as follows:

1. Elixir – Alcohol solution that is sweet and aromatic. Example: Phenobarbital Elixir.

2. Suspension – One or more drugs finely divided into a liquid such as water. Example: Penicillin suspension.

3. Syrup – Medication dissolved in concentrated solution of sugar and water. Example: Colace.

Liquid medications also come as tincture and extract preparations for oral use. Even though oral liquids may be administered by means other than p.o. as already discussed, they should never be given by any other route such as intravenously or by injection.

In solving problems that involve oral liquids, the methods presented in Chapters 13 and 14 can be used. The difference is you must calculate the volume or amount of liquid that contains the dosage of the medication. This information is usually indicated on the medication label and can be expressed per milliliter, cc, ounce, etc., for example 25 mg per mL. The amount may also be expressed in terms of multiple milliliters (mL) or cubic centimeters (cc). Example: 80 mg per 2 mL, 125 mg per 5 mL.

When calculating liquid medications the stock or what you have available is in liquid form, therefore the label on your answer will always be expressed in liquid measures such as mL, cc, m, etc.

Measuring Oral Liquids

The measurement of liquid medications can be done in several ways:

a) Using the standard measuring cup (plastic), which is calibrated in metric, apothecary, and household measures. When pouring liquid medications, they should be poured at eye level and read at the meniscus (a curvature made by the solution) (Figure 15.5).

b) Calibrated droppers are also used for the measurement of liquid medications (Figure 15.6).

c) Syringes may also be used to measure medications. The medication is poured in a medication cup and drawn up in the syringe without the use of a needle. This is often done when the amount desired cannot be measured accurately in a cup. There are some syringes called *oral syringes* that are designed for this purpose (Figure 15.7).

Before we proceed to calculate liquid medications, let's review some helpful pointers.

1. The label on the medication container must be read carefully to determine the dosage strength in the volume of solution, since it varies. Do not confuse dosage strength with the total volume. Example: the label on a medication may indicate a total volume of 100 cc, but the dosage strength may be 125 mg per 5 cc. Figure 15.8 illustrates sample labels on oral medications.

2. Answers are labeled using liquid measures. Example: cc, mL.

3. Calculations can be done using the same methods (formula, ratio-proportion) and the same steps as with solid forms of oral medications.

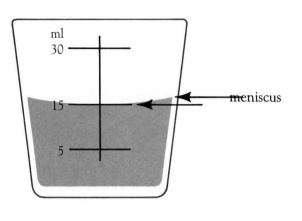

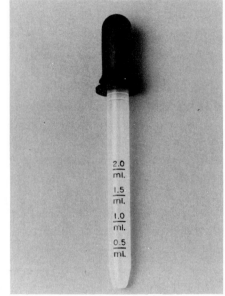

Figure 15.5 Measuring container (From Clayton/Stock: *Basic pharmacology for nurses*, ed 10, St Louis, 1993, Mosby.)

Figure 15.6 Medicine dropper (From Clayton/Stock: *Basic pharmacology for nurses*, ed 10, St Louis, 1993, Mosby.)

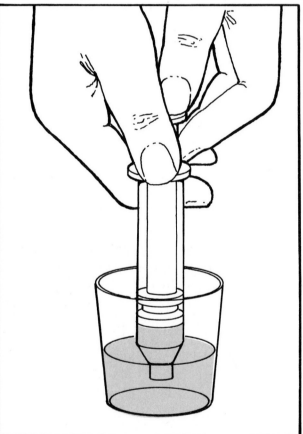

Figure 15.7 Filling a syringe directly from medicine cup (From Clayton/Stock: *Basic pharmacology for Nurses*, ed 9, St Louis, 1989, Mosby.)

A

C

B

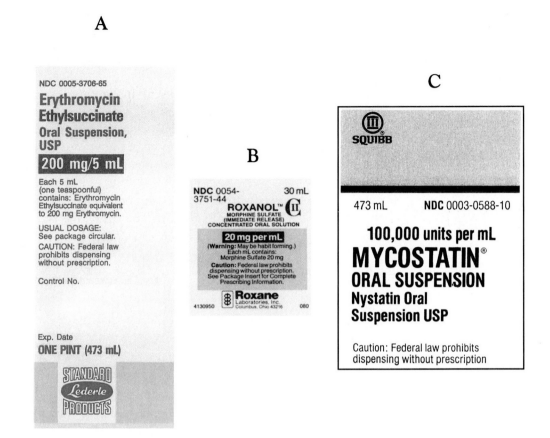

Figure 15.8 A, B, C, Drug labels. **A** = Erythromycin 200 mg, **B** = Roxanol 20 mg, **C** = Mycostatin. (From Dison: *Simplified drugs and solutions for nurses*, ed 10, St Louis, 1992, Mosby.)

Now let's look at some sample problems that involve the calculation of oral liquids.

Example 1:   Doctor's Order: Dilantin 200 mg p.o. t.i.d.
Available: Dilantin suspension labeled 125 mg per 5 cc.

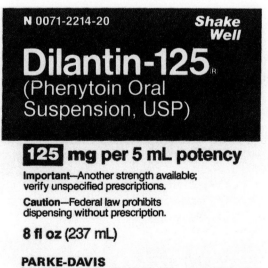

Set-up: 1. No conversion is required. Everything is in the same units of measure and the same system.
Doctor's Order: 200 mg.
Available: 125 mg per 5 cc.

2. Think: What would be a logical answer? In looking at Example #1 you can assume the answer will be greater than 5 cc.

3. Set up the problem using ratio-proportion or formula method.

4. Label the final answer with the correct unit of measure. In this case the label will be cc. Remember: The answer has no meaning without the appropriate label.

Solution Using Ratio-Proportion:

$$125 \text{ mg} : 5 \text{ cc} = 200 \text{ mg} : x \text{ cc}$$
$$\text{(Known)} \qquad \text{(Unknown)}$$

$$125 \, x = 200 \times 5$$

$$125 \, x = 1000$$

$$x = \frac{1000}{125} = 8 \text{ cc}$$

Solution Using Formula Method:

$$\frac{D}{H} \times Q = \frac{200 \text{ mg}}{125 \text{ mg}} \times 5 \text{ cc} = \frac{1000}{125} = 8 \text{ cc}$$

Note: When possible, reduction of the numbers can be done to make them smaller and easier to deal with.

Example 2:   Doctor's Order: Lactulose 30 g p.o. b.i.d.
Available: Lactulose labeled 10 g = 15 mL.

Solution Using Ratio-Proportion:

$$10 \text{ g} : 15 \text{ mL} = 30 \text{ g} : x \text{ mL}$$

$$10 \, x = 450$$

$$x = 45 \text{ mL}$$

Solution Using Formula:

$$\frac{D}{H} \times Q = \frac{30 \text{ g}}{10 \text{ g}} \times 15 \text{ ml} = 45 \text{ ml}$$

Example 3:   Doctor's Order: Elixir of Phenobarbital gr iss p.o. o.d.
Available: Elixir of Phenobarbital labeled 20 mg per 5 mL.

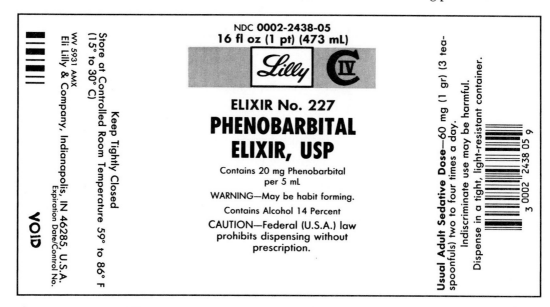

Note: A conversion is necessary before calculating the dosage.
What the doctor has ordered is different from what's available.

Doctor's Order: gr iss
Available: 20 mg per 5 mL.
Equivalent: 60 mg = gr 1.

60 mg : gr 1 = x mg : gr 1 1/2   (3/2)

60 mg : gr 1 = x mg : gr 3/2

$$x = \frac{180}{2}$$

x = 90 mg

Solution Using Ratio-Proportion:

20 mg : 5 mL = 90 mg : x mL

20 x = 450

$$x = \frac{450}{20}$$

x = 22.5 mL or 22 1/2 mL.

There are some medication orders that may be written by the doctor in both solid and liquid form that state the specific amount to be given, therefore requiring no calculation. Example Milk of Magnesia ℥ i p.o. h.s., Robitussin 15 mL p.o. q4h p.r.n., Multivitamin 1 tab p.o. o.d., Ferinsol 0.2 cc p.o. o.d.

Points to Remember:

✔ Liquid medications can be calculated using the same methods as those used for solid forms (tabs, caps).

✔ Read labels carefully on medication containers; identify the dosage strength contained in a certain amount of solution.

✔ Administration of accurate dosages of liquid medications may require the use of droppers, calibrated droppers, or the use of a syringe.

✔ The use of ratio-proportion or a formula is a means of validating an answer, however it still requires thinking in terms of the dosage you will administer and applying principles learned to calculate dosages that are sensible and safe.

Practice Problems

Calculate the following dosages for oral liquids. Don't forget to label your answer. Labels have been included where possible.

32.   Doctor's Order: Colace Syrup 100 mg by jejunostomy tube t.i.d.
    Available: Colace 20 mg per 5 mL.

NDC 0087-0720-01

SYRUP

COLACE®

DOCUSATE SODIUM
STOOL SOFTENER

8 FL OZ (½ PT)

Mead Johnson

Do not use if carton overwrap was missing or broken.
COLACE is used for prevention of dry, hard stools.
Usual daily dose
Infants and children under 3: As prescribed by physician.
Children 3 to 6: 1 to 3 teaspoons.
Children 6 to 12: 2 teaspoons one to three times daily.
Adults and older children: 1 to 3 tablespoons.
Keep this and all medication out of reach of children.

•P7169-09
•P7169-09
•P7169-09

The effect of COLACE on the stools may not be apparent until 1 to 3 days after first oral dose.

WARNING: As with any drug, if you are pregnant or nursing a baby, seek the advice of a health professional before using this product.

Each teaspoon (5 ml) contains 20 mg docusate sodium; each tablespoon (15 ml) contains 60 mg. Contains not more than 1% alcohol.

Store at room temperature. Protect from excessive heat.

MEAD JOHNSON
PHARMACEUTICALS
Bristol-Myers
U.S. Pharmaceutical and Nutritional Group
Evansville, IN 47721
Made in U.S.A.

33.   Doctor's Order: Ascorbic Acid 1 g by nasogastric tube b.i.d.
    Available: Ascorbic Acid solution 500 mg = 10 mL.

34. Doctor's Order: Kaon Chloride 40 mEq p.o. o.d.
    Available: Potassium oral solution 40 mEq = 15 mL.

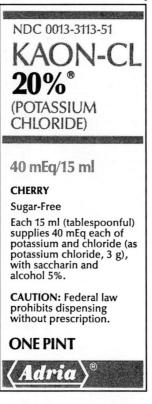

35. Doctor's Order: Theophylline Elixir 120 mg p.o. b.i.d.
    Available: Theophylline Elixir 80 mg/15 mL.

36. Doctor's Order: Erythromycin Oral Suspension 250 mg
    Available: Erythromycin suspension. Use the label below to determine how much
    solution is needed to administer the dose.

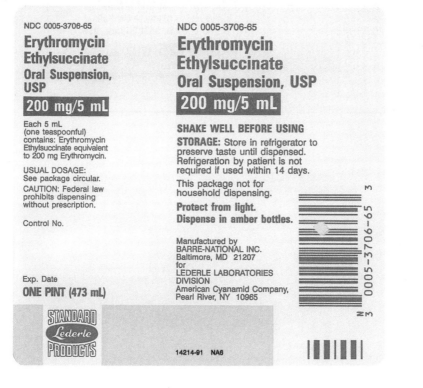

37.   Doctor's Order: Dilantin 100 mg p.o. t.i.d.
      Available: Dilantin suspension. Use the label below to determine how much solution
      is needed to administer the dose.

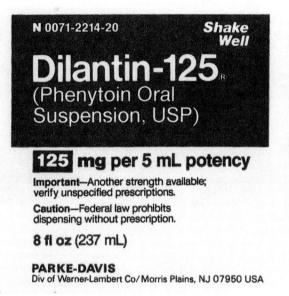

N 0071-2214-20   Shake
                                  Well

Dilantin-125®
(Phenytoin Oral
Suspension, USP)

125 mg per 5 mL potency

Important—Another strength available;
verify unspecified prescriptions.

Caution—Federal law prohibits
dispensing without prescription.

8 fl oz (237 mL)

PARKE-DAVIS
Div of Warner-Lambert Co/Morris Plains, NJ 07950 USA

Shake well before using.
Each 5 mL contains phenytoin,
125 mg with a maximum alcohol
content not greater than 0.6
percent.

Usual Dose—Adults, 1 teaspoonful three times daily;
Children, see package insert.

See package insert for complete
prescribing information.

**Store below 30° C (86° F).
Protect from freezing.**

Keep this and all drugs out of
the reach of children.

Exp date and lot

6505-00-890-1110

2214G013

38.   Doctor's Order: Digoxin 125 mcg p.o. o.d.
      Available: Digoxin Elixir labeled 0.05 mg per mL.

39.   Doctor's Order: Keflex 250 mg p.o. q6h.
      Available: Keflex oral suspension 125 mg/5 mL.

NDC 0777-2321-97
60 mL (When Mixed)   M-201

KEFLEX®
CEPHALEXIN FOR
ORAL SUSPENSION, USP
125 mg per 5 mL

40. Doctor's Order: Amoxicillin 0.5 g p.o. q6h.
    Available: Amoxicillin Oral Suspension.
    Using the label below, calculate the dosage you will administer.

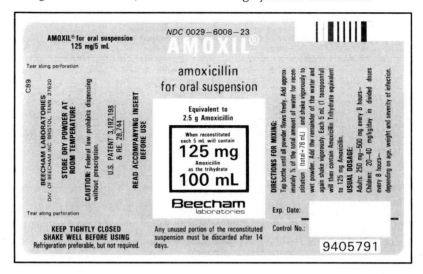

41. Doctor's Order: Phenobarbital 60 mg p.o. h.s.
    Available: Phenobarbital Elixir. Use the label below to calculate the dosage you
    will administer.

42.   Doctor's Order: Mellaril 150 mg p.o. b.i.d.
      Available: Mellaril concentrate.
      Using the label below, calculate the dosage you will administer.

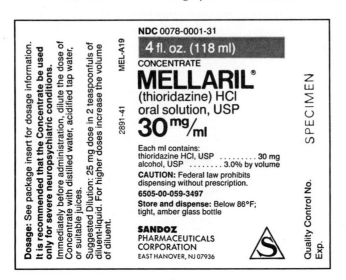

43.   Doctor's Order: Diphenhydramine HCl 25 mg p.o. b.i.d. p.r.n. for agitation.
      Available: Diphenhydramine Hydrochloride Elixir.
      Using the label below calculate the amount of medication you will administer.

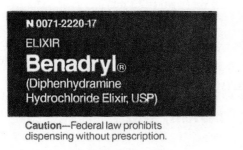

44.   Doctor's Order: Lithium Carbonate 600 mg p.o. h.s.
       Available: Lithium Citrate Syrup. Each 5 ml contains Lithium Carbonate 300 mg.
       a) How many mL are needed to administer the required dose?
       b) How many containers of the drug will you need to prepare the dose?

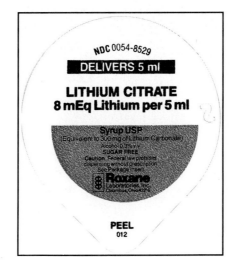

45.   Doctor's Order: Haldol 10 mg p.o. b.i.d.
       Available: Haldol concentrate labeled 2 mg/mL.

46.   Doctor's Order: Dicloxacillin Sodium 0.5 g by gastrostomy tube q6h.
       Available: Dicloxacillin Suspension 100 mL, labeled 62.5 mg per 5 mL.

47.   Doctor's Order: V-Cillin K Suspension 500,000 U. p.o. q.i.d.
       Available: V-Cillin K oral solution. Using the label below calculate the dose you
       would administer.

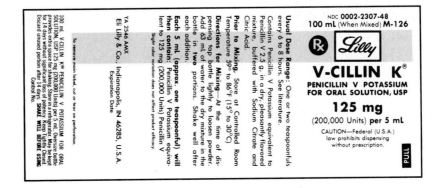

48. Doctor's Order: Keflex 1 g by nasogastric tube q6h.
    Available: Keflex oral suspension. Use the label below to calculate the dose you will
    administer.

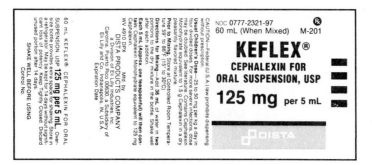

49. Doctor's Order: Trilafon 24 mg p.o. b.i.d.
    Available: Trilafon concentrate labeled 16 mg/5 mL.

50. Doctor's Order: Tylenol Elixir 650 mg by nasogastric tube q4h p.r.n. for temperature
    greater than 101°F.
    Available: Tylenol Elixir labeled 325 mg/10.15 mL.

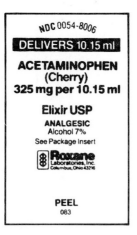

51.   Doctor's Order: Tagamet 400 mg p.o. q6h.
       Available: Tagamet labeled 300 mg/5 mL.

16 Parenteral and Liquid Medications

Objectives

After reviewing this chapter the student will be able to do the following:

1. Identify the various types of syringes used for parenteral administration
2. Read and measure dosages on a syringe
3. Read medication labels on parenteral medications
4. Calculate dosages of parenteral medications already in solution
5. Identify appropriate syringes to administer dosages calculated

The term *parenteral* is used to indicate medications that are administered by any route other than through the digestive system. However the term parenteral is commonly used to refer to the administration of medications by injection with the use of a needle and syringe. Examples of common parenteral routes are: Intramuscular (I.M.), Subcutaneous (S.C.), Intradermal, and Intravenous (I.V.). Medications that are administered by the parenteral route act quicker than oral medications because they are absorbed more rapidly into the bloodstream. The parenteral route may be desired when a rapid action of a drug is necessary, for a client who is unable to take a medication orally due to emesis (vomiting), or if a client is in an unconscious state. This route may also be desired for the client who is displaying irrational behavior and refuses medications by the oral route. Medications for parenteral use are available in liquid (solution) or powder. When medications are available in powder form they must be diluted with a liquid or solvent (reconstituted) before they can be used. Reconstitution of drugs in powder form will be covered in another chapter.

Packaging of Parenteral Medications

Parenteral medications are packaged in various forms:

1. Ampules – Sealed glass container usually designed to hold a single dose of medication. Ampules have a particular shape to them with a constricted neck. They are designed to snap open. The neck of the ampule may be scored or have a darkened line or ring around it to indicate where it should be broken to withdraw medication (Figure 16.1).

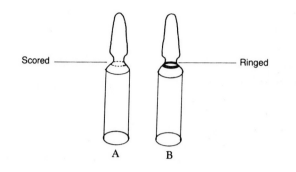

Figure 16.1 Ampules, scored and ringed (From Clayton/Stock: *Basic pharmacology for nurses,* ed 10, St Louis, 1993, Mosby.)

To withdraw the medication from an ampule the neck is snapped off by grasping the neck with an alcohol wipe or sterile gauze and breaking it off. An aspiration (filter) needle is inserted to withdraw the medication.

2. Vials – These are plastic or glass containers that have a rubber stopper (diaphragm) on them. The rubber stopper is covered with a metal lid until use to maintain sterility (Figure 16.2). Vials are available in different sizes. Multidose vials contain more than one dose of the medication. The label on the vial will specify the amount of medication in a certain amount of solution, for example 60 mg per mL, 0.2 mg per 0.5 mL. Single-dose vials contain a single dose of medication for injection. Most of the vials are multi-dose size. The medication in a vial may be in liquid (solution) form, or it may contain a powder that has to be reconstituted before administration.

To withdraw medication from a vial, the top is wiped with alcohol, air equal to the amount of solution being withdrawn is injected into the vial through the rubber stopper, the vial is inverted, and the desired volume of medication is withdrawn (Figure 16.3). Withdrawal of large amounts of medication may require less air to be injected.

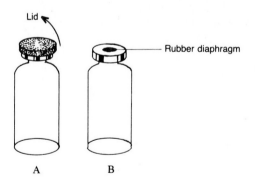

Figure 16.2 **A,** Metal lid, **B,** Rubber diaphragm vials (From Clayton/Stock: *Basic pharmacology for nurses,* ed 10, St Louis, 1993, Mosby.)

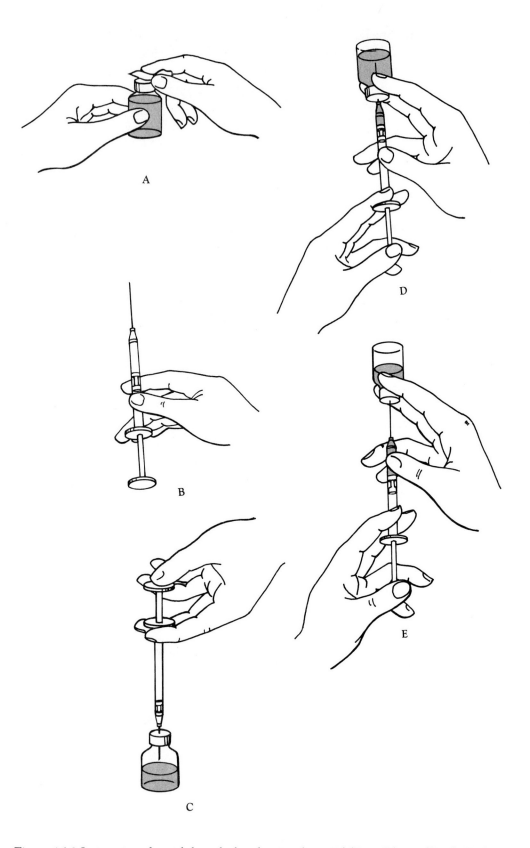

Figure 16.3 Instructions for withdrawal of medication from vial (From Clayton/Stock: *Basic pharmacology for nurses*, ed 10, St Louis, 1993, Mosby.)

3. Mix-O-Vials – Some medications come in mix-o-vials, for example Solu-Medrol, Solu-Cortef. These vials usually contain a single dose of medication. The mix-o-vial contains two compartments that are separated by a rubber stopper. The top compartment contains the sterile liquid (diluent), and the bottom compartment contains the powdered medication. When pressure is placed on the top of the vial the rubber stopper that separates the medication and liquid is released. This allows the liquid and medication to be mixed, thereby dissolving the drug. A needle is inserted to withdraw the medication (Figure 16.4).

4. Cartridge – Some medications come in a prefilled glass or plastic container. The cartridge is clearly marked indicating the amount of medication in it. Certain cartridges require a special holder called a *Tubex* or *Carpuject* to release the medication from the cartridge. The cartridge usually contains a single dose of medication. The unused portion of medication is discarded (Figure 16.5).

5. Prepackaged Syringes – The medication comes prepared for administration in a syringe with the needle attached. A specific amount of medication is contained in the syringe. The amount desired is administered, and the remainder is disposed of. These syringes are for single use only. Example: Valium comes in prepackaged syringes.

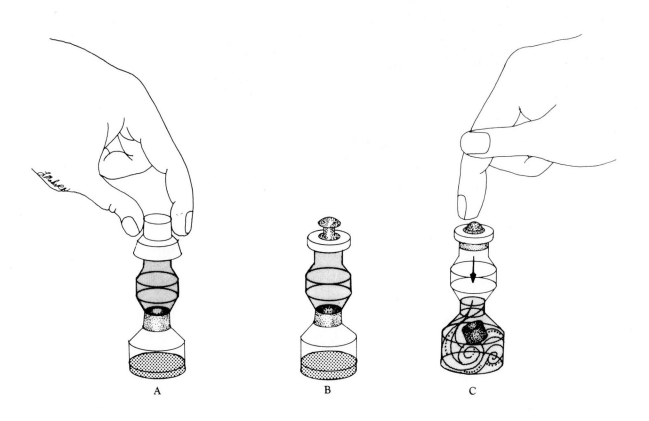

Figure 16.4 Mix-O-Vial Directions (From Clayton/Stock: *Basic pharmacology for nurses*, ed 10, St Louis, 1993, Mosby.)

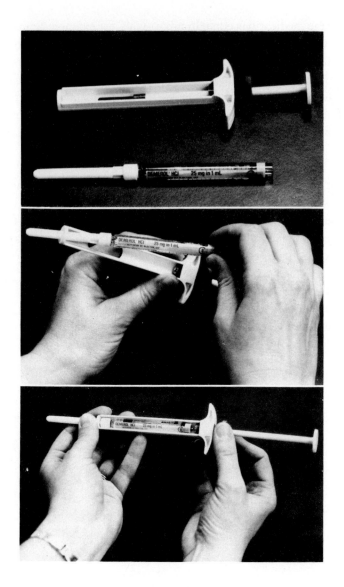

Figure 16.5 Cartridge Syringe (From Clayton/Stock: *Basic pharmacology for nurses*, ed 10, St Louis, 1993, Mosby.)

Syringes

There are various size syringes available for use. They have different capacities and specific calibrations. Syringes are made of plastic and glass. The plastic syringes are used most frequently. They are disposable and designed for one time use only. Syringes have three parts. Parts of a syringe include the following:

A) The barrel – The outer portion that has the calibrations of the syringe on it.

B) The plunger – The inner device that is pushed to eject the medication from the syringe.

C) The tip – The end of the syringe that holds the needle. The tip can be plain or LuerLok (Figure 16.6).

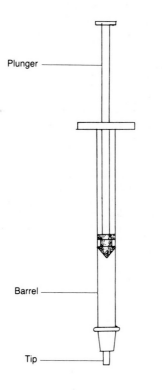

Figure 16.6 Parts of a Syringe (From Clayton/Stock: *Basic pharmacology for nurses*, ed 10, St Louis, 1993, Mosby.)

Types of Syringes

The three types of syringes are hypodermic, tuberculin, and insulin.

1. Hypodermic Syringes – Hypodermic syringes come in a variety of sizes. The syringes are calibrated differently and hold varying capacities. The smaller capacity syringes (2, 2 1/2, 3 cc) are used more often for the administration of medication, however hypodermic syringes are also available in larger sizes (10, 20, 50 cc). Syringes are labeled in cc and mL. The smaller capacity syringes (2, 2 1/2, 3 cc) are calibrated in minims (m) (Figure 16.7).

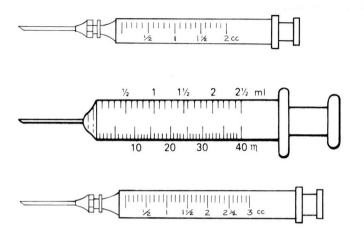

Figure 16.7 Hypodermic Syringes (From Dison: *Simplified drugs and solutions for nurses*, ed 10, St Louis, 1992, Mosby; Richardson: *The Mathematics of Drugs and Solutions*, ed 5, St Louis, 1994, Mosby; and Smith: *Dosages and solutions calculations*, St Louis, 1989, Mosby.)

Notice the side that indicates cc or mL. There are 10 spaces between the largest markings. This indicates the syringe is marked in tenths of a cc. Each of the lines is 0.1 cc. The longer lines indicate 1/2 (0.5) and full cc measures. On the other side of the syringe there are minim (m) markings. Each small line counts as 1 minim, and the longer lines represent 5 minim increments, for example, 5, 10, etc.

When looking at the syringe shown in Figure 16.8 notice the black rubber ring. When measuring medications and reading the medication withdrawn, the forward edge of the plunger head indicates the amount of medication withdrawn. The point where the rubber plunger tip makes contact with the barrel is the spot that should be lined up with the amount desired.

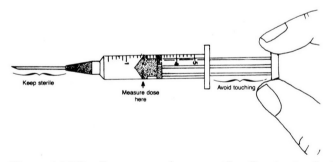

Figure 16.8 Reading measured amount of medication in plastic syringe (From Clayton/Stock: *Basic pharmacology for nurses*, ed 10, St Louis, 1993, Mosby.)

Let's examine the syringes below to illustrate specific amounts in a syringe.

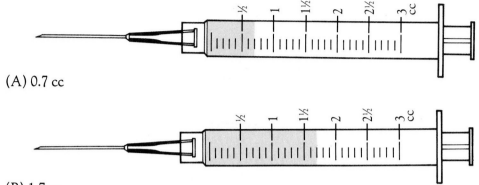

(A) 0.7 cc

(B) 1.7 cc

Since the smaller capacity syringes are used most often for the administration of medications it is very important to know how to read them to draw up amounts accurately.

Point to Remember:

✔ Small capacity hypodermics (2, 2 1/2, 3 cc) are calibrated in 0.1 of cc and minims. Dosages administered with them must correlate to the calibration.

Practice Problems

Shade the following amounts in on the syringes as indicated.

1. 0.8 cc

2. 1.2 cc

3. m 10

4. 1.5 cc

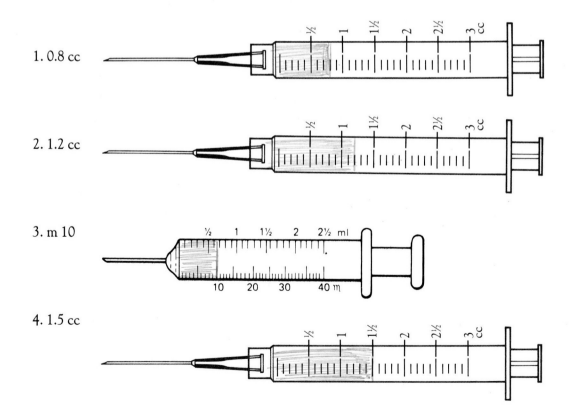

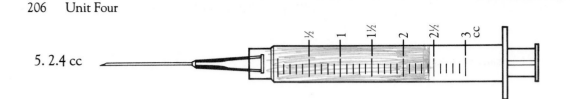

5. 2.4 cc

Identify the number of m shaded in on the syringe in Problem 6 and the number of cc shaded in on the syringes in Problems 7 - 10.

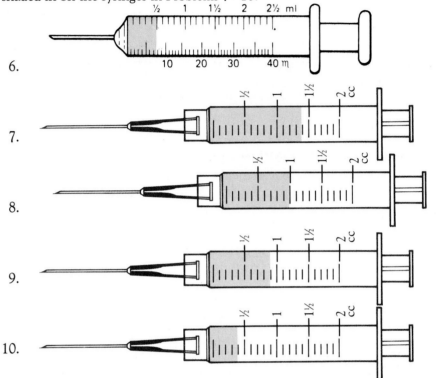

6.

7.

8.

9.

10.

1. Large Size Hypodermics: The larger size hypodermics (5, 6, 10, 12 cc) are used when volumes larger than 3 cc are desired. These syringes are used to measure whole numbers of cc as opposed to smaller units such as a tenth of a cc. There are no minim markings on the larger size syringes. Syringes that range from 5 to 12 cc in size are calibrated in 0.2 cc increments with whole number indicated by the long lines. See Figure 16.9 with 3.6 cc of medication drawn up.

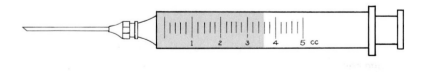

Figure 16.9 5 cc Syringe filled w/3.6 cc (From Dison: *Simplified drugs and solutions for nurses,* ed 10, St Louis, 1992, Mosby.)

A 10 cc syringe shown below indicates 6.6 cc (Figure 16.10).

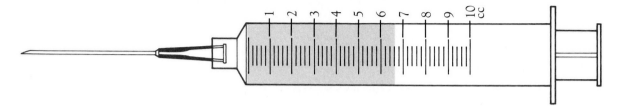

Figure 16.10 10 cc Syringe filled to 6.6 cc (From Dison: *Simplified drugs and solutions for nurses*, ed 10, St Louis, 1992, Mosby.)

Practice Problems

Indicate the number of ccs shaded in on the following syringes.

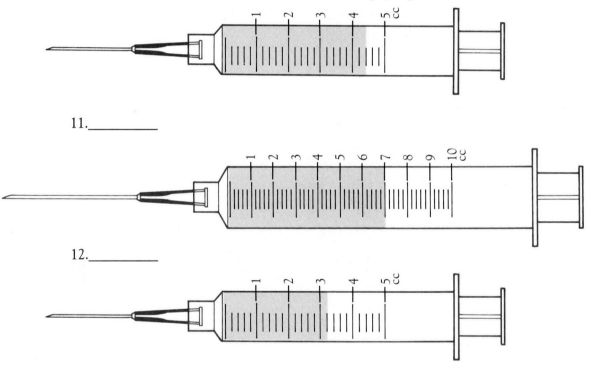

11._____

12._____

13._____

2. Tuberculin Syringe – This is a narrow syringe that has a total capacity of 1 cc. The volume of a tuberculin syringe can be measured on the cc or the minim scale. On the minim side of the syringe, the lines represent 1 minim. On the cc side of the syringe the syringe is calibrated in hundredths of a cc. The markings on the syringe (lines) are closer together to indicate how small the calibrations are (Figure 16.11).

Tuberculin syringes are used to accurately measure medications that are given in very small volumes (for example, Heparin). This syringe is also frequently used in pediatrics. Dosages such as 0.42 cc and 0.37 cc could be measured accurately using a tuberculin syringe. When using a tuberculin syringe, it is important to read it carefully to avoid error.

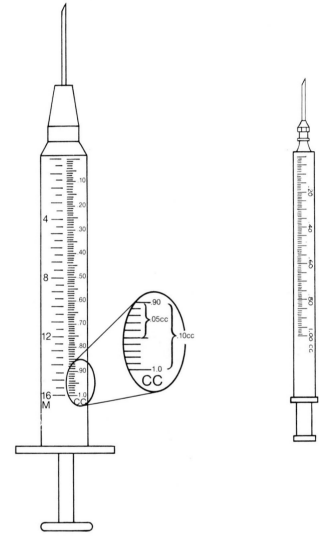

Figure 16.11 Tuberculin Syringes (From Dison: *Simplified drugs and solutions for nurses*, ed 10, St Louis, 1992, Mosby and Clayton/Stock: *Basic pharmacology for nurses*, ed 10, St Louis, 1993, Mosby.)

3. Insulin Syringes – These syringes are designed for the administration of insulin. Insulin dosages are measured in Units (U.). Insulin syringes are calibrated to match the dosage strength of the insulin being used. They are marked U-100 and are designed to be used with insulin that is marked U-100. There are two types of insulin syringes.

a) The Lo-Dose syringe is used to measure small doses and is 0.5 mL in size. It may be used for clients receiving 50 U. or less of U-100 insulin. It has a capacity of 50 U. The scale on the Lo-Dose syringe is easy to read. Each calibration (shorter lines) measures 1 U., and each 5-U. increment is numbered (long lines) (Figure 16.12).

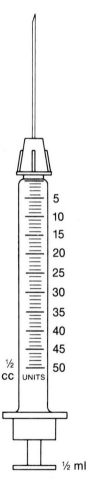

Figure 16.12 Lo-Dose Syringe (From Brown/Mulholland: *Drug calculations: process and problems for clinical practice*, ed 4, St Louis, 1992, Mosby.)

b) The 1 mL size syringe – This syringe is designed to hold 100 U. There are currently two types on the market. One type of 1 cc (100 U.) capacity has each 10 U. increment numbered. This syringe is calibrated in 2 U. increments. Odd numbered units are therefore measured between the even calibrations (Figure 16.13). Use of this syringe should be avoided if possible since accuracy of dosage is questionable. The second type of 1 cc capacity syringe has two scales on it. The odd numbers are on the left of the syringe and the even are on the right. The calibrations are in 1 U. increments. The best method to use when using this type of syringe is the following: Measure uneven dosages on the left, and even dosages are measured using the scale on the right (Figure 16.14). The calculation of insulin dosages and reading of the calibrations are discussed in more detail in Chapter 18.

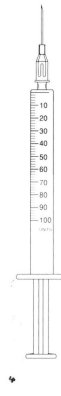

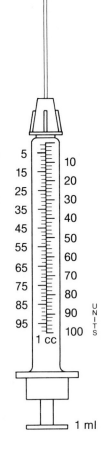

Figure 16.13 1 cc Capacity Syringe (From Dison: *Simplified drugs and solutions for nurses*, ed 10, St Louis, 1992, Mosby.)

Figure 16.14 1 cc Capacity Syringe-Insulin Units (From Brown/Mulholland: *Drug calculations: process and problems for clinical practice*, ed 4, St Louis, 1992, Mosby.)

Points to Remember:

✔ Hypodermic Syringes – 2, 2 1/2, and 3 cc are marked in minims and 0.1 of a cc. These small capacity syringes are most often used for medication administration.

✔ Hypodermic Syringes – 5 to 12 cc are marked in increments of 0.2 cc and whole numbers of cc.

✔ Hypodermic Syringes – 20 cc and larger are marked in 1 cc increments and may have other markings such as ounces.

✔ Tuberculin Syringe – small syringe that is marked in minims and hundredths of a cc. They are used for the administration of small doses.

✔ Insulin Syringes – are marked U-100 for administration with U-100 Insulin. Insulin is measured in units.

Before proceeding to discuss calculation of parenteral doses it is necessary to review some specifics in terms of reading labels. The reading of the label and understanding what information is essential is important in determining the correct dosage to administer.

Reading Parenteral Labels

The information contained on the parenteral label is similar to the information on an oral liquid label. It contains total volume of the container and the dosage strength (amount of medication in solution) expressed in cc or mL. It is important to read the label carefully to determine the dosage strength and volume. Example 25 mg per mL.

Let's examine some labels. In examining the Vistaril label below notice the total size of the vial is 10 cc. The dosage strength is 50 mg per mL.

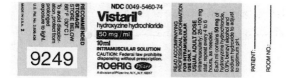

The atropine label shows that the total vial size is 20 mL, however there are 0.4 mg per mL. It is important to realize that although there is a total of 20 mL, each mL contains 0.4 mg.

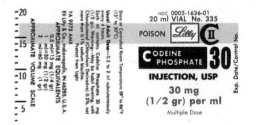

The Codeine label has a combination of two systems of measurement: grains, which is Apothecary, and mg and mL, which are metric. The vial size is 20 mL. Notice it states 30 mg (1/2 gr) per mL. If 60 mg = gr 1, then gr 1/2, which is 30 mg, is contained in 1 mL.

As you can see the dosage strength on parenteral labels can be expressed in metric, apothecary, or a combination of both.

Practice Problem

Refer to the Aminophylline label below, and answer the following questions.

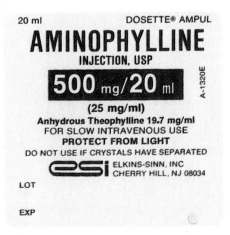

14. What is the total volume of the ampule?

15. What is the dosage strength?

16. If 250 mg was ordered, how many mL would this be?

Parenteral labels can also express medications in percentage strengths, as well as Units and Milliequivalents.

Drugs Labeled in Percentage Strengths

Drugs that are labeled as percentage solutions give information such as the percentage of the solution and the total volume of the vial or ampule. Although percentage is used, metric measures are used as well. Example: The figure below, which shows a label of Lidocaine 1%. Notice there are 10 mg/mL.

```
⊐ 5 mL   NDC 0074-4713-02
1% Lidocaine
HCl Inj., USP
50 mg (10 mg/mL)
              06-5915-2/R5-6/86
Abbott Laboratories
N. Chicago, IL60064, USA
```

Often no calculation is necessary when giving medications expressed in percentage strength. The doctor usually states the number of cc or mL to prepare or may state it in the number of ampules or vials. Example: Calcium Gluconate 10% may be ordered as, administer one vial of 10% Calcium Gluconate or 10 cc of 10% Calcium Gluconate (see label).

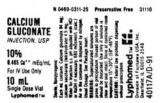

Solutions Expressed in Ratio Strength

A medication commonly expressed in terms of ratio strength is Epinephrine. Drugs expressed this way include metric measures as well and are often ordered by the number of cc and mL. Example Epinephrine may state 1:1000 and indicate 1 mg/mL.

Parenteral Medications Measured in Units

Some medications measured in units for parenteral administration are Heparin, Pitocin, Insulin, and Penicillin. Notice the labels indicate how many units per mL. Example Pitocin 10 Units/mL, Heparin 1000 Units per mL.

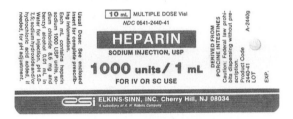

Parenteral Medications in Milliequivalents

Potassium and Sodium Bicarbonate are drugs that are expressed in milliequivalents. Like Units, Milliequivalents are specific measurements that have no conversion to another system and are specific to the medication used.

Practice Problem

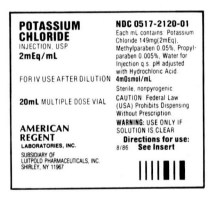

Using the label above, answer the following questions.

17. What is the total volume of the vial? _____

18. What is the dosage in mEq/mL? _____

Remember: It is important to read the label on parenteral medications carefully. Labels on parenteral medications include a variety of units to express dosage strengths. To calculate dosages to administer it is important to know the strength of the medication in solution per mL or cc.

Calculating Parenteral Dosages

The calculation of parenteral dosages can be done using the same rules and methods that were used in computing oral dosages. The ratio-proportion and formula methods have been presented in earlier chapters. There are some guidelines that will help to calculate a dosage that is logical, reasonable, and accurate.

Guidelines for Calculating Parenteral Dosages

1. Use ratio-proportion or formula method to calculate the dosage to be administered.

2. The rules and the steps for calculating parenteral dosages are the same as those used for computing oral dosages.

3. Remember the stock volume varies and is not always per 1 mL or cc. Read the label carefully to determine the dosage strength contained in a certain volume of solution.

4. Accuracy in calculating parenteral dosages depends on the syringe used. Therefore it is important to be able to understand syringes.

5. Small capacity syringes 2, 2 1/2, 3 cc are marked in minims and tenths (0.1) of a mL. These syringes are used most often for the administration of intra-muscular medications.

6. Tuberculin syringes are used for small dosages and are calibrated in hundredths (0.01) of a mL. Tuberculin syringes have a total capacity of one milliliter; they are designed to administer small doses and potent medications They frequently are used in pediatrics.

7. Insulin syringes are designed for insulin only. Measurement of insulin in an insulin syringe requires no calculation or conversion. In an emergency situation or when insulin syringes are not available, the tuberculin syringe may be used to administer insulin. This is possible because 100 units of insulin equals 1 milliliter. It is safest to measure insulin with an insulin syringe! Insulin will be discussed in more detail in Chapter 18.

Calculating Injectable Medications According to the Syringe

Now that you have an understanding of syringes, let's discuss obtaining an answer that is measurable according to the syringe being used.

Points to Remember:

✔ cc (mL) are never rounded off to a whole unit.

✔ Minims are only expressed as whole numbers.

✔ When using a 2, 2 1/2, 3 cc syringe answers in milliliters are rounded to the nearest tenth or expressed in minims.

    a) For an answer in milliliters (mL), math is carried two decimal places and rounded to the nearest tenth.

    Example: 1.75 mL = 1.8 mL

    b) To calculate minims, the math is carried out to the tenths place and rounded to the nearest whole number.

    Example: 16.9 = m 17

Using the equivalent m 16 = 1 cc is preferred and gives a more accurate answer. The maximum number of minims on a syringe is 40. A dose greater than 40 minims can't be measured.

Remember: Minims is an apothecary measure and is not exact. It is better to express answers in metric measures such as mL or cc.

✔ When using a tuberculin syringe to calculate a dose in mL, math is carried to the thousandths place and rounded to the nearest hundredth because the syringe is marked in hundredths (0.01) of a mL.
Example: 0.876 mL = 0.88 mL.

    a) When calculations come to the hundredths place evenly, rounding off is not necessary. Example: 0.53 mL can be drawn up accurately without rounding off.

    b) To calculate minims on this syringe, math is carried to the nearest hundredth and rounded to the nearest minim. Example: 9.28 = m 9. (9.28 rounds off to 9.3, because 0.3 is less than 0.5 it is dropped.)

✔ For injectable medications there are guidelines as to the amount of medication that can be administered. When the dosage exceeds these guidelines the dosage should be questioned and calculation double checked.

a) I.M. (Intramuscular) – the range is between 1 and 3 mL. According to Potter and Perry, *Fundamentals of Nursing* (1989) a healthy well-developed client can tolerate as much as 3 mL in large muscles. For the elderly or thin client and young children the dose is less than 2 mL. Whaley and Wong (1989) recommend giving no more than 1 mL to small children and older infants. The maximum dose that can be given to an adult is 4 cc.

b) s.c. (Subcutaneous) – The volume that can be administered safely is 1 mL or less.

✔ In administering medications by injection the absorption and consistency of the medication is also considered. For example, a dose of 3 cc of a thick oily substance may be divided into two injections of 1.5 mL each.

✔ Dosages administered are measured in mL, cc, and minims, therefore the answer is labeled accordingly.

✔ Proceed with calculations in a logical and reasonable manner.

✔ Injectables that are added to I.V. solution may have a volume greater than 5 mL.

Now with the guidelines in mind, let's look at some sample problems. Regardless of what method you use to calculate, the following steps are used.

Steps:

1. Check to make sure everything is in the same system and unit of measure.

2. Think or take a guess at what the answer should logically be.

3. Consider the type of syringe that is being used. The cardinal rule should always be any dose given must be able to be measured accurately in the syringe you are using.

4. Use the ratio-proportion or formula method to calculate the dosage.

Let's look at some sample problems calculating parenteral dosages.

Example 1:   Doctor's Order: Gentamicin 75 mg I.M. q8h.
Available: Gentamicin labeled 40 mg = 1cc.

Note: No conversion is necessary here. Think – The dosage ordered is going to be more than 1 cc but less than 2 cc. Set up and solve.

Solution Using Ratio-Proportion

$$40 \text{ mg} : 1 \text{ cc} = 75 \text{ mg} : x \text{ cc}$$

$$40x = 75$$

$$x = 1.87 \text{ cc.}$$

Answer: 1.9 cc.

The answer here is rounded to the nearest tenth of a mL (cc). Remember the syringe you are using is marked in tenths of a mL and minims.

Solution Using Formula

$$\frac{75 \text{ mg}}{40 \text{ mg}} \times 1 \text{ cc} = x$$

$$\frac{75}{40} = x$$

$$x = 1.87 \text{ cc}$$

Remember: The answer has to be rounded off to the nearest tenth of a cc. Therefore the answer is 1.9 cc.

The above answer could also be expressed as minims. When changing to minims do not round off the number of cc to the nearest tenth. Change the answer to minims by multiplying the value obtained for cc before it is rounded off. Use m 16 = 1cc. Remember however it is always preferred to express the answer in metric measures, since apothecary measures are not exact. To convert to minims use any of the methods presented in Chapter 8. In the above problem we would change to minims as follows:

$$m\ 16 : 1 \text{ cc} = x\ m : 1.87 \text{ cc}$$

$$x = 1.87 \times 16$$

$$x = m\ 29.92 \quad \text{(Answer: m 30)}$$

Remember: Minims are expressed as whole numbers, therefore the answer to the nearest whole number is m 30.

Look at the syringes below, illustrating the amounts shaded in on a syringe.

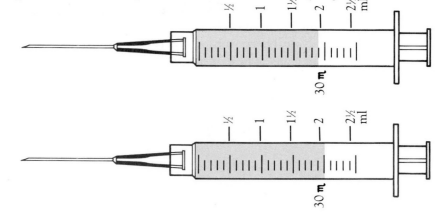

Example 2:   Doctor's Order: Kantrex 500 mg I.M. q12h.
Available: Kanamycin (Kantrex) labeled 0.5 g per 2 cc.

In this problem a conversion is necessary. Equivalent: 1000 mg = 1g. Convert what is ordered to what is available. 500 mg = 0.5 g. To get rid of the decimal convert what's available to what's ordered. 0.5 g = 500 mg. Remember either way will net the same final answer.

Think – The dosage you will need to give is greater than 1 cc, and it's being given I.M. The dosage therefore should fall within the range that is safe for I.M. The solution after making conversion is as follows:

Solution Using Ratio-Proportion

$$0.5\,g \,:\, 2cc = 0.5\,g \,:\, x\,cc$$

$$0.5x = 1.0$$

$$x = \frac{1.0}{0.5}$$

$$x = 2\,cc.$$

Solution Using Formula

$$\frac{0.5\,g}{0.5\,g} \times 2\,cc = x$$

$$\frac{0.5 \times 2}{0.5 \times 1} = x$$

$$\frac{1.0}{0.5} = x$$

$$x = 2\,cc$$

Look at the syringe illustrating this amount drawn up.

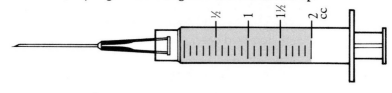

2 cc in syringe.

Example 3:   Doctor's Order: Morphine Sulfate gr 1/2 I.M. stat.
Available: Morphine Sulfate in a 20 mL vial, labeled
15 mg per mL.

1. A conversion is necessary. Convert gr 1/2 to mg using the
   equivalent 60 mg = gr 1, gr 1/2 therefore is 30 mg.

2. Think – You will need more than 1 mL to administer the dose.

3. Set up the problem, and calculate the dose to be administered.

Solution Using Ratio-Proportion

$$15 \text{ mg} : 1 \text{ mL} = 30 \text{ mg} : x \text{ mL}$$

$$15x = 30$$

$$x = 2 \text{ mL}$$

Solution Using Formula

$$\frac{30 \text{ mg}}{15 \text{ mg}} \times 1 \text{ mL} = x$$

$$\frac{30}{15} = x$$

$$x = 2 \text{ mL}$$

Note: Refer to the above example (#2) to visualize 2 cc in a syringe.

Example 4:   Doctor's Order: Atropine Sulfate gr 1/100 I.M. stat.
Available: Atropine Sulfate in 20 mL vial labeled 0.4 mg
per mL.

1. Conversion is necessary. Use the equivalent 60 mg = gr 1.
   gr 1/100 = 0.6 mg

2. Think – The dosage will be greater than 1 mL to administer the
   required dose.

3. Set up the problem to solve for the dosage to administer.

Solution Using Ratio-Proportion

$$0.4 \text{ mg} : 1 \text{ mL} = 0.6 \text{ mg} : x \text{ mL}$$

$$0.4x = 0.6$$

$$x = \frac{0.6}{0.4}$$

$$x = 1.5 \text{ mL or } 1\ 1/2 \text{ mL}$$

Solution Using Formula

$$\frac{0.6 \text{ mg}}{0.4 \text{ mg}} \times 1 = x$$

$$\frac{0.6}{0.4} = x$$

$$x = 1.5 \text{ mL}, \ 1\ 1/2 \text{ mL}$$

Let's look at this amount shaded in on a syringe.

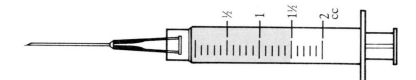

Calculating Dosages for Medications in Units

There are certain drugs that are measured in Units. Some medications measured in units include vitamins, antibiotics, insulin, and Heparin. The calculation of insulin will be discussed in Chapter 18. In determining the dosage to administer when medications are measured in Units, the same steps are used as with other parenteral medications. Dosages of certain medications such as Heparin are administered with a tuberculin syringe, as opposed to a hypodermic (2, 2 1/2, 3 cc). Heparin because of its effects is never rounded off, but rather exact doses are given. Heparin will also be discussed in more detail in a Chapter 21. Let's look at sample problems with Units.

> **Example 1:**   Doctor's Order: Heparin 750 U. s.c. o.d.
> Available Heparin 1000 U. per mL.
> Using a 1 cc syringe calculate the dose to be administered.

Problem Set-up:

1. No conversion is required. There is no conversion that exists for Units.

2. Think – The dosage to be given is less than 1 cc. This dose can be accurately measured in a 1 cc tuberculin syringe. To administer in a hypodermic (2, 2 1/2, 3 cc) the dosage would have to be expressed to the nearest tenth of a mL or expressed as minims.

3. Set up the problem, and calculate the dose to be given.

Solution Using Ratio-Proportion

$$1000 \text{ U.} : 1 \text{ mL} = 750 \text{ U.} : x \text{ mL}$$

$$1000\,x = 750$$

$$x = \frac{750}{1000}$$

$$x = 0.75 \text{ mL}$$

Solution Using Formula

$$\frac{750 \text{ U.}}{1000 \text{ U.}} \times 1 \text{ mL} = x$$

$$\frac{750}{1000} = x$$

$$x = 0.75 \text{ mL}$$

1 cc (1 mL) syringe illustrating 0.75 mL shaded in.

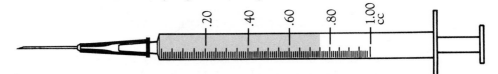

Example 2:   Doctor's Order: Penicillin G 500,000 U. I.M. b.i.d.
Available: Penicillin G labeled 300,000 U. per mL

Problem Set-up:

1. No conversion is required.

2. Think – The dosage ordered is more than what is available. Therefore more than 1 cc would be required to administer the dose.

3. Set up the problem in ratio-proportion or formula to calculate the dosage.

Solution Using Ratio-Proportion

$$300,000 \text{ U.} : 1 \text{ mL} = 500,000 \text{ U.} : x \text{ mL}$$

$$300,000\,x = 500,000$$

$$x = \frac{500,000}{300,000}$$

$$x = 1.66 \text{ mL}$$

Note: The division here is carried two decimal places. This answer is then rounded off to 1.7 mL. Remember the hypodermic syringe (2, 2 1/2, 3 cc) is marked in tenths of a mL.

Solution Using Formula

$$\frac{500,000 \text{ U.}}{300,000 \text{ U.}} \times 1 \text{ mL} = x$$

$$\frac{500,000}{300,000} = x$$

$$x = 1.66 \text{ mL}$$

$$x = 1.7 \text{ mL}$$

Illustration of the dosage calculated in a hypodermic syringe.

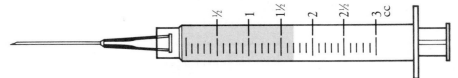

Chapter Review

Calculate the dosages for the problems below, and shade the dosage in on the syringe provided. Labels have been provided for some problems. Express your answers to the nearest tenth except where indicated.

1.   Doctor's Order: Sandostatin 0.05 mg s.c. o.d.
     Available: Sandostatin labeled 1 mL = 100 mcg.

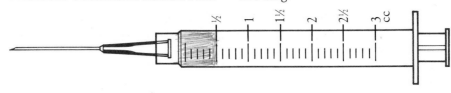

2.   Doctor's Order: Demerol 50 mg I.M. and Vistaril 25 mg I.M. q4h p.r.n. for pain.
       Available: Demerol labeled 75 mg/mL.
                        Vistaril labeled 50 mg/mL.

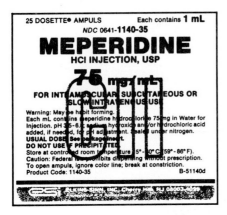
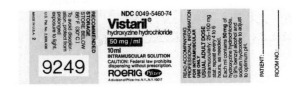

What is the total amount of cc you will administer?
Shade the total number of cc on the syringe provided.

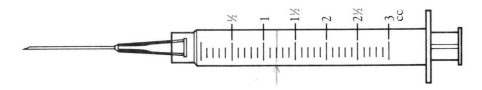

3.   Doctor's Order: Reglan 5 mg I.M. b.i.d. 1/2 hour a.c.
       Available: Reglan labeled 10 mg per 2 mL.

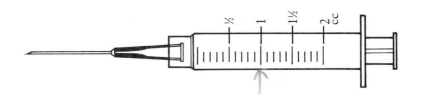

4.   Doctor's Order: Heparin 5000 U. s.c. b.i.d.
       Available: Heparin labeled 20,000 U. per mL
       Express your answer in hundredths.

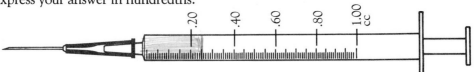

5. Doctor's Order: Morphine Sulfate gr 1/4 I.M. q4h p.r.n.
   Available: Morphine with the following label. Use the label below to calculate the dosage.

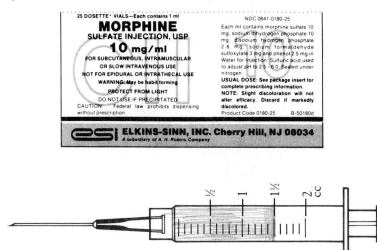

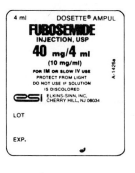

6. Doctor's Order: Lasix (Furosemide) 20 mg I.M. stat.
   Available: Lasix with the following label. Use the label below to calculate the dosage.

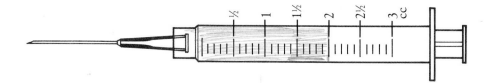

7. Doctor's Order: Clindamycin 0.3 g I.M. q6h.
   Available: 4 mL vial labeled 150 mg per mL.

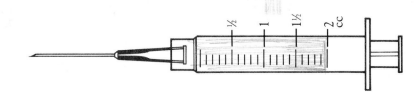

8. Doctor's Order: Atropine gr 1/150 I.M. stat.
    Available: Atropine labeled 0.4 mg per mL.

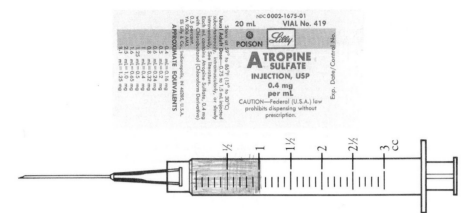

9. Doctor's Order: Kefzol 0.5 g I.M. q6h.
    Available: Vial labeled 225 mg per mL.

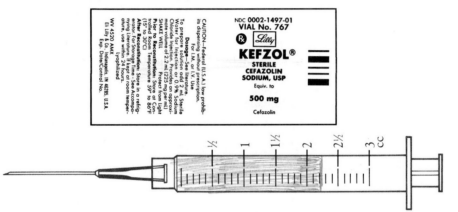

10. Doctor's Order: Digoxin 100 mcg I.M. q.d.
    Available: Digoxin injection with the label below.

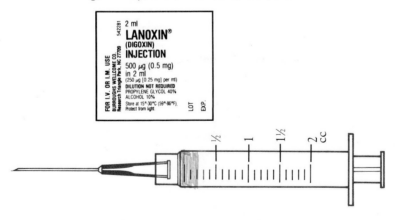

11. Doctor's Order: Phenobarbital labeled gr 1/2 I.M. b.i.d.
    Available: Phenobarbital labeled 120 mg per mL.

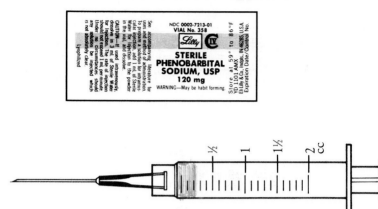

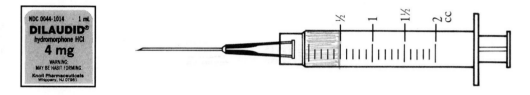

12. Doctor's Order: Dilaudid 2 mg s.c. q4h p.r.n. for pain.
    Available: Vial 1 mL in size labeled 4 mg.

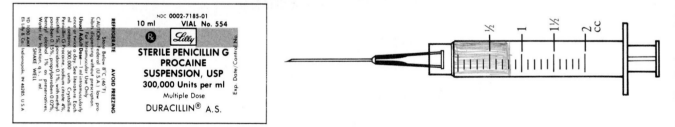

13. Doctor's Order: Penicillin G 250,000 U. I.M. q6h.
    Available: Penicillin G labeled 300,000 U. per mL.

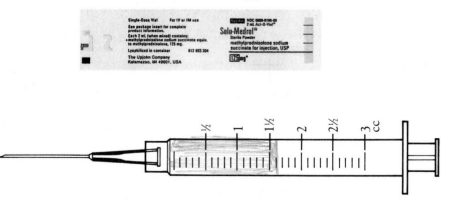

14. Doctor's Order: Solu-Medrol 100 mg I.M. q8h x 2 doses.
    Available: Solu-Medrol labeled 125 mg per 2 mL

15.   Doctor's Order: Methergine 0.4 mg I.M. q4h x 3 doses.
       Available: Methergine labeled 0.2 mg/mL.

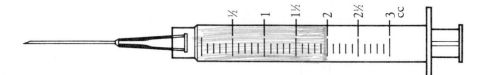

16.   Doctor's Order: Heparin 8000 U. s.c. q12h.
       Available: Heparin labeled 10,000 U. per mL.

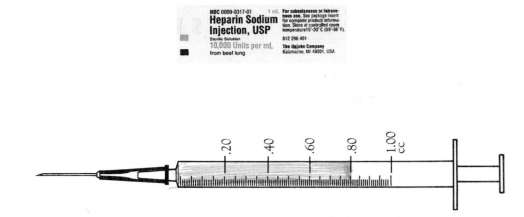

17.   Doctor's Order: Morphine Sulfate 4 mg I.M. q4h p.r.n.
       Available: Morphine labeled 10 mg per mL

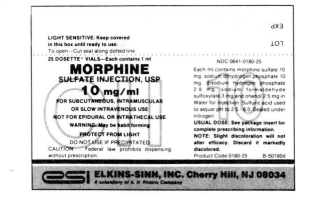

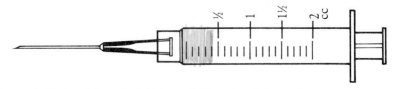

18.   Doctor's Order: Vitamin K 10 mg I.M. q.d. x 3 days.
       Available: Vitamin K labeled 5 mg per mL.

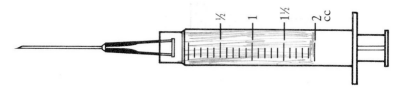

19.   Doctor's Order: Codeine gr 1/4 I.M. q4h p.r.n. for pain.
       Available: Codeine Phosphate. Use the label below to calculate the dosage.

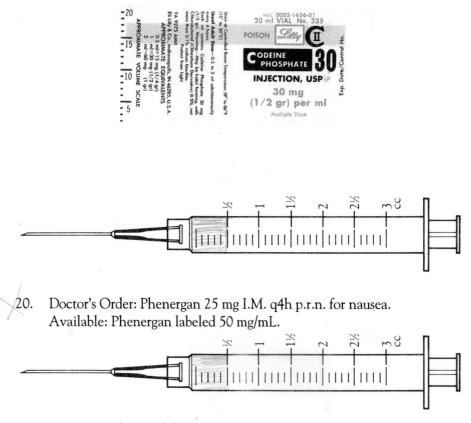

20.   Doctor's Order: Phenergan 25 mg I.M. q4h p.r.n. for nausea.
       Available: Phenergan labeled 50 mg/mL.

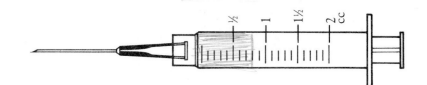

21.   Doctor's Order: Stadol 1.5 mg I.M. q3-4h for pain.
       Available: Stadol labeled 2 mg/mL.

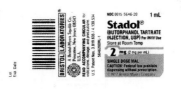

22.   Doctor's Order: Dilaudid 3 mg I.M.
       Available: Dilaudid 4 mg per mL.

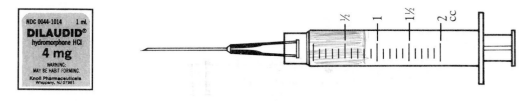

23.   Doctor's Order: Scopolamine gr 1/300 s.c. stat.
       Available: Scopolamine labeled 0.4 mg/mL.

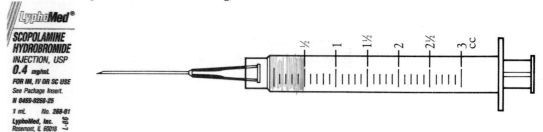

24.   Doctor's Order: Haldol 3 mg I.M. q6h p.r.n.
       Available: Haldol 5 mg/mL.

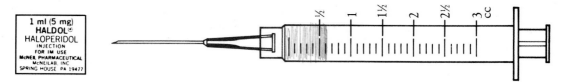

25.   Doctor's Order: Seconal Sodium 90 mg I.M. h.s. p.r.n.
       Available: Seconal Sodium 50 mg/mL.

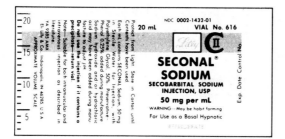

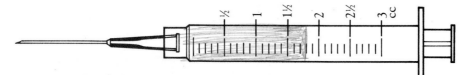

26.   Doctor's Order: Solucortef 400 mg I.V. o.d. for a severe inflammation.
       Available: Solucortef 250 mg per 2 mL.

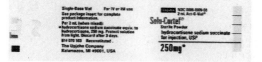

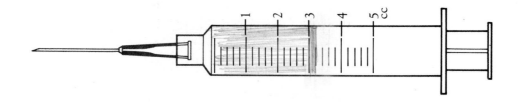

27. Doctor's Order: Solumedrol 40 mg I.V. q6h x 3 days.
     Available: Solumedrol 125 mg/2 mL.

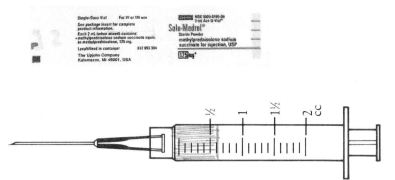

Directions: Use the medication labels provided to calculate the volume necessary to administer the dosage ordered. Fill in the syringes to indicate the amount of solution you will draw up.

28. Doctor's Order: Robinul 200 mcg I.M. preop on call
     Available:

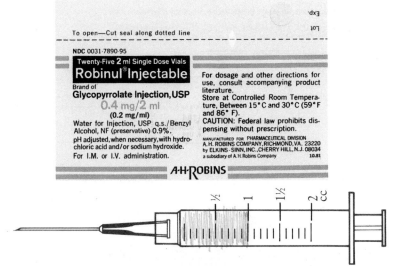

29. Doctor's Order: Heparin 2500 U. s.c. o.d.
     Available:

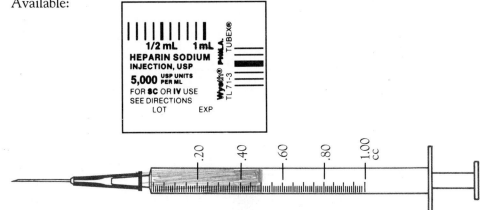

30. Doctor's Order: Vistaril 35 mg I.M. stat.
     Available:

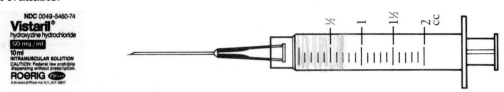

31. Doctor's Order: Meperidine 60 mg I.M. q3-4h p.r.n. for pain.
     Available:

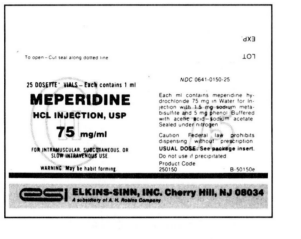

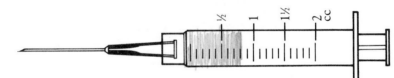

32. Doctor's Order: Bicillin 400,000 U. I.M. q4h.
     Available:

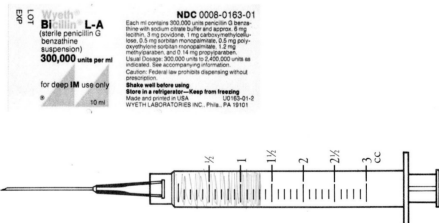

33.   Doctor's Order: Lanoxin 0.4 mg I.M. stat.
       Available:

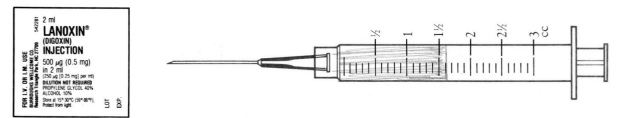

34.   Doctor's Order: Amikin 100 mg I.M. q8h.
       Available:

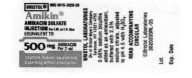

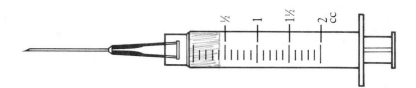

35.   Doctor's Order: Depo-Medrol 60 mg I.M. b.i.d. x 3 days.
       Available:

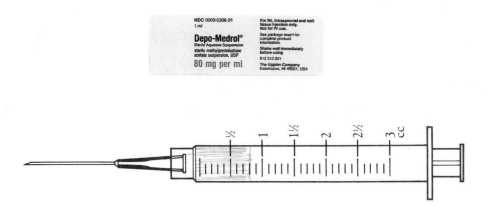

17 Powdered Drugs

Objectives

After reviewing this chapter the student will be able to do the following:

1. Prepare a solution from a powdered medication according to directions on the vial or other resources
2. Identify essential information to be placed on the vial of a medication after it is reconstituted
3. Determine the best concentration strength for medications ordered, when there are several directions for mixing
4. Calculate dosages from reconstituted medications

Some drugs are unstable in liquid form for long periods of time and therefore are packaged in powdered form. When medications come in powdered form, they must be diluted with a liquid referred to as a *diluent* or *solvent* before they can be administered to a client. Once a liquid is added to a powdered drug, the solution may only be used for 1 to 14 days depending on the type of the medication.

The process of adding a solvent or liquid to a medication that is in the form of a powder is called *reconstitution*. If you think about it, this process is something you do in everyday situations. For example, when you make Kool-Aid or ice tea (powdered form), what you're doing in essence is reconstituting. The Kool-Aid for example is the powder, and the water you add to it is considered the diluent, or solvent. Medications requiring reconstitution can be for oral or parenteral use. (Figure 17.1)

Basic Principles for Reconstitution

The initial step in preparing a powdered medication is to carefully read the information on the vial or the package insert since directions for reconstituting would be indicated.

1. The drug manufacturer provides directions for reconstitution. They provide information regarding the number of mL of diluent or solvent that should be added, as well as the type of solution that should be used to reconstitute the medication. The concentration (or strength) of the medication after it has been reconstituted according to the directions is also indicated on some medications. The directions for reconstituting must be read carefully and followed.

234

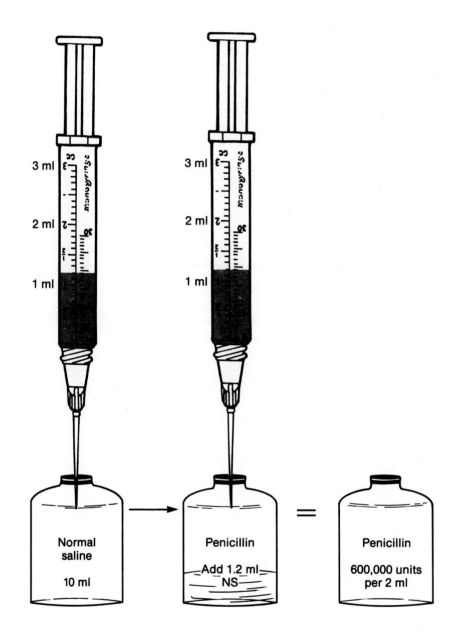

Figure 17.1 Showing Reconstitution (From Brown/Mulholland: *Drug calculations: process and problems for clinical practice*, ed 4, St Louis, 1992, Mosby.)

2. The diluents (solvents, liquids) commonly used for reconstitution are sterile water or sterile normal saline, prepared for injection. Other solutions that may be used are 5% dextrose and water and bacteriostatic water. Some powdered medications for oral use may be reconstituted with tap water. The manufacturer's directions will tell you which solution to use. If the medication requires a special solution for reconstitution, it is usually supplied by the drug manufacturer and packaged with the medication. When the solution for reconstitution is not indicated most solutions can be safely mixed with sterile water.

3. Once you have located the directions on the label for reconstitution of the medication you need to identify the following information:
   a) The type of diluent to use for reconstitution.
   b) The amount of diluent to add.
   c) The length of time the medication is good for once it is reconstituted.
   d) Directions for storing the medication after mixing.
   e) The strength or concentration of the medication after it's reconstituted.

4. If there are no directions for reconstitution on the label or on a package insert, or if any of the information (listed in # 3) is missing consult appropriate resources such as the PDR (Physician's Desk Reference), pharmacology text, hospital drug formulary, or the pharmacy.

5. After mixing the powdered drug, you must place the following information on the medication vial.
   a) Your initials.
   b) The date and time prepared and the expiration date and time. Note: If all of the solution is used that is mixed, this information is not necessary. Information regarding the date and time of preparation and date and time for expiration is crucial when all of the medication is not used. Powdered medications once reconstituted must be used within a certain time period. For example, Ampicillin once reconstituted must be used within an hour.

6. When reconstituting medications that are in multiple dose vials or have several directions as to how it can be prepared, information regarding the dosage strength or final concentration (what the medication's strength or concentration is after you mixed it) must be on the label, for example 500 mg/mL. This is important since others using the medication after you need to know this in determining the dosage to administer.

7. After adding the diluent to the powdered medication, the total reconstituted volume will be greater than the amount of diluent. The reconstituted material represents the diluent plus the powder. For example, you may add 1.5 mL of diluent to a powder and have a total volume of 2.5 mL.

Let's examine some labels of powdered medications by looking first at the reconstitution instructions for a single strength solution. Examine the label for Ampicillin 1 gram.

Practice Problems

NDC 0015-7404-20
6505-00-993-3518
Polycillin-N®
STERILE AMPICILLIN
SODIUM For I.M. or I.V. Use
EQUIVALENT TO

1 gram AMPICILLIN

CAUTION: Federal law prohibits
dispensing without prescription.

BRISTOL LABORATORIES
Div. of Bristol-Myers Company
Syracuse, New York 13201

For I.M. use, add 3.5 ml diluent (read accompanying circular). Resulting solution contains 250 mg ampicillin per ml. **Use solution within 1 hour.** This vial contains ampicillin sodium equivalent to 1 gram ampicillin.

Usual Dosage: Adults—250 to 500 mg I.M. q. 6h.

READ ACCOMPANYING CIRCULAR for detailed indications, I.M. or I.V. dosage and precautions.

740420DRL-14
© 1977 Bristol Laboratories

Lot
Exp. Date

Use the above label to answer the following questions.

1. How much diluent is added to the vial to prepare the drug for I.M. use?_____

2. What kind of solution can be used for the diluent?_____

3. What is the final concentration of the prepared solution for I.M. administration?

   _____

4. How long will reconstituted material retain its potency?_____

5. The doctor ordered 500 mg I.M. q6h. How many mL will you give? Shade the amount on the syringe provided.

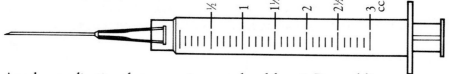

Another medication that comes in a powdered form is Prostaphlin.

NDC 0015-7979-20
6505-00-900-0901
Prostaphlin®
OXACILLIN SODIUM
FOR INJECTION
Buffered—For I.M. or I.V. Use
EQUIVALENT TO

500 mg OXACILLIN

BRISTOL LABORATORIES
A Bristol-Myers Company
Evansville, IN 47721

This vial contains oxacillin sodium monohydrate equivalent to 500 mg oxacillin, and 10 mg dibasic sodium phosphate. • Add 2.7 ml Sterile Water for Injection, U.S.P. • Each 1.5 ml contains 250 mg oxacillin. • **Usual Dosage:** Adults—250 mg to 500 mg intramuscularly every 4 to 6 hours. See circular for intravenous use.

READ ACCOMPANYING CIRCULAR
Discard solution after 3 days at room temperature or 7 days under refrigeration.
CAUTION: Federal law prohibits dispensing without prescription.
©Bristol Laboratories
7979200RL-9

LN 7979-99

Lot
Exp. Date

Using the above label answer the following questions.

6. How many mL of diluent are needed to prepare the solution?_____

7. What kind of solution is used as the diluent?_____

8. What is the dosage strength of the prepared solution?_____

9. How long does the medication retain its potency at room temperature?_____

10.   How long does the medication retain its potency if it is refrigerated?_____

11.   The doctor ordered 400 mg I.M. q6h. How many mL will you give? Shade the amount in on the syringe provided.

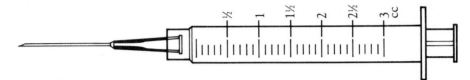

Using the label for Kefzol answer the following questions.

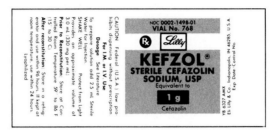

12.   How much diluent must be added to the vial to prepare an I.M. dose?

13.   What kind of solution is used as the diluent?

14.   What is the dosage strength of the prepared solution?

15.   How long will the reconstituted solution maintain its potency if refrigerated?

16.   The doctor ordered Kefzol 500 mg I.M. q6h. How many mL will you give? Shade the amount in on the syringe provided.

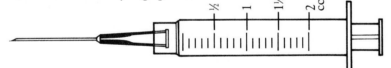

Refer to the label for Cefobid, and answer the following questions.

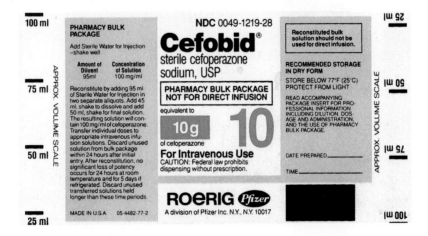

17. What route of administration is the medication indicated for? _____

18. How much diluent must be added to prepare the solution? _____

19. What type of solution is used for the diluent? _____

20. What is the dosage strength of the prepared solution? _____

21. How long does the medication maintain its potency at room temperature?

    _____

22. How long does the medication maintain its potency if refrigerated? _____

23. The doctor ordered 1 g I.V. q6h. How many mL will you give? Shade the amount in
    on the syringe provided.

Reconstituting Medications with More than One Direction for Mixing

Some medications come with a choice of how to reconstitute them therefore providing a choice of dosage strengths. In this case the nurse must choose the concentration or dosage strength appropriate for the dosage ordered. A common medication that has a choice of dosage strengths is Penicillin. When a medication comes with several directions for preparation or offers a choice of dosage strengths the following guidelines may be used.

Guidelines for Choosing Appropriate Concentrations

1. Consider the route of administration.

   a) I.M. – You are concerned that the amount does not exceed the maximum allowed I.M. However you don't want to choose a concentration that will result in irritation when injected into a muscle. When a choice of strengths can be made do not choose an amount that would exceed the amount allowed I.M. or that is very concentrated.

   b) I.V. – Keep in mind that this medication is usually further diluted because once reconstituted, the reconstituted material is then placed in additional fluid of 50 to 100 cc depending on the medication being administered. Example: Erythromycin requires the reconstituted solution be placed in 250 cc of fluid before administration to a client. In pediatrics a medication may be given in a smaller volume of fluid depending on the age, the child's size, and the medication.

2. Choose the concentration or dosage strength that comes closest to what the doctor has ordered. The dosage strengths are given for the amount of diluent used.

Example: If the Doctor orders 300,000 Units of a particular medication I.M. and the choices of strength are 200,000 U./mL, 250,000 U./mL, and 500,000 U./mL; the strength that is closest to 300,000 U./mL is 250,000U./mL. It allows you to administer a dosage within the range for I.M. and it is not the most concentrated.

3. The word respectively may be used sometimes on a medication label for directions on reconstitution. For example, reconstitute with 23 mL, 18 mL, 8 mL of diluent to provide concentrations of 200,000 U., 250,000 U., 500,000 U. per mL respectively. The word *respectively* means in the order given. In terms of the directions for reconstitution this means if you add 23 mL diluent, it will provide 200,000 U. per mL, 18 mL diluent will provide 250,000 U. per mL, etc. In other words the amounts of diluent correspond to the order in which the concentrations are written. Remember: When you are mixing a medication that is a multiple strength solution, the dosage strength that you prepare must be written on the vial.

Let's look at a sample label that shows a multiple strength solution.

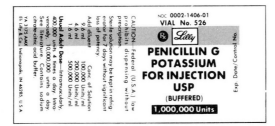

When looking at the Penicillin label, notice it states 1,000,000 Units. This means there is a total of 1,000,000 Units of Penicillin in the vial. The directions for reconstitution and the dosage strengths that can be obtained are listed on the left side of the label. If the dosage ordered for the client was for example 200,000 U. q6h, the most appropriate strength to mix would be 200,000 U. per mL. When reading the directions if you look across next to the dosage strength, you will notice that 4.6 mL of diluent must be added to obtain a concentration of solution 200,000 Units per mL. Since this is a multiple strength solution the dosage strength you choose must be indicated on the vial after you reconstitute it. Since the type of diluent is not indicated on the label, other resources such as those recommended previously in our discussion must be consulted.

Using the above label answer the following questions.

24. What concentration strength would be obtained if you added 1.6 mL of diluent? _____ .

25. How long can the potency of the medication be obtained if it is refreigerated? _____ .

Using the label below for Penicillin G Potassium answer the following questions.

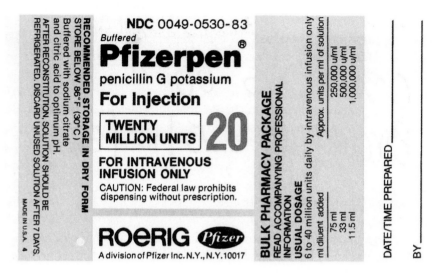

26.   What is the total number of Units of Penicillin contained in the vial? _____.

27.   If you add 33 mL of diluent to the vial, what dosage strength will you print on the label? _____.

28.   If the doctor ordered 2,000,000 U. IV, which dosage strength would be appropriate to use? _____.

29.   How long will the medication maintain its potency if refrigerated? _____.

Calculation of Medications When the Final Concentration (Dosage Strength) is Not Stated

Sometimes medications come with directions for only one way to reconstitute them, and the label does not indicate the final dosage strength after its mixed, such as "becomes 250 mg per cc." Example: A particular medication is available in 1 gram in powder. Directions tell you that adding 2.5 cc of sterile water yields 3 cc of solution. When you add 2.5 cc of sterile water the solution expands to 3 cc. The concentration is not changing; you will get 3 cc of solution, however it will be equal to 1 gram.

The problem is therefore calculated using 1 g = 3 cc.

Before we proceed to calculate dosages let's review the steps to use with medications that have been reconstituted.

1. The formula or the ratio-proportion method may be used to calculate the dosage. What's available becomes the dosage strength you obtain after mixing the medication according to the directions.

2. Powdered medications expand when a liquid is added (diluent + powder).

3. The volume the medication expands to must be considered when calculating the problem.

4. When the final concentration is not stated, the total weight of the medication in powdered form is used and the number of ccs produced is indicated after the solvent or liquid has been added.

5. As with all calculation problems check to make sure that the ordered and the available medication's are in the same system of measurement and the same units.

6. Don't forget to label your answer.

Calculation of Dosages to Administer

To calculate the dosage to administer after reconstituting a medication, the ratio-proportion or formula method may be used, as with other forms of medication. However the (H) have or what's available is the dosage strength you obtain when you mix the medication according to the directions. If using ratio-proportion therefore the known ratio is also the dosage strength obtained when you mix the medication. In the formula $\frac{D}{H} \times Q = X$, the Q is the volume of solution that contains the dosage strength.

To illustrate the above, let's calculate the dosage you would administer if you mixed the Penicillin and made a solution containing 1,000,000 Units per mL. The doctor has ordered 2,000,000 U. I.M.

Ratio-Proportion

$$1,000,000 \text{ U.} : 1 \text{ mL} = 2,000,000 \text{ U.} : x \text{ mL}$$
$$\text{(Known)} \qquad\qquad \text{(Unknown)}$$

$$\frac{1,000,000}{1,000,000} x = \frac{2,000,000}{1,000,000}$$

$$x = \frac{2,000,000}{1,000,000}$$

$$x = 2 \text{ mL}$$

Formula

$$\frac{2,000,000 \text{ U.}}{1,000,000 \text{ U.}} \times 1 \text{ mL} = x$$

$$\frac{2,000,000}{1,000,000} = x$$

$$x = 2 \text{ mL}$$

Sample Problem: Doctor orders 0.5 g of an antibiotic I.M. q4h. Available: 1 g of the drug in powdered form that reads add 1.7 mL of sterile water, each mL will then contain 500 mg.

Solution:

1. A conversion is necessary. Equivalent 1000 mg = 1 g. Convert what's ordered into the available units. This will eliminate a decimal point.

2. Think: What would a logical answer be?

Using Ratio-Proportion

$$500 \text{ mg} : 1 \text{ mL} = 500 \text{ mg} : x \text{ mL}$$
$$\text{(Known)} \qquad \text{(Unknown)}$$

$$\frac{500}{500}\,x = \frac{500}{500}$$

$$x = \frac{500}{500}$$

$$x = 1 \text{ mL}$$

Using Formula

$$\frac{500 \text{ mg}}{500 \text{ mg}} \times 1 \text{ mL} = x$$

$$\frac{500}{500} = x$$

$$x = 1 \text{ mL}$$

Points to Remember:

✔ If the medication is not used entirely after it is mixed, any medication remaining for use must have the following information clearly written on the label.

a) Initials of the preparer.
b) The dosage strength (final concentration) per volume of solution (cc, mL).
c) Date and time of preparation and the date and time of expiration.

Note: If there is no area on the vial for this information to be indicated the information can be written directly on the vial in an area that can be read clearly.

✔ Read all directions carefully; if there are no instructions on the vial the package insert, the pharmacy, or other reliable resources may be used to find the necessary information for reconstitution.

✔ When directions on the label are for I.M. and I.V. reconstitution, read the label carefully for the solution you are preparing.

✔ Read directions relating to storage and the time period for maintaining potency relating to how the medication is stored (room temperature, refrigeration).

Chapter Review

In the following problems, calculate the amount you will prepare to administer. Use the labels where provided to obtain the necessary information, and shade the dosage you calculated in on the syringe provided.

1.   Doctor's Order: Ampicillin 400 mg I.M. q4h.
      How many mL will you administer? Shade the amount in on the syringe provided.

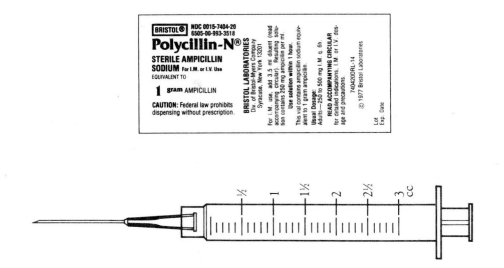

2.   Directions state the following for I.V. administration: Reconstitute with 10 mL of diluent. The vial contains Ampicillin 1 g.
      Doctor's Order: Ampicillin 1 g I.V. q6h.
      How many mL will you administer? Shade the amount in on the syringe provided.

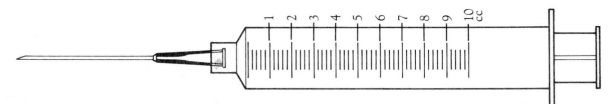

3. Doctor's Order: Oxacillin 300 mg I.M. q6h.
How many mL will you administer? Shade the amount in on the syringe provided.

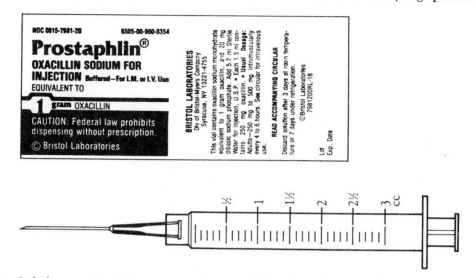

4. Label states: For I.V. use reconstitute with 30 mL sterile water for injection.
Each 30 mL of reconstituted solution will contain 3 g Mezlocillin.
Doctor's Order: Mezlocillin 1.5 g I.V. q6h.
How many mL will you administer?

5. Doctor's Order: Ticar 1 g I.M. q6h.
a) How many mL of diluent must be added?
b) What type of diluent is used?
c) What is the dosage strength of the reconstituted solution?
d) How many mL will you administer? Shade the amount in on the syringe provided.

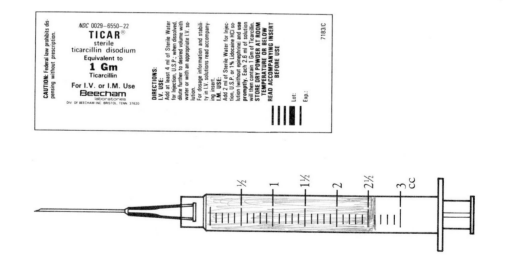

6. Doctor's Order: 600,000 U. I.V. q4h.
    a) Which dosage strength would be best to choose?
    b) How many mL of diluent would be needed to make the dosage strength?
    c) How many mL will you administer? Shade the amount in on the syringe provided.

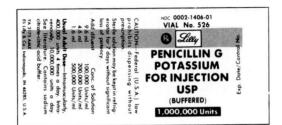

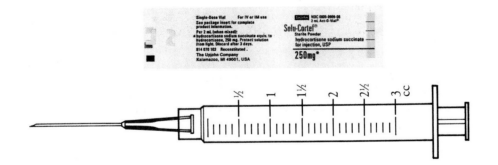

7. Doctor's Order: Solu-Cortef 200 mg I.V. q6h x 1 week.
    a) How many mg per mL is the reconstituted material?
    b) How many mL will you administer? Shade the amount in on the syringe provided.

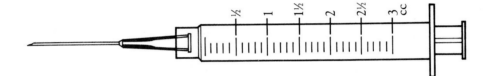

8. Doctor's Order: Carbenicillin 1 g I.M. q6h.
    a) What type of diluent is used?
    b) If you reconstitute with 9.5 mL of diluent, how many mL will you administer? Shade the amount in on the syringe provided.

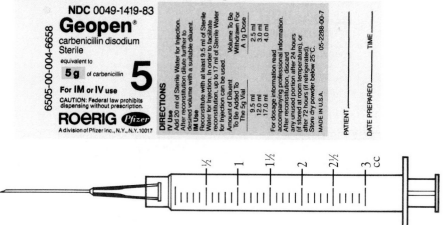

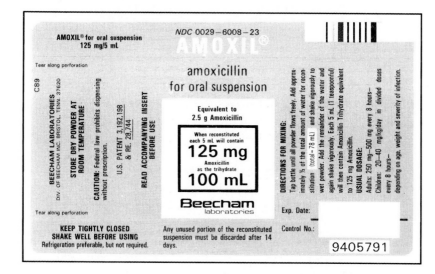

9. Doctor's Order: Amoxicillin 500 mg p.o. q6h.
    a) How many mL of diluent must be added?
    b) What is the dosage strength after reconstitution?
    c) How many mL are needed to administer the required dosage?

10.   Doctor's Order: Staphcillin 1g I.M.
       a) How much diluent must be added for I.M.?
       b) How many mL will you administer? Shade the amount in on the syringe provided.

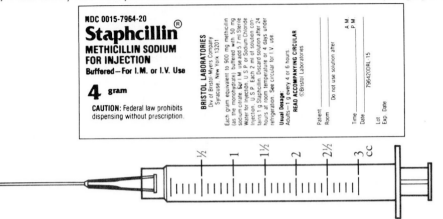

Directions: Use the labels where provided to answer the questions for each situation.

11.   Doctor's Order: Ancef 500 mg I.M. q8h.

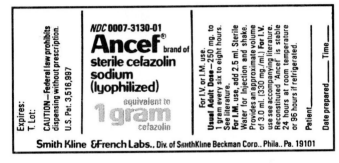

       a) How many mL of diluent should be used to reconstitute?
       b) What will be the dosage strength of the reconstituted Ancef?
       c) How many mL will you administer? Shade the amount in on the syringe provided.

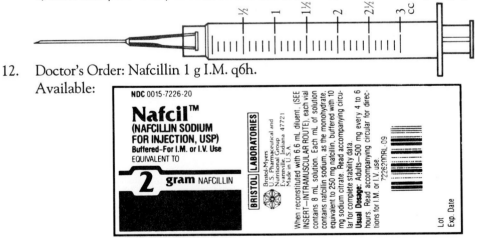

12.   Doctor's Order: Nafcillin 1 g I.M. q6h.
       Available:

       a) What is the dosage strength of the reconstituted Nafcillin?
       b) How many mL will you administer? Shade the amount in on the syringe provided.

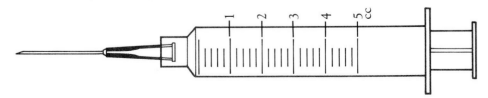

13. Doctor's Order: Cefotaxime 750 mg I.M. q8h
    Available: Cefotaxime with the following package insert.

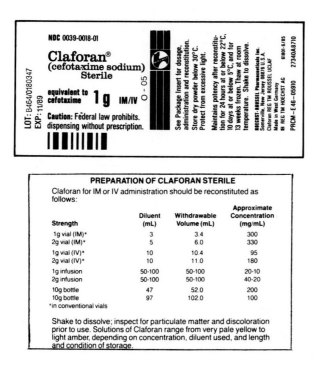

Strength	Diluent (mL)	Withdrawable Volume (mL)	Approximate Concentration (mg/mL)
1g vial (IM)*	3	3.4	300
2g vial (IM)*	5	6.0	330
1g vial (IV)*	10	10.4	95
2g vial (IV)*	10	11.0	180
1g infusion	50-100	50-100	20-10
2g infusion	50-100	50-100	40-20
10g bottle	47	52.0	200
10g bottle	97	102.0	100

PREPARATION OF CLAFORAN STERILE

Claforan for IM or IV administration should be reconstituted as follows:

*in conventional vials

Shake to dissolve; inspect for particulate matter and discoloration prior to use. Solutions of Claforan range from very pale yellow to light amber, depending on concentration, diluent used, and length and condition of storage.

a) What is the total grams of Cefotaxime in the vial?
b) According to the package insert, what volume of diluent is used for I.M. reconstitution?
c) What is the dosage strength of the reconstituted Cefotaxime?
d) How many mL will you administer to give 750 mg I.M.? Shade the amount in on the syringe provided.

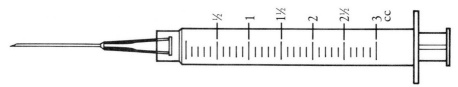

14.   Doctor's Order: Streptomycin 0.5 g I.M. q6h.

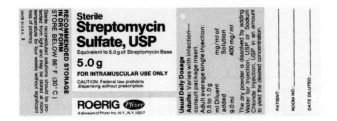

a) What is the total grams of Streptomycin in the vial?
b) What is the volume of diluent used for reconstitution?
c) What is the dosage strength of the reconstituted Streptomycin?
d) How many mL will you administer? Shade the amount in on the syringe provided.

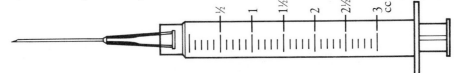

15.   Doctor's Order: Chloromycetin 0.5 g I.V. q6h

N 0071-4057-03
Chloromycetin®
Sodium Succinate
(Sterile Chloramphenicol
Sodium Succinate, USP)

Each vial delivers the equivalent of
1 GRAM chloramphenicol
100 mg per mL when reconstituted

PARKE-DAVIS
Div of Warner-Lambert Co
Morris Plains, NJ 07950 USA

a) What is the volume of diluent used for reconstitution?
b) What is the dosage strength of the reconstituted Chloromycetin?
c) How many mL will you administer? Shade the amount in on the syringe provided.

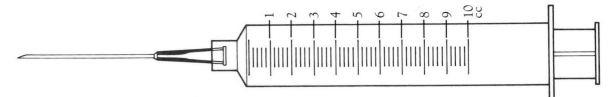

16.   Doctor's Order: Penicillin G 400,000 U. I.M. q4h.
       Available: Penicillin G 5,000,000 Units. Directions state add 8 mL diluent to provide
       500,000 U/mL.
       How many mL will you administer? Shade the amount in on the syringe provided.

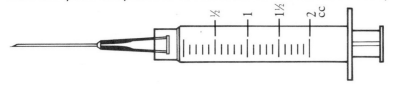

17.   Doctor's Order: Penicillin G Potassium 600,000 U. I.M. o.d.

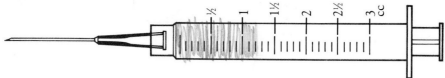

a) What would be the best strength to reconstitute?
b) How many mL of diluent would be used?
c) How many mL of the medication will you give? Shade the amount in on the syringe
   provided.

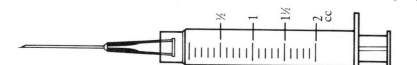

18.   Doctor's Order: Ceftazidine 250 mg I.M. q12h.
       Available: Ceftazidime 600 mg. Directions for I.M. use state add 1.5 mL of an
       approved diluent to provide 300 mg/mL.
       How many mL will you administer? Shade the amount in on the syringe provided.

19.   Doctor's Order: Ticar 0.5 g I.M. q6h.

a) How many mL of diluent would be used to reconstitute?
b) What is the dosage strength of the reconstituted Ticar?
c) How many mL will you administer? Shade the amount in on the syringe provided.

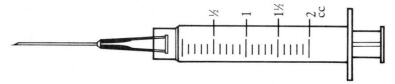

20.   Doctor's Order: Staphcillin 1 g I.M. q6h.

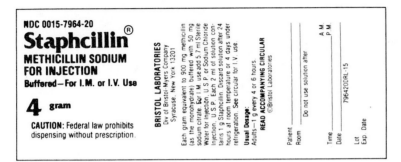

NDC 0015-7964-20

Staphcillin®
METHICILLIN SODIUM
FOR INJECTION
Buffered—For I.M. or I.V. Use

4 gram

CAUTION: Federal law prohibits
dispensing without prescription.

BRISTOL LABORATORIES
Div of Bristol-Myers Company
Syracuse, New York 13201

Each gram equivalent to 900 mg methicillin
(as the monohydrate) buffered with 50 mg
sodium citrate. For I.M. use add 5.7 ml Sterile
Water for Injection, U.S.P. or Sodium Chloride
Injection, U.S.P. Each 2 ml of solution contains 1 g Staphcillin. Discard solution after 24
hours at room temperature or 4 days under
refrigeration. See circular for I.V. use.

Usual Dosage:
Adults—1 g every 4 or 6 hours.
READ ACCOMPANYING CIRCULAR
©Bristol Laboratories

Patient
Room

Do not use solution after

Time   A.M. P.M.
Date

Lot
Exp. Date

7964200RL-15

a) How many mL of diluent would be used to reconstitute ?
b) What is the dosage strength of the reconstituted Staphcillin?
c) How many mL will you administer? Shade the amount in on the syringe provided.

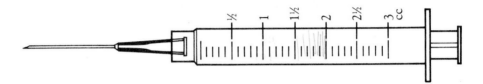

18 Insulin

Objectives

After reviewing this chapter the student will be able to do the following:

1. Identify important information on insulin labels
2. Read calibrations on U-100 insulin syringes
3. Measure insulin in single dosages
4. Measure combined insulin dosages
5. Convert insulin Units to milliliters

Insulin is used in the treatment of diabetes mellitus. Insulin is a hormone secreted by the Islets of Langerhan in the pancreas. It is a necessary hormone for glucose use by the body. Individuals who do not produce adequate insulin experience an increase in their blood sugar (glucose) level. These individuals may require the administration of insulin. Accuracy in insulin administration is extremely important since inaccurate dosages can lead to serious or life-threatening effects. Insulin dosages are measured in Units (U.) and administered with syringes that correspond to insulin U-100. U-100 insulin means 100 Units per/mL.

Types of Insulin

There are different types of insulin available today. Choice of dosage and which insulin preparation to use is dependent on the needs of the client. Insulin is obtained from human and animal sources. The origin of insulin is indicated on the label. Human insulin is identified as semi-synthetic, while the animal sources are identified by use of pork or beef on the label. Due to the variations, the doctor should specify the origin of insulin when writing insulin orders. Be sure to read the label carefully to administer insulin of the correct origin. The other information that can be found on the label is the type of insulin. This is indicated by a letter that follows the trade name (Figures 18.1 and 18.2).

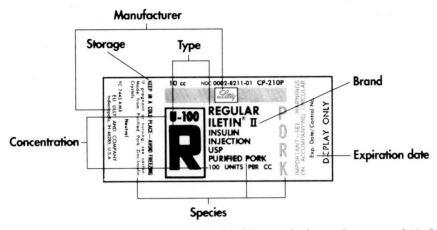

Figure 18.1 Regular insulin (From Dison: *Simplified drugs and solutions for nurses*, ed 10, St Louis, 1992, Mosby.)

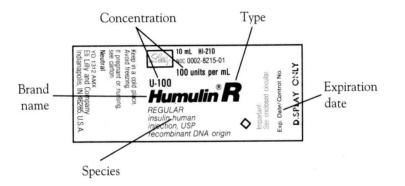

Figure 18.2 Humulin (From Dison: *Simplified drugs and solutions for nurses*, ed 10, St Louis, 1992, Mosby.)

The letter that follows the trade name on insulin labels for example Humulin (R), tells you the type and action time. Nurses must be familiar with onset of action, peak, and duration, which vary depending on the type of insulin. Insulins are classified as rapid acting (Regular insulin), intermediate acting (NPH), and long acting (PZI). The expiration date is also indicated on the label and is important to check, as well as the concentration 100 U/mL. On insulins manufactured under the trade name of Humulin an international symbol is also indicated on the label, so insulins can be identified worldwide.

Example: (◇) = Regular, (▢) = NPH. See insulin labels below.

Notice that both labels shown are Humulin (trade name), but they are followed by the letters N and R. N = NPH (intermediate acting), R = Regular (rapid acting). Note the international symbols on the label as well.

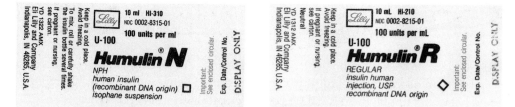

Practice Problems

Using the labels below, identify the type of insulin and its origin. Note the left side of the labels indicates whether made from beef or pork.

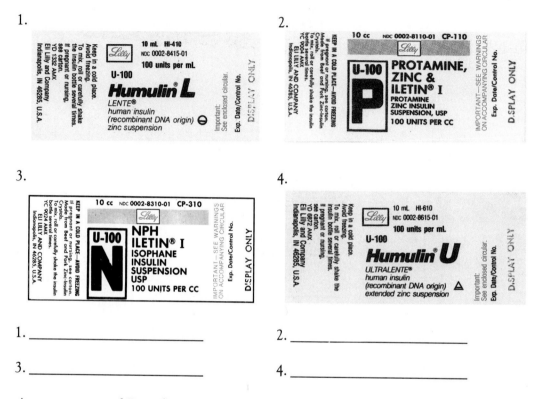

1.

2.

3.

4.

1. _____

2. _____

3. _____

4. _____

Appearance of Insulin

Regular insulin is clear in appearance and is the only insulin that may be given I.V. Other insulin is cloudy in appearance and must be rotated between the hands to mix.

U-100 Syringe

The U-100 syringe was discussed in Chapter 16. As a review insulin is administered subcutaneously, usually with a syringe marked U-100. There are different types of U-100 syringes: The different types are as follows:

1. Lo-Dose Syringe – has a capacity of 50 Units (0.5 cc). Each calibration on the syringe measures 1 Unit.

2. 1 cc (100 U.) capacity – There are two types of 1 cc syringe in current use.

   a) Single scale that is calibrated in 2 U. increments. Any dose measured on this syringe that is an odd number of units would be measured between the even calibrations. This would not be the desired syringe for clients with vision problems.

   b) Double scale has odd number of units on the left and even units on the right. To avoid confusion the scale on the left should be used for odd units (for example 13 U.) and the scale on the right for even number of units (for example 26 U.). When measuring even number of units, each calibration then is measured as two units.

As a review of what the syringes look like refer to Figure 18.3, which shows the three types of insulin syringes discussed.

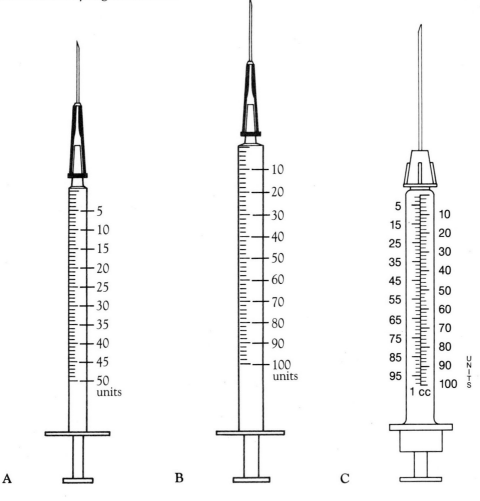

Figure 18.3 A, Lo-Dose Insulin Syringe (From Dison: *Simplified drugs and solutions for nurses,* ed 10, St Louis, 1992, Mosby.) **B,** Single Scale Syringe (From Dison: *Simplified Drugs and Solutions for Nurses,* ed 10, 1992, Mosby.) **C,** Double-Scale Insulin Syringe (From Brown/Mulholland: *Drug calculations process and problems for clinical practice,* ed 4, 1992, Mosby.)

Let's look at some insulin dosages measured in the syringes to help you visualize the amounts in a syringe.

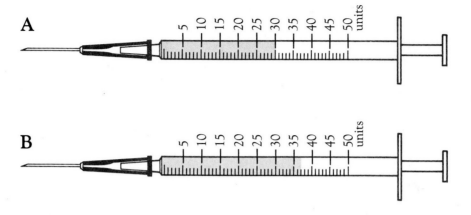

Syringe A shows 30 Units and syringe B shows 37 Units on a Lo-Dose syringe.

Indicate the dosages on the Lo-Dose syringes indicated by the arrows.

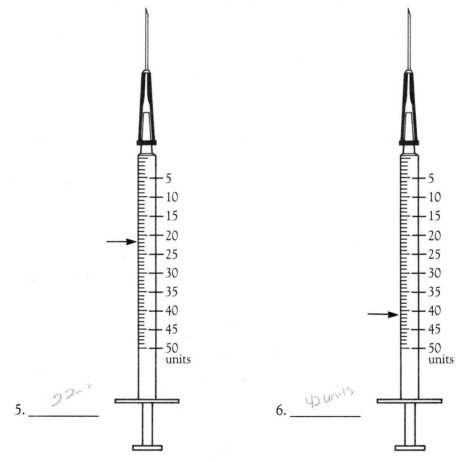

5. _____

6. _____

Using the syringes below measure the following doses. Use an arrow to indicate the dosages. Check your answers at the end of the book.

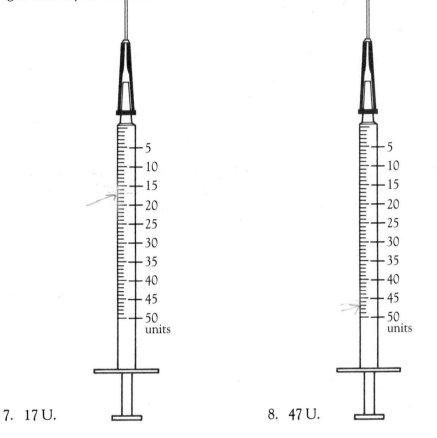

7. 17 U.   8. 47 U.

Now let's look at what dosages would look like on a single scale 1 cc capacity syringe.

The syringes below show 25 U. in syringe **A** and 55 U. in syringe **B**. Notice the dosages are drawn up in between the even calibrations.

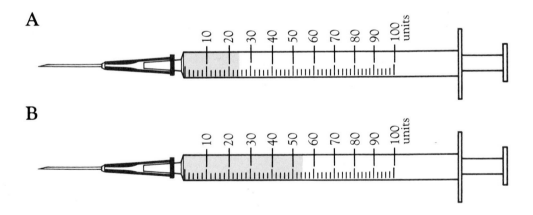

Now let's look at the dosage indicated on a double scale insulin syringe. Below syringe C shows 37 U.; notice the scale on the left is used. Syringe D shows 54 U.; notice the scale on the right is used.

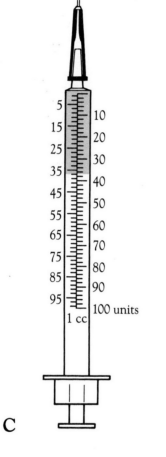

C

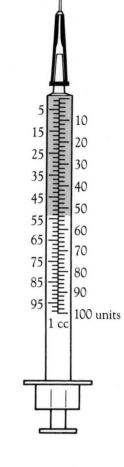

D

Read the following dosages indicated by the arrows on the U-100 (1 cc) syringe.

9._____

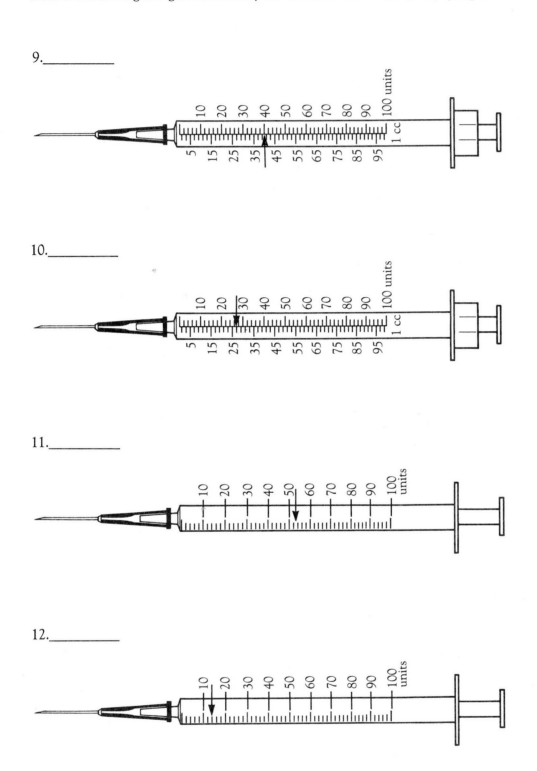

10._____

11._____

12._____

Draw an arrow on each U-100 syringe below to indicate the following dosages.
13. 88 U.   14. 44 U.   15. 30 U.

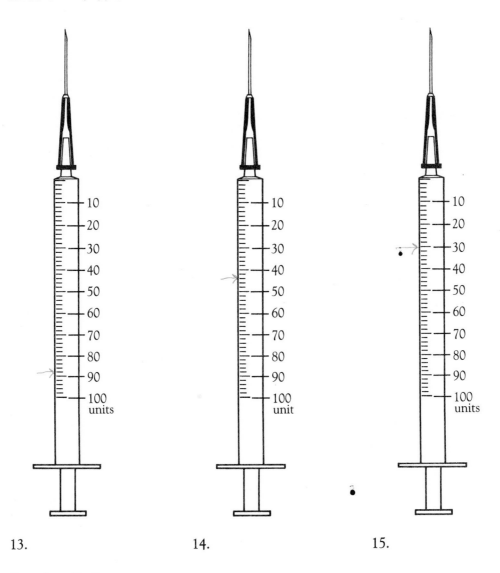

13.   14.   15.

Insulin Orders

Like any medication order that is written, insulin orders must be written clearly and contain certain information to prevent errors in administration. An error in administration can cause harmful effects to a client. Insulin orders should contain the following information:

a) The name of the insulin, including the origin. Example: Humulin Regular; Humulin NPH.

b) The number of Units to be administered. Example: 20 U., Humulin Regular.

c) The route (subcutaneous). Insulin is usually administered s.c., however Regular insulin can be administered I.V. as well.

d) The time it should be given. Example 1/2 hour before meals.

e) The strength of the insulin to be administered should also be indicated. Example U-100.

Example of Insulin Order: Regular Humulin insulin U-100 20 U. s.c. before breakfast.

Coverage Orders (sometimes referred to as sliding scale) – Sometimes in addition to standing insulin orders a client may have additional insulin ordered to "cover" their increased blood sugar levels. Regular insulin is used because of its immediate action and short duration. A coverage order is written specifying the dose of insulin according to the blood sugar and the frequency. The amount of insulin and the blood sugar level should be specific. A sample coverage order (sliding scale) for example would be:

Humulin Regular U-100 according to finger stick q8h.

0–180 no coverage

181–240 2 U. s.c.

241–300 4 U. s.c.

301–400 6 U. s.c.

Greater than 401, 8 U. s.c., notify M.D. Repeat finger stick in 2 hours.

Note: The above sliding scale is an example used in one patient . It is not a standard scale. Sliding scales are individualized for clients.

Preparing a Single Dose of Insulin in an Insulin Syringe

The measurement of insulin in an insulin syringe requires no calculation or conversion.

Example 1:   To measure 40 Units, withdraw U-100 insulin to the 40 mark on the U-100 syringe. A Lo-Dose syringe can also be used to draw up this dose as shown below.

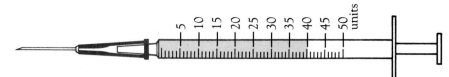

Example 2:   Doctor's Order: Humulin NPH 70 U. s.c. o.d.
Available: Humulin NPH labeled 100 U.

There is no calculation or conversion required here, draw up the required amount using a U-100 (1 cc) syringe.

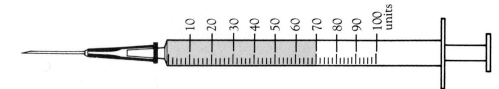

Measuring Two Types of Insulin in the Same Syringe

Sometimes individuals may require two different types of insulin for control of their blood sugar.

Example NPH and Regular. To decrease the number of injections it is common to mix two insulins in a single syringe. To mix insulin in one syringe remember:

Regular Insulin is Always Drawn Up in the Insulin Syringe First!

Drawing Regular insulin up first prevents contamination of the Regular insulin with other insulin.

To prepare insulin in one syringe (mixing insulin) the following steps are done:

1. Inject air equal to the amount being withdrawn into the vial of cloudy insulin first. When injecting the air the tip of the needle should not touch the solution.

2. Remove the needle from the cloudy insulin.

3. Using the same syringe, inject the amount of air into the Regular insulin (clear) equal to the amount to be withdrawn, invert or turn the bottle up in the air and draw up the desired amount.

4. Remove the syringe from the Regular insulin, and check for air bubbles. If air bubbles are present gently tap the syringe to remove them.

5. Next go back to the cloudy insulin, and withdraw the desired dosage.

6. The total number of Units in the syringe will be the addition of the two insulin orders.

See Figure 18.4, illustrating the technique of mixing two insulins in the same syringe.

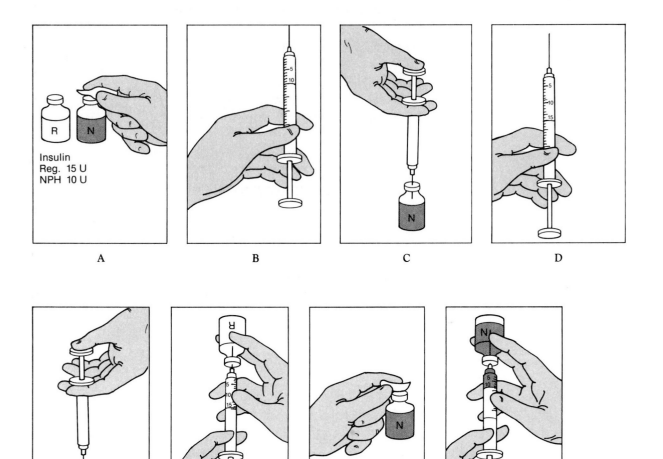

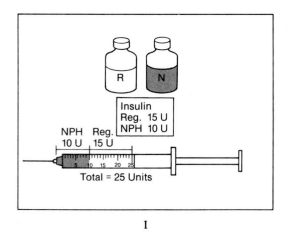

Figure 18.4 Preparing two drugs in one syringe (From Clayton/Stock: *Basic pharmacology for nurses*, ed 10, St Louis, 1993, Mosby.)

Example: The order is to administer 18 U. of Regular and 22 U. of NPH.

The total amount of insulin is 40 U. (18 U. + 22 U. = 40 U.)

To administer this dose a Lo-Dose syringe can be used, as well as the U-100 (1 cc) syringe. However since the dose is 40 U. the Lo-Dose would be more desirable. (See syringe below illustrating this dosage in a syringe.)

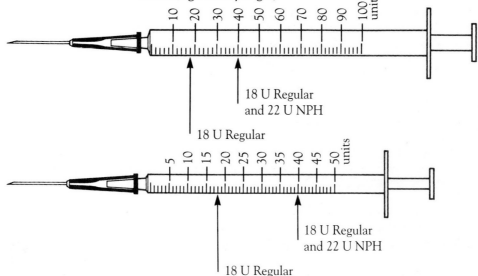

18 U Regular
and 22 U NPH

18 U Regular

18 U Regular
and 22 U NPH

18 U Regular

When mixing insulins it is important to follow the steps outlined to prevent the contamination of Regular insulin with other insulins. To help you remember the steps recall: The last one injected into is drawn up first or run fast first (Regular), then slow down (NPH).

Measuring Insulin When an Insulin Syringe is Not Available

Dosages of insulin must be exact and therefore should always be measured and administered with an insulin syringe. Only in an emergency, or when an insulin syringe is not available should any other type of syringe be used. A Tuberculin syringe or 1 mL size syringe can be used to measure insulin, because 100 Units of insulin = 1 mL.

Example: Doctor's Order: Humulin NPH 40 U. s.c. od
Available: Humulin NPH 100 U. No insulin syringes are available. You have a Tuberculin syringe.

1. Note: no conversion is necessary in terms of Units.

2. Think: What answer would be logical based upon the syringe you have.

3. Set up in a proportion or formula and solve.

Solution Using Ratio Proportion:

100 U. : 1 mL = 40 U. : x mL

$$\frac{100}{100}\,x = \frac{40}{100}$$

$$x = \frac{40}{100} = 0.4 \text{ mL}$$

Solution Using Formula:

$$\frac{40 \text{ U.}}{100 \text{ U.}} \times 1 \text{ mL} = x$$

$$x = \frac{40}{100} = 0.4 \text{ mL}$$

Tuberculin syringe illustrating this amount:

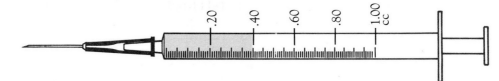

Note: A U-40 strength of insulin is still available, although it is not often used. To administer this insulin you need a syringe calibrated U-40 to measure the dosage.

Points to Remember:

✔ U-100 means 100 U/mL.

✔ To ensure accuracy insulin should be given only with an insulin syringe. When no insulin syringe is available a Tuberculin syringe may be used.

✔ Insulin dosages must be exact.

✔ Lo-Dose syringes are desirable for small doses up to 50 Units.

✔ A U-100 (1 cc capacity) syringe is desirable when the dose exceeds 50 Units.

✔ When mixing insulin, Regular insulin is always drawn up first.

✔ The total volume when mixing insulins is the addition of the two insulin amounts.

Chapter Review

Using the syringes below indicate the dose you would prepare. Indicate the dosage on the syringe with an arrow.

1. Doctor's Order: Regular Humulin insulin 35 U. s.c. o.d.
   Available: Regular Humulin U-100.

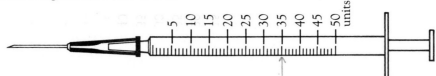

2. Doctor's Order: Humulin NPH 56 U. s.c. o.d.
   Available: Humulin NPH U-100.

3. Doctor's Order: Humulin Regular 18 U. s.c. and NPH 40 U. s.c. o.d.
   Available: Humlin Regular U-100, Humulin NPH U-100.

4. Doctor's Order: Regular pork insulin 9 U. s.c. o.d.
   Available: Regular pork insulin labeled U-100.

Directions: Indicate the number of units measured in the following syringes.

5. Units Measured_____

6. Units Measured_____

7. Units Measured_____

8. Units Measured_____

9. Units Measured_____

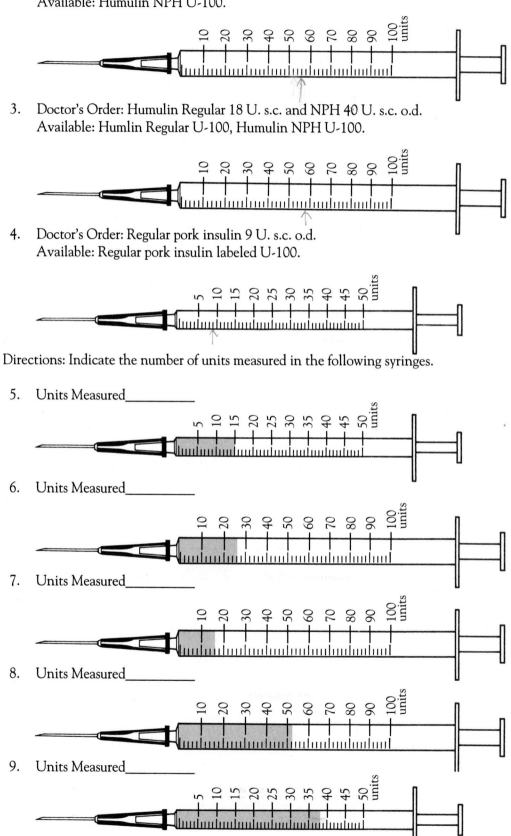

10.   Units Measured_____

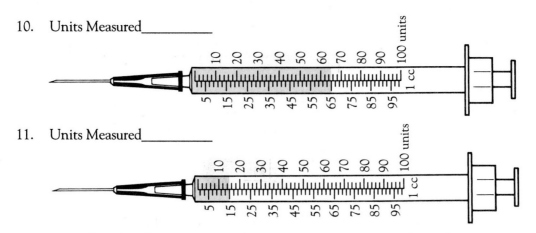

11.   Units Measured_____

Directions: Calculate the dosage of insulin where necessary, and shade the dose in on the syringe provided. Insulin labeled 100 U/mL is available for all problems regardless of the type of insulin.

12. Doctor's Order: Humulin Regular 10 U. s.c. a.c. 7:30 AM

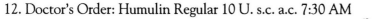

13. Doctor's Order: Humulin Regular 16 U. s.c. and 24 U. s.c. Humulin NPH a.c. 7:30 AM

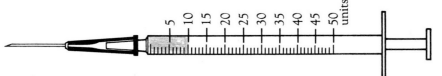

14. Doctor's Order: Lente insulin 75 U. s.c. a.c. 7:30 AM

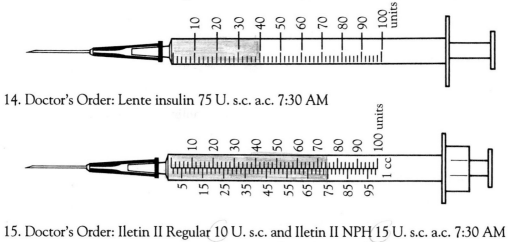

15. Doctor's Order: Iletin II Regular 10 U. s.c. and Iletin II NPH 15 U. s.c. a.c. 7:30 AM

16. Doctor's Order: Humulin Regular 5 U. s.c. and Humulin NPH 25 U. s.c. a.c. 7:30 AM

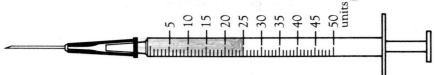

17. Doctor's Order: Humulin Lente 40 U. s.c. and Humulin Regular 10 U. s.c. at 7:30 AM

18. Doctor's Order: Humulin NPH 48 U. s.c. and Humulin Regular 30 U. s.c. a.c. 7:30 AM

19. Doctor's Order: Humulin Regular 16 U. s.c. and Humulin Lente 12 U. s.c. at 7:30 AM

20. Doctor's Order: Humulin Regular 17 U. 5 PM

21. Doctor's Order: Iletin II NPH 15 U. s.c. 10 PM

22. Doctor's Order: Humulin Regular 26 U. s.c. and Humulin NPH 48 U. s.c. q.d.

23. Doctor's Order: Iletin Regular II 27 U. s.c. at 5 PM

24. Doctor's Order: Iletin Regular I 21 U. s.c. and Iletin II NPH 35 U. s.c. od.

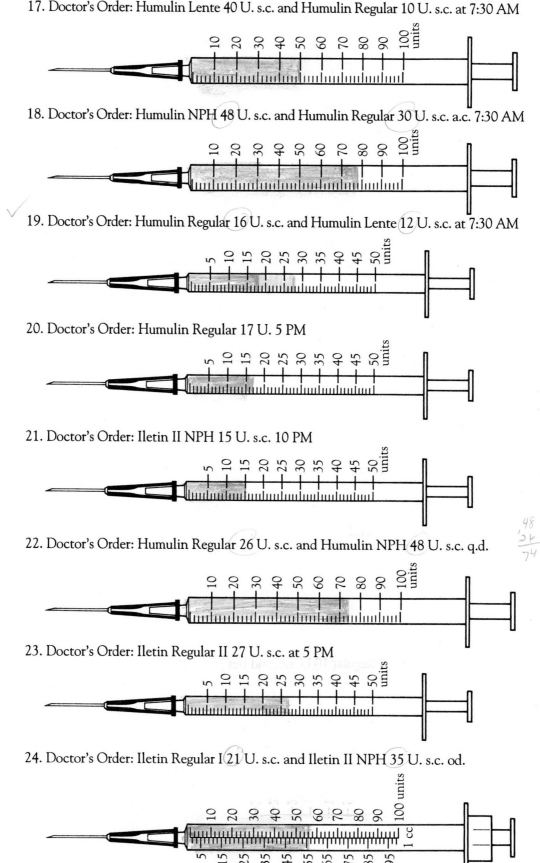

25. Doctor's Order: Novolin Regular 5 U. s.c. and Novolin Lente 35 U. s.c. 7:30 AM

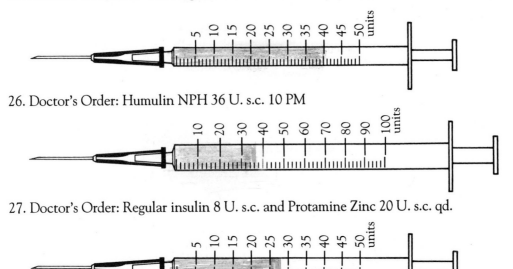

26. Doctor's Order: Humulin NPH 36 U. s.c. 10 PM

27. Doctor's Order: Regular insulin 8 U. s.c. and Protamine Zinc 20 U. s.c. qd.

28. A client is on a sliding scale for insulin dosages. The doctor ordered Humulin Regular insulin q6h as follows.

finger stick   0–180   no coverage
                 181–240   2 U. s.c.
                 241–300   4 U. s.c.
                 301–400   6 U. s.c.
                 > 400   8 U. s.c. and repeat finger stick in 2 hours.

At 11:30 AM the client's finger stick is 364. Shade the syringe in to indicate the dosage that should be given.

29. Doctor's Order: Humulin NPH 66 U. s.c. 10 PM

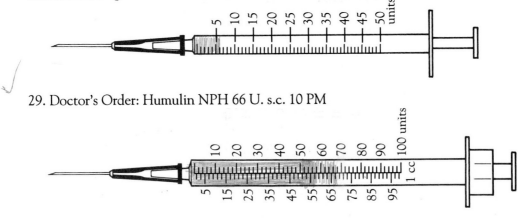

30. Doctor's Order: UltraLente insulin 32 U. s.c. q AM

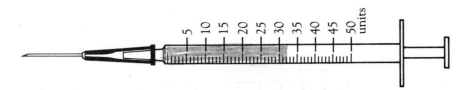

Calculate the amount of insulin to administer in a Tuberculin syringe using U-100 insulin (100 U. per mL).

Shade the dose in on the Tuberculin syringe.

DON'T ROUND OFF

31. Doctor's Order: Humulin NPH 38 U. s.c. 10 PM

32. Doctor's Order: Humulin Regular 12 U. s.c. at 5 PM

33. Doctor's Order: Lente insulin 60 U. s.c. q.d.

34. Doctor's Order: NPH 64 U. s.c. at 7:30 AM

Shade the dose in on the insulin syringe.

35. Doctor's Order: Lente II insulin 35 U. s.c. q.d.

36. Doctor's Order: Humulin Regular 9 U. s.c. 5 PM

37. Doctor's Order: Humulin NPH 24 U. s.c. 10 PM

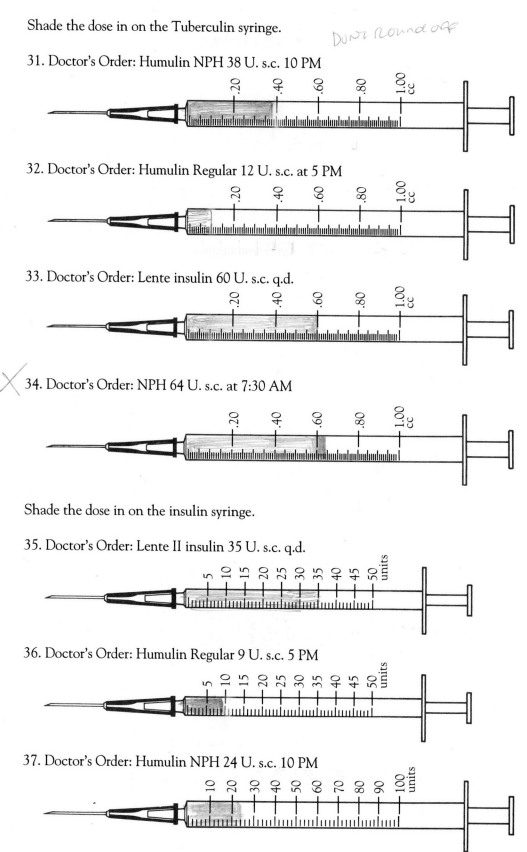

19 Pediatric Dosage Calculation

Objectives

After reviewing this chapter the student will be able to do the following:

1. Convert body weight from 1b to kg
2. Convert body weight from kg to lb
3. Calculate dosages based on mg per kg
4. Determine whether a dosage is safe
5. Determine BSAs (body surface area) using the west Nomogram
6. Calculate dosages using BSA

Introduction

The safe administration of medications to infants and children requires knowledge of the methods used in calculating dosages. Exact, accurate doses are especially important since even small discrepancies can be dangerous because of the size of pediatric clients.

The two methods currently being used to calculate pediatric dosages are as follows:

⚡ 1) According to the weight of the child (mg per kg).

⚡ 2) According to the child's body surface area (BSA).

Principles Relating to Basic Calculations

Before beginning calculation of medications for the child or infant, there are some guidelines that are helpful to know.

1. Calculation of pediatric dosages, like adult dosages, involves the use of ratio-proportion or the formula $\dfrac{D}{H} \times Q = X$ to determine the amount of medication to administer.

2. Pediatric dosages are much smaller than those for an adult. Micrograms are used a great deal, as well as minims. The Tuberculin syringe (1 cc capacity) is used for the administration of very small dosages.

3. I.M. doses are usually not more than 1 cc; however, this can vary with the size of the child.

4. Dosages that are less than 1 cc may be measured in minims, tenths of a cc, or with a Tuberculin syringe in hundredths of a mL. However, as with adults the preference is to express an answer using metric measures such as mL or cc instead of minims.

5. Medications in pediatrics generally are not rounded off to the nearest tenth but may be administered with a Tuberculin syringe to ensure accuracy. Again answers may be changed to minims, but the preference is for metric measures since they are more accurate.

6. All answers must be labeled.

Calculation of Dosages Based on Body Weight

Let's begin our discussion with calculation of dosages according to mg/kg of body weight. Before calculating dosages according to mg/kg of body weight it is essential that you be able to convert a child's weight. Most drug references state dosages in terms of kg. Therefore the most common conversion you will encounter will involve the conversion of lb to kg. To do this remember the conversion 1 kg = 2.2 lb.

Remember the following when converting weights:

1. 2.2 lb = 1 kg.

2. To convert from lb to kg divide the number of lb by 2.2. Carry the division out to the hundredth place, and round off the answer to the nearest tenth. Calculations based on body weight can be rounded off to the nearest tenth.

3. To convert from kg to lb multiply by 2.2, and express the answer to the nearest tenth.

Note: Students should know that although pounds are an apothecary measure, a decimal may be seen when expressing weight, for example 65.8 lb.

Let's do some sample problems with the conversion of weights.

Example 1:   Convert 30 lb to kg.

2.2 lb = 1 kg.

2.2 lb : 1 kg = 30 lb : x kg.

$$\frac{2.2}{2.2} x = \frac{30}{2.2}$$

$30 \div 2.2 = 13.63$ (rounded to the nearest tenth = 13.6 kg.)

Practice Problems

Convert the following weights in lb to kg.

1. 20 lb   =   _9.1_ kg

2. 64 lb   =   _29.1_ kg

3. 22 lb   =   _10_ kg

4. 52 lb   =   _23.6_ kg

5. 71 lb   =   _32.3_ kg

Converting kg to lb

Example 1:   Convert 24 kg to lb.

2.2 lb = 1 kg

2.2 lb : 1 kg = x lb : 24 kg

x = 24 × 2.2

x = 52.8 lb

Practice Problems

Convert the following weights in kg to lb.

6.   20 kg   =   _44_ lb

7.   46 kg   =   _101.2_ lb

8.   22 kg   =   _48.4_ lb

9.   15 kg   =   _33_ lb

10. 34 kg   =   _74.8_ lb

Once you have determined the child's weight in kg you are ready to calculate the medication dose. The calculation of dosage involves three steps:

1) Calculation of the daily dose.

2) Division of the daily dose by the number of doses to be administered.

3) Use of either ratio-proportion or the formula method to calculate the number of tablets or capsules or the volume to give to administer the ordered dose.

Example 1:   Refer to label.

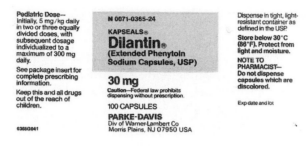

A child weighs 18 kg and requires Dilantin. The recommended dose is 5 mg/kg/daily in two or three equally divided doses. Now that we have the dosage information and the child's weight we can calculate the dosage for this child. Note: The child's weight is in kg (5 mg/kg). No conversion of weight is required.

Step 1:   Start by calculating the safe total daily dose for this child.

$$5 \text{ mg} \times 18 \text{ kg} = 90 \text{ mg/day.}$$

The safe dose for this child (total) = 90 mg/day.

Step 2:   Now determine the amount of each dose.

The dose is to be given in three equally divided doses. Therefore:

$$\frac{90 \text{ mg}}{3} = 30 \text{ mg per dose}$$

After calculating the safe dose for a child you can assess whether what the doctor ordered is a safe dose.

The doctor ordered 20 mg q8h. Is this a safe dose?

$$q8h = 24 \div 8 = 3 \text{ doses.}$$

$30 \times 3 = 90$ mg. Compare the ordered daily dose with the safe daily dose you calculated in Step 1. A daily dose of 90 mg is safe.

Step 3:   Use the ratio-proportion or formula method to determine the number of capsules to give.

Dilantin is supplied in 30 mg capsules (refer to label). The ordered dose is 30 mg per dose.

$$30 \text{ mg} : 1 \text{ capsule} = 30 \text{ mg} : x \text{ capsules}$$

$$30x = 30$$

$$x = 1 \text{ capsule} \quad \text{or} \quad \frac{30 \text{ mg}}{30 \text{ mg}} = 1 \text{ capsule}$$

You would give 1 capsule q8h to administer the ordered dose.

Example 2:   Doctor orders Gentamicin 50 mg IVPB q8h for a child weighing 40 lb. The pediatric drug handbook states the recommended dose for a child is 6 to 7.5 mg/kg/24 h divided q8h.

First a weight conversion is necessary since you have the child's weight in lb, the reference is in kg. Convert the child's weight in lb to kg to the nearest tenth.

$$\frac{2.2 \text{ lb}}{40 \text{ lb}} = \frac{1 \text{ kg}}{x \text{ kg}}$$

$$\frac{2.2 \, x}{2.2} = \frac{40}{2.2}$$

$$x = 18.18 \text{ kg}$$

The weight is 18.2 kg.

Now that you've converted the weight we can calculate the safe dose. You must calculate and obtain a range. (The recommended dose is 6 to 7.5 mg/kg/24 h)

Therefore calculate the low and high range:

$$6 \text{ mg} \times 18.2 \text{ kg} = 109.2 \text{ mg} \qquad 7.5 \text{ mg} \times 18.2 \text{ kg} = 136.5 \text{ mg}$$

The safe range for the child weighing 18.2 kg is 109.2 mg to 136.5 mg.

Now divide the total daily dose by the number of times the drug will be given in a day.

$$q8h = 24 \div 8 = 3$$

$$109.2 \div 3 = 36.4 \text{ mg per dose} \qquad 136.5 \div 3 = 45.5 \text{ mg per dose}$$

The dose range is 36.4 mg to 45.5 mg per dose q8h. The ordered dose of 50 mg q8h exceeds the dose of 109.2 mg to 136.5 mg total dose for 24 hours.

50 mg q8h = 50 × 3 = 150 mg.

Remember that factors such as the child's medical condition might have warranted a larger dose. Call the doctor to verify the dose.

Example 3: The recommended dose for Dicloxacillin Sodium for oral suspension is 12.5 mg/kg/day for children weighing less than 40 kg (88 lb) in equally divided doses q6h. What is the dosage for a child weighing 36 lb?

First convert the child's weight in lb to the nearest tenth of a kg.

2.2 lb : 1 kg = 36 lb : x kg (or state ratio as a fraction).   16.4kg

$$\frac{2.2}{2.2}x = \frac{36}{2.2}$$

x = 16.36 kg. To the nearest tenth the weight is 16.4 kg.

Now that you've converted the weight to kg we can calculate the safe dose for this child.

$$\frac{12.5 \text{ mg}}{x \text{ mg}} = \frac{1 \text{ kg}}{16.4 \text{ kg}}$$

x = 16.4 × 12.5

x = 205 mg

205 mg/day is the safe dose for a child weighing 16.4 kg

If 50 mg is ordered q6h, is this a safe dose?

24 h ÷ 6 h = 4 doses per day

50 mg × 4 doses = 200 mg per day

The ordered dose is safe.

Next calculate the amount of medication to give to administer the ordered dose. Dicloxacillin Sodium oral suspension is available in a dosage strength of 62.5 mg per 5 mL. Use either ratio-proportion or formula method as follows:

62.5 mg : 5 mL = 50 mg : x mL

62.5x = 250 mg

x = 4 mL

or

$$\frac{50 \text{ mg}}{62.5 \text{ mg}} \times 5 \text{ ml}$$

$$\frac{250}{62.5} = 4\text{ml}$$

You would give 4 mL to administer the ordered dose of 50 mg.

When information concerning a pediatric dosage is not present on the drug label, refer to the package insert, the PDR, or other reference text. Now try the following practice problems. Some labels or portions of package inserts have been included for some problems.

Practice Problems

11.   Refer to the label and answer the following. The child weighs 35 lb.

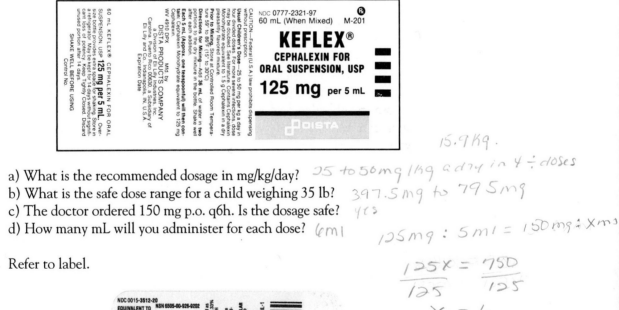

a) What is the recommended dosage in mg/kg/day?   *15.9 kg.*   *25 to 50 mg /kg a day in 4 ÷ doses*
b) What is the safe dose range for a child weighing 35 lb?   *397.5 mg to 795 mg*
c) The doctor ordered 150 mg p.o. q6h. Is the dosage safe?   *yes*
d) How many mL will you administer for each dose?   *6 ml*   *125 mg : 5 ml = 150 mg ÷ X ms*

12.   Refer to label.

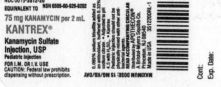

125X = 750
125   125
X = 6

The PDR indicates 15 mg/kg/day q8h of Kanamycin. The doctor ordered 200 mg I.V. q8h for a child weighing 35 kg.
a) What is the maximum dose for 24 hours?   *525*
b) What is the divided dose?   *175*
c) Is the dosage ordered safe?   *No - check order c̄ Dr.*

13. The recommended dose of Clindamycin oral suspension is 8 to 25 mg/kg/day in four divided doses. A child weighs 40 kg.

NDC 0009-0760-04

Keep Container Tightly Closed

DO NOT REFRIGERATE SOLUTION

Store solution at room temperature

NDC 0009-0760-04   100 mL (when mixed)

Cleocin Pediatric®
Flavored Granules
clindamycin palmitate hydrochloride for oral solution, USP

75 mg per 5 mL

Equivalent to 75 mg per 5 mL clindamycin when reconstituted

Upjohn   Caution : Federal law prohibits dispensing without prescription.

Shake well before each use

Discard any unused portion two weeks after reconstitution
Date of reconstitution _____

LOT

Usual child dosage-5 mL (1 teaspoonful) four times daily.
See package insert for complete product information.
WARNING - NOT FOR INJECTION
Store unreconstituted product at controlled room temperature 15°-30° C (59°-86° F) Reconstitute with a total of 75 mL of water as follows : add a large portion of the water and shake vigorously ; add remaining water and shake until solution is uniform. Each 5 mL (teaspoonful) of the solution contains clindamycin palmitate HCl equiv. to 75 mg clindamycin. Each bottle contains the equivalent of 1.5 grams clindamycin.

810 898 106   EXP

Made in Belgium for
The Upjohn Company
Kalamazoo, MI 49001, USA

320mg — 1000mg

a) What is the maximum dose for 24 hours? *1000mg*
b) What is the divided dose? *80mg — 250mg*

14. The doctor orders Phenobarbital 10 mg q12h for a child weighing 9 lb. The Pediatric Drug handbook states maintenance dose is 3 to 5 mg/kg/day q12h.
a) What is the child's weight in kg to the nearest tenth? *4.1 kg*
b) What is the range of dosage that is safe for this child? *12.3 mg — 20.5mg*
c) Is the dose ordered safe? *yes*
d) Phenobarbital Elixer is available in a dosage strength of 20 mg per 5 mL. What will you administer for one dose? *2.5 ml*   *20mg : 5ml = 10mg : xml*

$$\frac{20x}{20} = \frac{50}{20} = 2.5\,ml$$

15. The doctor orders Morphine Sulfate 7.5 mg s.c. q4h p.r.n. for a child weighing 84 lb. The recommended maximum dose for a child is 0.1 to 0.2 mg/kg/dose. Is the dosage ordered safe? How many mL would you administer for one dose?

LOT

EXP

25 DOSETTE® VIALS--Each contains **1 mL**

MORPHINE
SULFATE INJECTION, USP

15 mg/mL

FOR SUBCUTANEOUS, INTRAMUSCULAR OR SLOW INTRAVENOUS USE
NOT FOR EPIDURAL OR INTRATHECAL USE
WARNING: May be habit forming
PROTECT FROM LIGHT
DO NOT USE IF PRECIPITATED
CAUTION: Federal law prohibits dispensing without prescription.

ELKINS-SINN, INC. Cherry Hill, NJ 08003-4099
A subsidiary of A. H. Robins Company

NDC 0641-**0190-25**
Each mL contains morphine sulfate 15 mg, monobasic sodium phosphate, monohydrate 10 mg, dibasic sodium phosphate, anhydrous 2.8 mg, sodium formaldehyde sulfoxylate 3 mg and phenol 2.5 mg in Water for Injection, pH 2.5-6.5; sulfuric acid added, if needed, for pH adjustment. Sealed under nitrogen.
USUAL DOSE: See package insert.
Store at 15°-30° C (59°-86° F). Avoid freezing.
NOTE: Slight discoloration will not alter efficacy. Discard if markedly discolored.
Product Code: 0190-25   B-50190g

LIGHT SENSITIVE: Keep covered in this box until ready to use. To open—Cut seal along dotted line

38.2 kg

3.8mg to 7.6mg

yes the dose is safe

15mg : 1ml = 7.5mg : xml

$$\frac{15x}{15} = \frac{7.5}{15}$$

0.5 mL

16.   The recommended dose of Dilantin is 4 to 8 mg/kg/day q12h. The doctor ordered
       15 mg p.o. q12h for a child weighing 11 lb. Is the dosage ordered safe? *yes*
       What would you administer for one dose? *0.6 ml*

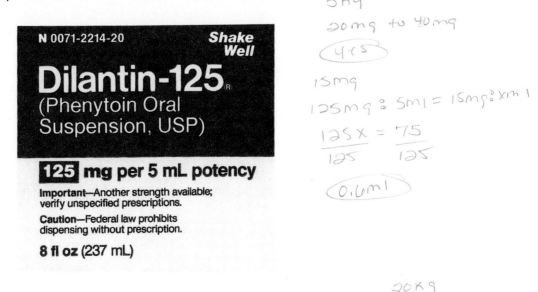

5 Kg

20mg to 40mg

yes

15mg

125mg : 5ml = 15mg : xml

$$\frac{125x}{125} = \frac{75}{125}$$

0.6ml

20Kg

17.   The recommended initial dose of Mercaptopurine is 2.5 mg/kg/daily p.o. What
       would the recommended daily dose be for a child weighing 44 lb?   *no more than 50mg*

18.   The recommended dose for a child I.V. of Vancomycin is 40 mg/kg/24h divided q6h.
       The doctor ordered 200 mg I.V. q6h for a child weighing 38 lb.
       a) What is the child's weight in kg to the nearest tenth? *17.3 Kg*
       b) What is the maximum dose for this child in 24 hours? *692 mg*
       c) What is the divided dose? *173 mg*
       d) Is the dosage ordered safe? *No*

       order
       200mg × 4 = 860
       Is it safe? No!

Points to Remember:

✔ To convert lb to kg divide by 2.2.

✔ To convert kg to lb multiply by 2.2.

✔ To calculate dosages the child's weight must be converted to the reference.

✔ To calculate dosage:

    1. Determine the child's weight in kg if needed.

    2. Multiply the child's weight in kg by the dose kg/day.

    3. Divide the total daily dose by the number of doses needed to administer.

    4. Calculate the number of tablets or volume to administer for each dose by use of ratio-proportion or the formula method.

✔ When the recommended dose is given as a range calculate based on the low and high for each dose.

✔ Question any discrepancies in dosages ordered, and remember factors such as age, weight, and medical conditions can cause discrepancies. Ask the doctor to clarify the order when a discrepancy exists.

✔ Use appropriate resources to determine the safe range for a child's dosage.

Calculation of Pediatric Dosages Using Body Surface Area

A child's BSA is determined by comparing a child's weight and height with what is considered average or the norm. Many pediatric dosages are prescribed based on the child's BSA. The BSA is determined from the height and weight of a child and the use of the West Nomogram (Figure 19.1).

This information is then applied to a formula for dosage calculation. Remember all children are not the same size at the same age, therefore the West Nomogram can be used to determine the BSA of a child.

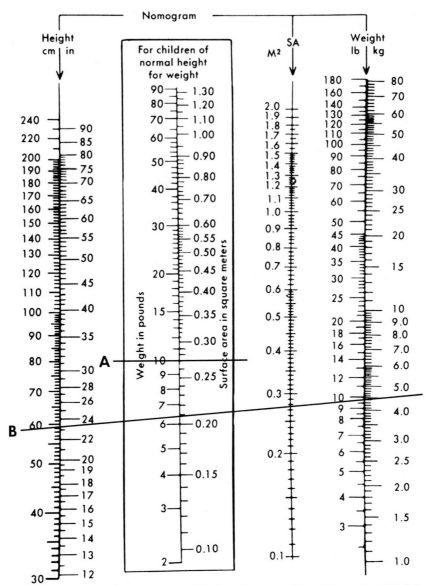

Figure 19.1 West Nomogram for estimation of body surface area (From Dison: *Simplified drugs and solution for nurses*, ed 10, 1992, Mosby, and Behran RE, Vaughn VC, editors: *Nelson's textbook of peds*, ed 13, Philadelphia, 1987, WB Saunders.)

The BSA is used to calculate dosages for infants and children up to 12 years of age. It is also possible to determine the BSA from weight alone, if the child is of normal height and weight.

Reading the West Nomogram Chart

Refer to the chart in Figure 19.1. Note: The height is on the left hand side of the chart, and the weight is on the right hand side. To identify the correct values on the BSA chart you must be able to read it. This entails reading the numbers and determining what the calibration between them is measuring. For example, look at the column indicated by weight, and study how it's marked. Looking at the bottom of the chart notice there are four calibrations between 0.10 and 0.15; those numbers in between are read as 0.11, 0.12, etc. Notice the calibrations between 15 and 20 are 1-lb increments.

Practice Problems

Refer to the BSA chart and determine the BSA from the column marked "Surface Area in Square Meters."

19. For a child weighing 30 lb _____

20. For a child weighing 10 lb _____

21. For a child weighing 52 lb _____

In addition to determining the BSA based on weight it can also be calculated using both height and weight. If you refer to the chart notice the column for height and weight. This chart also includes the weight in lb and kg. Notice the column for height (in cm and inches). To determine the surface area a ruler is used and placed on the graph from the height to the weight column. The surface area (M^2) is indicated where the line crosses the BSA column second from right of the Nomogram.

Practice Problems

Using the nomogram calculate the following BSAs.

22. A child who is 90 cm long and weighs 50 lb.

23. A child who is 60 cm long and weighs 10 lb.

24. A child who is 100 cm long and weighs 10 kg.

25. A child who is 30 inches long and weighs 20 lb.

Dosage Calculation Based on BSA

If you know the child's BSA the dosage calculation is done by multiplying the recommended dose (M^2) by the child's BSA.

Example 1: The recommended dosage is 3 mg per M^2. The child has a BSA of 1.2 M^2.

1.2 × 3 mg = 3.6 mg

Example 2: The recommended dosage is 30 mg per M^2. The child has a BSA of 0.75 M^2.

0.75 × 30 = 22.5 mg.

Calculating Using the Formula

The BSA is expressed in square meters (M^2). The child's BSA is then inserted into the following formula.

Formula:

$$\frac{\text{BSA of child (M}^2)}{1.7 \ (\text{M}^2)} \times \text{adult dose} = \text{child's dose}$$

The formula uses the average adult dose, BSA $(1.7 \ \text{M}^2)$

Example 1: The doctor has ordered a medication for which average adult dosage is 125 mg. What will the dose for a child with a BSA of $1.4 \ \text{M}^2$?

$$\frac{1.4}{1.7} \times 125 \ \text{mg} = 102.94 \ \text{mg} = 102.9 \ \text{mg}$$

Example 2: The adult dose for a medication is 100 to 300 mg. What will the dosage be for a child with a BSA $0.5 \ \text{M}^2$?

$$\frac{0.5}{1.7} \times 100 = 29.4 \ \text{mg}$$

$$\frac{0.5}{1.7} \times 300 = 88.2 \ \text{mg}$$

The dosage range is 29.4 to 88.2 mg

Practice Problems

Using the West Nomogram Chart when indicated, calculate the child's dosage for the following drugs. Express your answer to the nearest tenth.

26. Child's height 32 in.
     Child's weight 25 lb.
     a. What is the child's BSA?
     b. The recommended adult dose is 25 mg.
     c. What is the child's dose?

27. Child's height 100 cm.
     Child's weight 10 kg.
     Adult dosage 200 to 400 mg.
     a. What is the child's BSA?
     b. What is the child's dose?

28. The normal adult dosage of a drug is 5 to 15 mg. What will the dosage be for a child whose BSA is $1.5 \ \text{M}^2$?

29. The doctor ordered 5 mg of a drug for a child with a BSA of 0.8 M^2. The average adult dose is 20 mg. Is this a correct dose?

30. The child's BSA = 0.92. The doctor ordered 7 mg of a drug. The average adult dose is 25 mg. Is this correct?

31. The child's BSA is 1.5 M^2. The doctor ordered an antibiotic for which average adult dosage is 250 mg. What will the child's dosage be?

32. The recommended dose is 20 to 30 mg per M^2. The child has a BSA of 0.74 M^2. What will the child's dosage be?

33. The child has a BSA of 0.67 M^2. Average adult dosage is 20 mg. The doctor ordered 8 mg. Is the dosage correct?

34. The child has a BSA of 0.94 M^2. The recommended adult dose is 10 to 20 mg. What will the child's dosage be?

35. Child's weight 20 lb.
    Child's height 30 in.
    Adult dose 500 mg.
    a. What is the child's BSA?
    b. What is the child's dosage?

Points to Remember:

✔ BSA is determined from a nomogram using the child's height and weight.

✔ When you know the child's BSA, the dosage is determined by multiplying the BSA by the recommended dose.

✔ To determine whether a child's dose is safe, a comparison must be made between what is ordered and the calculation of the dosage based on BSA.

✔ Formula for calculating child's dosage is as follows:

$$\frac{\text{child's BSA}}{1.7 \text{ M}^2} \times \text{adult dosage}$$

Chapter Review

Read the dosage information or label given for the following problems. Express body weight conversion to the nearest tenth where indicated and dosages to the nearest tenth.

1. The doctor orders Lasix 10 mg I.V. stat for a child weighing 22 lb. The Pediatric handbook states 1 mg/kg as an initial dose is safe. Is the dosage ordered safe for this child?

2. The doctor orders Amoxicillin 150 mg p.o. q8h for an infant weighing 23 lb. The Pediatric handbook states the maximum daily dosage for an infant is Amoxicillin p.o. 20 to 40 mg/kg/24h divided q8h. Is the dosage ordered safe?
    a) What is the child's weight to the nearest tenth?
    b) What is the maximum dose for 24 h?
    c) What is the divided dose?
    d) Is the dose ordered safe?

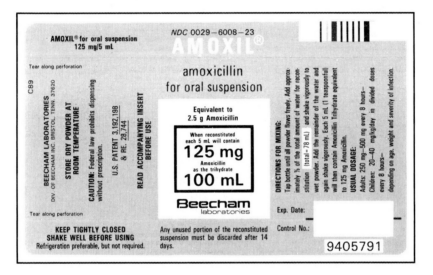

3. The doctor orders Furadantin oral suspension 25 mg p.o. q6h for a child weighing 17 kg. Round the child's weight to the nearest tenth. Refer to the Furadantin label below and determine:
    a) If this is a safe dosage.
    b) How many mL must be given per dose to administer the ordered dose.

4. The doctor orders 100 mg p.o. q6h of Dicloxacillin for a child weighing 35 kg. The Pediatric Reference indicates 12.5 mg/kg/day for children weighing less than 40 kg in equally divided doses q6h. Is the dosage ordered safe?

5. The doctor orders Vibramycin 75 mg p.o. q12h for a child weighing 30 lb. Refer to the label below, and determine if this is a safe dose.

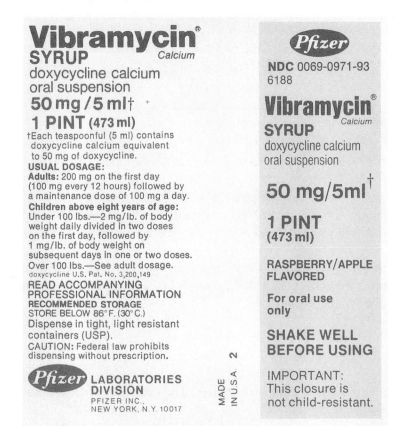

6. The doctor orders Oxacillin oral solution 250 mg p.o. q6h for a child weighing 42 lb. The Pediatric Reference states 60 mg/kg/day in equally divided doses q6h.

7. The doctor orders Cleocin suspension 150 mg p.o. q8h for a child weighing 36 lb. The Pediatric drug handbook states 10 to 25 mg/kg/24h divided q6 to 8h. Is the dosage ordered safe?

8. The doctor orders Keflex suspension 250 mg p.o. q6h for a child weighing 66 lb. Using the Keflex label below determine if the dosage ordered is safe. How many mL would you give to administer one dose?

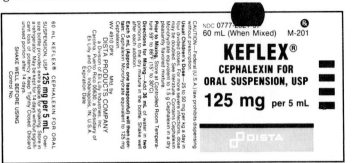

9. The doctor orders Streptomycin Sulfate 400 mg I.M. q12h for a child weighing 35 kg.
   a) The PDH recommends 20 to 40 mg/kg/day divided q12h I.M. Is the dosage ordered safe?
   b) A 1g vial of Streptomycin Sulfate is available in powdered form with the following instructions: Dilution with 1.8 mL of sterile water will yield 400 mg per mL. How many mL will you give to administer the ordered dose?

10. A child weighs 46 lb and has a mild infection. The doctor ordered Gantrisin oral suspension 250 mg p.o. q6h. The PDH states 120 mg/kg/24h in four equally divided doses. Is the dosage ordered safe?

Use the nomogram provided, determine the BSA, and calculate the child's dosage by using the formula. Express dosages to the nearest tenth.

11. Child's height 30 inches and weight 20 lb. The adult dose of an antibiotic is 500 mg.

    a. What is the BSA?_____

    b. What is the child's dose?_____

12. Child's height 32 inches and weight 27 lb. The adult dose for a medication is 25 mg.

    a. What is the BSA?_____

    b. What is the child's dose?_____

13. Child's height is 120 cm and weight 40 kg. The adult dose for a medication is 250 mg.

    a. What is the BSA?_____

    b. What is the child's dose?_____

14. Child's height is 50 inches and weight 75 lb. The adult dose for a medication is 30 mg.

    a. What is the BSA?_____

b. What is the child's dose?_____

15.   Child's height is 50 inches and weight 70 lb. The adult dose for a medication is 150 mg.

a. What is the BSA?_____

b. What is the child's dose?_____

Determine the child's dosage for the following drugs. Express answers to the nearest tenth.

16.   The adult dose of a drug is 50 mg. What will the dosage be for a child with a BSA of 0.70 M^2?

17.   The adult dose of a drug is 10 to 20 mg. What will the dosage range be for a child whose BSA is 0.66 M^2?

18.   The adult dose of a drug is 2000 U. What will the dosage be for a child with a BSA of 0.55 M^2?

19.   The adult dose of a drug is 200 to 250 mg. What will the dosage be for a child with a BSA of 0.55 M^2?

20.   The adult dose of a drug is 150 mg. What will the dosage be for a child with a BSA of 0.22 M^2?

Calculate the child's dosage in the following problems. Determine if the doctor's order is correct. If the order is incorrect give the correct dosage. Express answers to the nearest tenth.

21.   A child with a BSA of 0.49 M^2 has an order of 25 mg for a drug with an average adult dose of 60 mg.

22.   A child with a BSA of 0.32 M^2 has an order of 4 mg for a drug with an average adult dose of 10 mg.

23.   A child with a BSA of 0.68 M^2 has an order of 50 mg for a drug with an average adult dose of 125 to 150 mg.

24.   A child with a BSA of 0.55 M^2 has an order of 5 mg for a drug. The adult dose is 25 mg.

25.   A child with a BSA of 1.2 M^2 has an order for 60 mg of a drug. The adult dose is 75 to 100 mg.

Unit Five

Basic I.V., Heparin, and Critical Care Calculations

The ability to accurately calculate flow rates for I.V. medications provides the essentials needed for both heparin administration and critical care calculations.

CH 20

293 - 302

p. 813

STUDY

FOR

WED'S

LAB

10/9

20 Basic I.V. Calculations

Objectives

After reviewing this chapter the student will be able to do the following:

1. Identify from I.V. tubing packages the drop factor in gtt/mL
2. Calculate flow rates using a formula method
3. Calculate the flow rate for medications ordered intravenously over a specified time period

When clients are receiving intravenous (I.V.) therapy, it is important to make sure they are receiving the correct amount. The doctor is responsible for writing the I.V. order. The doctor's order must specify the following:

1. The type of I.V. fluid.

2. The amount (volume) to be administered.

3. The time period the I.V. is to infuse.

I.V. fluids are usually ordered on the basis of mL/hr. Example: 3000 cc/24 hours, 1000 cc in 8 hours. Smaller volumes of fluid are often used when the I.V. contains medications such as antibiotics. Rates for I.V. fluids are usually determined in gtt/mL.

I.V. Tubing

I.V. tubing has a drip chamber. The nurse determines the flow rate by adjusting the clamp and observing the drip chamber to count the drops per minute. The size of the drop depends on the type of I.V. tubing used. The calibration of I.V. tubing in gtt/mL is known as the *drop factor*, and is indicated on the box in which the I.V. tubing is packaged. This calibration is necessary to calculate flow rates (Figure 20.1).

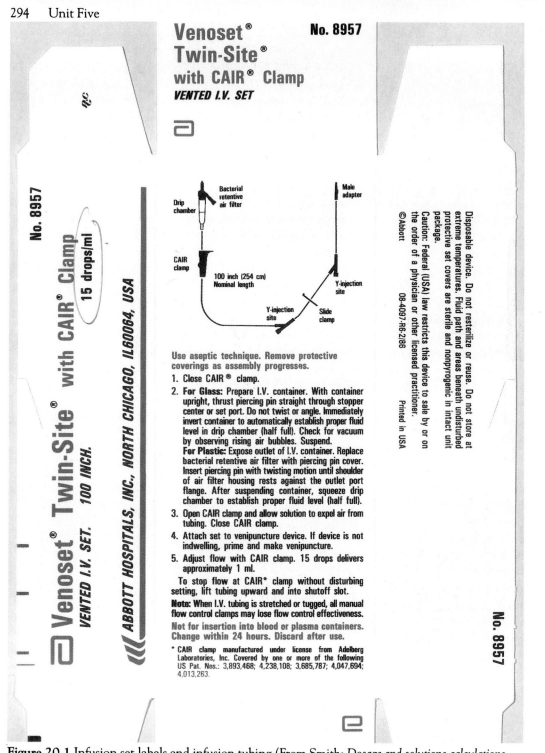

Figure 20.1 Infusion set labels and infusion tubing (From Smith: *Dosage and solutions calculations,* St Louis, 1989, Mosby.)

There are two types of tubing used to administer I.V. fluids. The two common types of tubing are as follows:

a. Macrodrop tubing – The standard type of tubing used for general I.V. administration. This type of tubing delivers a certain number of gtt/mL according to the manufacturer. Macrodrop tubing delivers 10, 15, or 20 gtts equal to 1 mL (cc). Macrodrops are large drops, therefore large amounts of fluid are administered in macrodrops.

b. Microdrip tubing – Delivers small tiny drops, which can be inferred from the word (micro). Microdrip tubing is used when small amounts and more exact measurements are needed, for example in pediatrics, the elderly, and in critical care settings. Microdrip tubing delivers 60 gtt, which is equal to 1 mL (cc). Since there are 60 minutes in an hour, the number of microdrops per minute is equal to the number of mL/hr. For example if a client is receiving 100 milliliters per hour, they are receiving 100 microdrops/minute.

Formula Method for Calculating I.V. Flow Rate

To calculate the flow rate or rate at which an I.V. is to infuse the nurse needs to know the following:

1. The volume or number of mL (cc) to infuse.

2. The drop factor.

3. The time element (minutes or hours). This information is placed in the following formula:

Formula:

$$\frac{V_1}{T_1} \times \frac{V_2}{T_2} = gtt\,/\,minute$$

Note: Numbers have been placed in the formula for the purpose of explanation.

$$\frac{Volume}{Time} \times \frac{Volume}{Time} = gtt\,/\,minute$$

Explanation of Formula

V_1 = volume (the total number of mL (cc) to infuse).

T_1 = time in hours (the number of hours the I.V. is to infuse).

V_2 = drop factor of the tubing used. For example 10 gtt = 1 cc; 60 gtt = 1 cc.

T_2 = time in minutes (since there are 60 minutes in an hour, the number is always 60, unless the I.V. is to infuse for a time period less than an hour, then you can place the number of minutes in this position.

Note: To place the number of minutes in the T_1 position the number of minutes must be expressed in hours by dividing the number of minutes by 60. It is easier to place the number of minutes directly into the formula in the T_2 position to avoid extra calculation.

Before calculating let's review some basic principles:

1.   Drops per minute are always expressed in whole numbers. You cannot regulate something at a half of a drop. Since drops are expressed in whole numbers, principles of rounding off are applied, for example 19.5 gtt = 20 gtt.

2.   Carry division of problem one decimal place to round to a whole number of drops.

3.   Answers must be labeled. The label is usually drops per minute, unless asked otherwise.

    Example: 100 gtt/min or 17 gtt/min.

To reinforce the differences in gtt factor the type of tubing is sometimes included as part of the label.

    Example: 100 microgtt/minute or 17 macrogtt/minute.

Let's look at a sample problem and the step by step method of using the formula to obtain the answer.

    Example 1: The doctor orders an I.V. to infuse at 100 mL/hr. The drop factor is 10gtt/mL. How many gtt/min should the I.V. infuse?

Steps:

1. Set up the problem, placing the information given in the correct position.

$$\frac{V_1}{T_1} \times \frac{V_2}{T_2} = \frac{100\ mL}{1\ hr} \times \frac{10\ gtt\ /\ mL}{60\ min}$$

2. Reduce where possible to make numbers smaller and easier to manage. Note: Labels are dropped when starting to perform mathematical steps.

$$\frac{100}{1} \times \frac{10}{60} = \frac{100}{1} \times \frac{1}{6} = \frac{100}{6}$$

3. Divide $\dfrac{100}{6}$ to obtain gtt/min.

    Carry division at least one decimal place, and round off to the nearest whole number.

$$\frac{100}{6} = 16.6$$

    Answer: 17 gtt/min

To deliver 100 mL/hr, with a drop factor of 10 drops per mL, the I.V. rate should be adjusted to 17 drops per minute.

This answer can also be expressed with the type of tubing as part of the label.

Example: 17 macrogtt/min.

Example 2:   Administer an I.V. of 50 cc in 20 minutes using a microdrip set (60 gtt/mL).

1. $50 \text{ mL} \times \dfrac{60 \text{ gtt/mL}}{20 \text{ (min)}}$

Note: Here the 20 minutes is placed in the T_2 position because it represents the time in minutes. The time period is less than an hour. A 1 could also be placed under 50, not to denote 1 hour, but because 50/1 is the same as 50.

or

$$\dfrac{50 \text{ mL}}{1} \times \dfrac{60 \text{ gtt/mL}}{20 \text{ (min)}}$$

2. $50 \times \dfrac{3}{1}$ or $\dfrac{50}{1} \times \dfrac{3}{1}$

3. Either way of setting the problem up gives 150 as an answer.

Answer: 150 gtt/min.

To deliver 50 cc in 20 minutes with a drop factor of 60 drops per mL, the I.V. rate should be adjusted to 150 gtt/min.

This may sound like a lot, however remember the tubing used is a microdrop. This answer may be expressed as 150 microdrops per minute.

The formula method may also be used to calculate gtt/min for a volume of fluid to be administered in more than 1 hour.

Example: 1000 cc D5W to infuse in 8 hours. The drop factor is 10 gtt/mL. How many gtt/min should the I.V. be regulated at?

Solution:

$$\dfrac{1000 \text{ ml}}{8 \text{ hr}} \times \dfrac{10 \text{ gtt/mL}}{60 \text{ min}}$$

$$\dfrac{1000}{8} \times \dfrac{1}{6} = \dfrac{1000}{48} = 20.8 \text{ or } 21 \text{ drops/min}$$

Another approach to doing this is to first find the cc per hour. Dividing the total volume to be infused by the number of hours equals mL/hr or:

$$\frac{V_1}{T_1} = \frac{\text{total volume}}{\text{time}} = \text{mL/hr}$$

$$\frac{1000 \text{ mL}}{8 \text{ hr}} = 125 \text{ ml/hr}$$

After determining the mL/hr you would place it into the formula and proceed to calculate gtt/min. This lessens the size of the numbers and makes math calculations easier.

$$\frac{125 \text{ mL/hr}}{1} \times \frac{10 \text{ gtt/mL}}{60 \text{ min}}$$

$$\frac{125}{1} \times \frac{1}{6} = \frac{125}{6} = 20.8 = 21 \text{ gtt/min}$$

As you can see the formula method can be used for calculating flow rates for less than an hour or for several hours.

Practice Problems

Calculate the flow rate in gtt/min.

1. Administer I.V. at 75 mL/hr. The drop factor is 10 gtt/mL.

2. Administer 30 mL/hr. The drop factor is a microdrop.

3. Administer 125 mL/hr. The drop factor is 15 gtt/mL.

4. Administer 1000 mL in 6 hours. The drop factor is 15 gtt/mL.

5. An I.V. medication with a volume of 60 mL is to be administered in 45 minutes using a microdrip set.

6. 1000 mL of Ringers Lactate is to infuse in 16 hours. The drop factor is 15 gtt/mL.

7. Infuse 150 mL of D5W in 2 hours. The drop factor is 20 gtt/mL.

8. Administer 3000 mL D51/2 NS in 24 hours. The drop factor is 10 gtt/mL.

9. Infuse 2000 mL D5W in 12 hours. The drop factor is 15 gtt/mL.

10. Administer 60 cc of I.V. medication in 30 minutes. The drop factor is a microdrip.

Calculating I.V. Flow Rates When Several Solutions are Ordered

Doctors often write I.V. orders for different amounts or types of fluid to be given in a certain time period. These orders are frequently written for a 24-hour interval and usually are split over three shifts. I.V. solutions may have medications added such as Potassium chloride or multivitamins.

Steps to calculating:

1. Add up the total amount of fluid.

2. Proceed as with other I.V. problem calculation.

Note: When medications such as Potassium chloride and vitamins are added to intravenous solutions, they are generally not considered in the total volume.

> **Example 1:**   The doctor orders the following I.V.s for 24 hours. The drop factor is 15 gtt/mL.
>
> 1000cc D_5W c̄ 10 mEq KCL (Potassium chloride)
>
> 500 cc D_5Ns c̄ 1 ampule MVI (multivitamin)
>
> 500 cc D_5W

Solution:

1. Add up total volume.

2. Place information given into formula.

3. Proceed to calculate.

$$\frac{V_1}{T_1} \times \frac{V_2}{T_2} = \frac{2000 \text{ mL}}{24 \text{ hr}} \times \frac{15 \text{ gtt/mL}}{60 \text{ min}}$$

$$\frac{500}{6} \times \frac{1}{4} = \frac{500}{24} = 20.8 = 21 \text{ gtt/min}$$

Remember this could have also been done by finding the mL/hr first and making the numbers smaller and easier to calculate. Calculating I.V. flow rate when there is more than one I.V. with the hourly rate indicated eliminates the step of adding up the solutions. The hourly rate becomes the total volume.

Example 2: The doctor orders the following I.V.s. The drop factor is
10 gtt/mL to infuse at 150 mL/hr.

1000 cc D5W

1000 cc NS

500 cc D51/2 NS

The hourly rate is 150 mL/hr. Calculation is done based on this:

$$\frac{150 \text{ mL}}{1 \text{ hr}} \times \frac{10 \text{ gtt/mL}}{60 \text{ min}} =$$

$$\frac{150}{1} \times \frac{1}{6} = \frac{150}{6} = 25 \text{ gtt/min}$$

Practice Problems

Calculate the flow rates in gtt/min.

11. Doctor's order: D5R/L c̄ 20 units Pitocin × 2 Liters at 125 cc/hr. The drop factor is 15 gtt/mL.

12. Doctor's order: For 16 hours the drop factor is 10 gtt/mL.

    D5W 500 cc c̄ 10 mEq KCl.

    D5W 1000 cc.

    D5W 1000 cc c̄ 1 ampule MVI.

13. Doctor's order: 1000 cc D5 0.9% NS × 3 liters at 100 mL/hr. The drop factor is a microdrop.

14. Doctor's order: D5W 1000 mL + 20 mEq KCl × 2 Liters. For 10 hours the drop factor is 15 gtt/mL.

Intravenous Medications

As previously discussed in the section on calculating I.V. flow rates, when several solutions are ordered, medications can be added directly to the intravenous solution.

Medications such as antibiotics can also be given by adding a secondary container of solution that contains the medication. The administration of medications by attaching it to a port on the primary line is referred to as "piggyback" (see Figure 20.2).

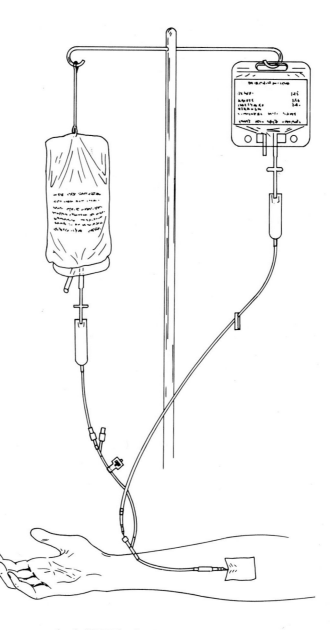

Figure 20.2 Intravenous piggyback (IVPB) administration set-up. Note that the smaller bottle is hung higher than the primary bottle.

The volume of the "piggyback" container is usually 50 to 100 cc and should infuse over 20, 30, or 60 minutes depending on the type and amount of medication added. The same formula used to calculate I.V. infusion times is used to calculate the gtt/min.

Sample Problem

The doctor ordered Keflin 2 g IVPB (piggyback) over 30 minutes. The Keflin is placed in 100 cc of fluid after it is dissolved. The drop factor is 15 gtt/mL. How many gtt/min should the I.V. be regulated at?

$$\frac{100}{1} \times \frac{15}{30}$$

$$30\overline{)1500}$$ 50

50 gtt/min

To calculate: The 100 cc of fluid the medication is placed in is used as the volume.

$$\frac{100 \text{ mL}}{1} \times \frac{15 \text{ gtt/ml}}{30 \text{ min}}$$

$$\frac{100}{1} \times \frac{1}{2} = \frac{100}{2} = 50$$

The I.V. would be regulated at 50 gtt/min.

As shown in Figure 20.2 the smaller bottle or bag (piggyback) is hung higher than the larger (primary) bottle. Since infusion flow is controlled by gravity, the primary bottle will resume infusion after the piggyback is empty. The drops per minute will then have to be reset to the correct amount calculated for the primary I.V.

Eletronic pumps can also be used for the administration of I.V. fluids and I.V. medications. The pumps are set to deliver a specific rate of flow per hour. The mechanisims of how the pump works will depend on the manufacturer. Special tubing is usually required for the pump, and calculations are based on that (Figures 20.3 and 20.4).

Practice Problems

15.   Mezlocillin 3 g IVPB in 130 cc NS over 1 hour. The drop factor is 15 gtt/mL.

16.   Erythromycin 250 mg in 100 cc D5W to infuse over 1 hour. The I.V. tubing delivers 20 gtt/mL.

17.   Ampicillin 1g in 50 cc D5W over 45 minutes. The drop factor is 10 gtt/mL.

18.   Clindamycin 900 mg in 75 cc D5W over 30 minutes. The drop factor is 10 gtt/mL.

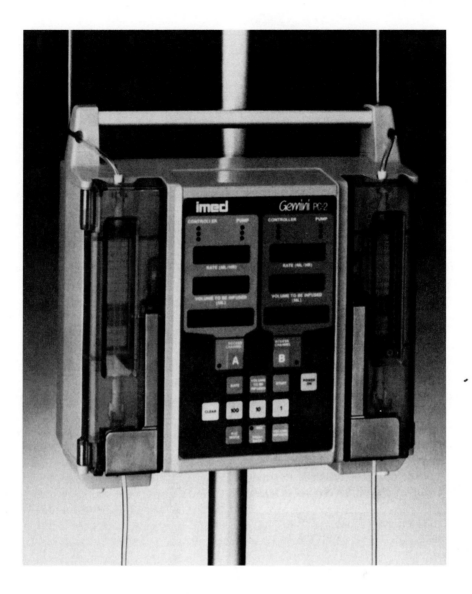

Figure 20.3 Intravenous controller for the simultaneous regulation or main I.V. infusion and a secondary, intermittent medication infusion. (From McKenry/Salerno: *Pharmacology in nursing,* ed 18, St Louis, 1992, Mosby.)

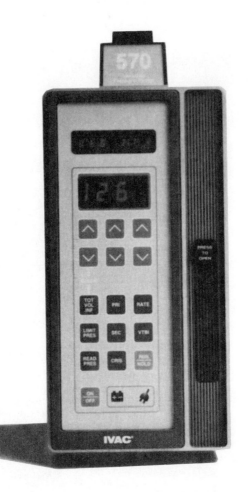

Figure 20.4 Infusion pump used when positive pressure provided by peristaltic action on the tubing produces the preset drop rate (From McKenry/Salerno: *Pharmacology in nursing*, ed 18, St Louis, 1992, Mosby.)

Heparin Locks

Heparin locks are used in various institutions. A heparin lock is an I.V. catheter that is inserted into a vein and left in place. It may be used when access to a vein is required for the administration of medications or fluids on an intermittent basis (Figure 20.5).

The drug heparin is instilled into the apparatus to prevent clotting at the insertion site. This is referred to as *heparinization*. Intravenous medications may be administered by the heparin lock "push" or by the drip method. Hospital protocol must be followed carefully for a heparin lock. The doctor prescribes the dose of heparin to be administered. Most heparin locks are flushed with 1 mL of solution containing 10 units of heparin, after a medication has been given (see following label). Heparin will be discussed in more detail in Chapter 21.

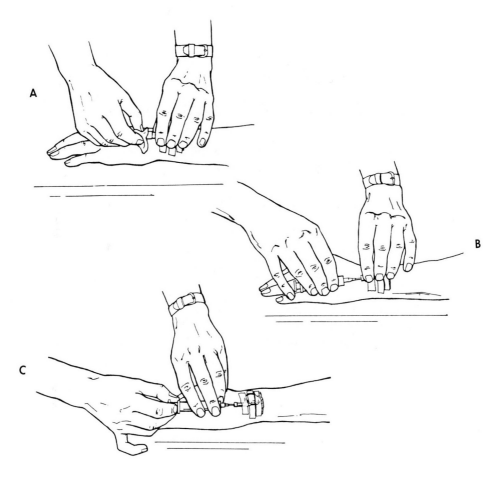

Figure 20.5 Heparin lock for injection of drug. **A,** Injection site is cleansed. **B,** A 25-gauge needle attached to a syringe containing prescribed drug is inserted into the heparin lock. **C,** Following gentle aspiration, the drug is injected slowly. Heparin is usually injected at a rate of no more than 1 mL per minute.

When medications are administered by a heparin lock, the lock must first be flushed with sterile normal saline before and after a medication is given, followed by a dilute solution of heparin. The letters "SISH" are used to remember the technique for medication administration: Saline, Intravenous medications, Saline, and Heparin. A heparin lock eliminates the need for venipuncture each time I.V. medication is to be given and removes the need for a continuously infusing I.V. Many clients can be discharged with a heparin lock in place and taught how to care for it. While heparin locks have many advantages, a major disadvantage is the bolusing of clients with doses of heparin (patent anticoagulants) despite dilute forms of heparin being used. Therefore many institutions now refer to the heparin lock as a med-lock, and heparin is used only when the catheter is initially inserted and for any subsequent flushings of the lock (for example, after the nurse administers medication with normal saline).

Determining the Amount of Drug in a Specific Amount of Solution

Sometimes medications are added to I.V. solutions and the doctor orders a certain amount of the drug to be given in a certain time period.

Example 1:   The doctor may order 20 mEq of Potassium to be placed in 1000 cc of fluid to be administered at a rate of 2 mEq of Potassium per hour. The flow rate (gtt/min) can be determined using the same formula as for other I.V.s, but first the volume to be infused must be calculated by use of ratio-proportion.

Step 1: Calculate the number of mL of solution needed to deliver 2 mEq of Potassium chloride.

what doctor ordered

$$20 \text{ mEq} : 1000 \text{ mL} = 2 \text{ mEq} : x \text{ mL}$$

total amount of drug in volume of solution   desired volume of solution

Solution:

$$20 : 1000 = 2 : x$$

$$20x = 1000 \times 2$$

$$20x = 2000$$

$$x = \frac{2000}{20}$$

$$x = 100 \text{ mL}$$

Therefore 100 mL of fluid would be needed to administer 2 mEq of Potassium chloride per hour.

Step 2: Determine the rate of flow by substituting this information into the formula if 100 mL of solution (containing 2mEq of Potassium chloride) is to be administered over 1 hour using 15 gtt $=$ 1 mL. The rate of flow is determined by:

$$\frac{100 \text{ mL}}{1 \text{ hr}} \times \frac{15 \text{ gtt/mL}}{60 \text{ min}}$$

$$\frac{100}{1} \times \frac{1}{4} = \frac{100}{4} = 25 \text{ gtt/min}$$

25 gtt/min would deliver 2mEq of Potassium chloride each hour from this solution.

Example 2: The doctor orders 100 U. of Regular insulin to be added to 500 cc of 0.45% saline to infuse at 10 U. per hour. The I.V. flow rate should be how many mL per hour?

Solution:

Step 1: Set up a proportion with the known on one side and the unknown on the other.

$$100 \text{ U. : } 500 \text{ cc} = 10 \text{ U. : } x$$

$$100 \, x = 500 \times 10$$

$$100 \, x = 5000$$

$$x = 50 \text{ cc/hr}$$

For the client to receive 10 U. of insulin per hour, 50 cc per hour must be administered.

Step 2: Determine the flow rate in gtt/min using 20 gtt $=$ 1mL.

$$\frac{50 \text{ cc}}{1 \text{ hr}} \times \frac{20 \text{ gtt/mL}}{60 \text{ min}} = \frac{50}{3} = 16.67 = 17 \text{ gtt/min}$$

17 gtt per minute would deliver 10 units of insulin per hour.

Practice Problems

Solve the following problems using the steps indicated.

19. 15 mEq of Potassium chloride is added to 1000 mL of D5 0.45% NS to be administered at a rate of 4 mEq per hour.
   a) How many mL of solution is needed to administer 4mEq per hour?

b) The administration set delivers 10 gtt/mL; calculate the gtt/min to deliver 4 mEq per hour.

20. Doctor's order: 10 U. of Regular insulin per hour. 50 U. of insulin is placed in 250 mL Normal Saline.
a) How many mL/hr should the I.V. infuse at?
b) Calculate the gtt/min if the administration set delivers 15 gtt/mL.

21. Doctor's order: 15 U. of Regular insulin per hour. 40 U. of insulin is placed in 250 mL of Normal Saline.
a) How many mL/hr should the I.V. infuse at?
b) Calculate the gtt/min if the administration set delivers 60 gtt/mL.

Determining Infusion Times and Volumes

You may need to calculate:

a)   Time in hours – How long it will take a certain amount of fluid to infuse or how long it may last.

b)   Volume – The total number of ccs a client will receive in a certain time period.

These unknown elements can be determined by use of the same formula and simple mathematics.

Remember the formula:

$$\frac{Volume}{Time} \; \frac{V_1}{T_1} \times \frac{V_2}{T_2} = gtt/min$$

Steps to Calculating a Problem with an Unknown

1. Take information given in problem and place in formula.

2. Place an x in the formula in the position of the unknown (for example, Volume V_1 position or in T_1 position [time in hours]).

3. Obtain an algebraic equation so that you can solve for x.

4. Solve equation.

5. Label answer in hours or ccs for volume.

Sample Problem

An I.V. is regulated at 20 microdrops per minute. How many hours will it take for 100 ccs to infuse?

Note: If it is regulated at 20 microdrops, then the drip factor or apparatus used was a microdrip. You cannot convert macrodrip into a microdrip and vice versa.

Note: In the sample problem, you are being asked the number of hours or T_1 so therefore when placing problem into formula, an x will go in T_1 position. 60 is in V_2 poition because if regulated at 20 microgtt/min, a microdrop set was used.

Problem Set Up In Formula

1. $\dfrac{V_1}{T_1} \times \dfrac{V_2}{T_2} = \dfrac{100\ cc}{x\ hr} \times \dfrac{60\ gtt/cc}{60\ min} = 20$ microdrops/min.

2. Reduce by cancellation of the fraction 60/60 and get 1.

$$\dfrac{100}{x} \times \dfrac{1}{1} = 20$$

3. Obtain an algebraic equation: (you must multiply so you can get rid of times sign [$\times$]).

a) $\dfrac{100}{x} \times 1 = 20$

b) $\dfrac{100}{x} = 20$ (after multiplication)

4. Solve for x by cross multiplying. Now you have the equal sign in between, which is necessary to solve for an unknown.

$$\dfrac{100}{x} = 20$$ (Note: placing 20 over 1 doesn't alter value.)

or

$$\dfrac{100}{x} = \dfrac{20}{1}$$

$$20x = 100$$

$$x = 5\ hours$$

Note: Label is hours since that's what you were being asked.

When calculating time intervals and time or answer comes out in hours and minutes, express the entire time in hours. For example 1 hour and 30 minutes = 1.5 hours or 1 1/2 hours; 1 1/2 hours is the preferred term.

When calculating volume, proceed with the problem in the same way as calculating time interval except x is placed in a different position (V_1).

Sample Problem

An I.V. is regulated at 17 macrodrops per minute. The drop factor is 15 gtt/cc. How much fluid volume in ccs will the client receive in 8 hours?

1. Place information into formula $\dfrac{\text{Volume}}{\text{Time}} \times \dfrac{\text{Volume}}{\text{Time}} = \text{gtt/min}$

    a) $\dfrac{x}{8} \times \dfrac{15}{60} = 17$ gtt/min

    b) $\dfrac{x \text{ cc}}{8 \text{ hr}} \times \dfrac{1 \text{ gtt/cc}}{4 \text{ min}} = 17$ after reducing 15/60

    c)   Multiply to obtain equation and get rid of × sign.

          $\dfrac{x}{32} = 17$

    d) $x = 32 \times 17$

Answer: 544 cc

Note: Label on this answer would be ccs.

Some of the problems illustrated in calculating an unknown may be solved without the formula; however, using the formula is recommended.

Practice Problems

Solve the following problems as indicated.

22. You find that there is 150 cc of fluid left in an I.V. The I.V. is infusing at 60 microdrops/min.
 How long will the fluid last?

23. An I.V. is infusing at 35 gtt/min.
 The administration equivalency is 15 gtt/cc.
 How many ccs of fluid will the client receive in 5 hours?

24. You find that there is 180 cc of fluid left in an I.V. that is infusing at 45 gtt/min. The drop factor is 15 gtt/cc.
How many hours will the fluid last?

25. An I.V. is infusing at 45 gtt/min. The drop factor is 15 gtt/mL. How many ccs will the client receive in 8 hours?

26. You find there is 90 cc of fluid left. The flow rate is 60 gtt/min. How long will the fluid last?

Recalculating an I.V. Flow Rate

Flow rates on I.V.s change when a client stands, sits, or is repositioned in bed. Therefore nurses must frequently check the flow rates. I.V.s generally are labeled with a start and finish time, as well as markings with specific time periods. Sometimes I.V.s infuse ahead or behind schedule if not monitored closely. When this happens the I.V. flow rate must be recalculated. To recalculate the flow rate the nurse uses the volume remaining and time remaining.

The recalculated flow rate should not vary from the original rate by more than 25%. It is recommended that if the recalculated rate varies more than 25% from the original, the doctor should be notified. The order may have to be revised.

Example: An I.V. of 1000 cc was to infuse in 8 hours at 31 gtt/min. The drop factor is 15 gtt/mL. After 4 hours you notice 700 mL of fluid left in the I.V. Recalculate the flow rate for the remaining solution.

Solution:

Time remaining = 4 hours

Volume of solution remaining = 700 mL

$$\frac{700 \text{ ml}}{4 \text{ hr}} \times \frac{15 \text{ gtt/mL}}{60 \text{ min}}$$

$$\frac{700}{4} \times \frac{1}{4} = \frac{700}{16} = 44 \text{ gtt/min}$$

In this situation the flow rate has to be increased from 31 gtt/min to 44 gtt/min. Always assess the client first to determine their ability to tolerate an increase in fluid. The doctor should be notified if there is doubt. This same method can be used if an I.V. is ahead of schedule. An alternate to doing this problem without first calculating mL/hr would be to use the total amount.

Example of I.V. Ahead:

An I.V. of 1000 mL D5W is to infuse from 8 AM to 4 PM (8 hr). The drop factor is 10 gtt/mL. The rate is set at 20 gtt/min. In 5 hours you notice 700 cc has infused. Recalculate the flow rate for the remaining solution.

Solution:

Time remaining = 3 hours
Volume of solution remaining = 300 cc

$$\frac{300 \text{ mL}}{3 \text{ hr}} \times \frac{10 \text{ gtt/mL}}{60 \text{ min}}$$

$$\frac{300}{3} \times \frac{1}{6} = 16.66$$

In this situation the flow rate has to be decreased from 20 gtt/min to 17 gtt/min. Although the I.V. is ahead of schedule, it also requires assessment of the client's ability.

Practice Problems

27. An I.V. of 500 cc was ordered to infuse in 8 hours using a drop factor of 15 gtt/mL. After 5 hours you find 250 cc of fluid left. Recalculate the flow rate in gtt/min.

28. 250 cc of I.V. fluid was to infuse in 3 hours using 15 gtt/mL. With 1 1/2 hours remaining, you find 200 cc left. Recalculate the flow rate in gtt/min.

This concludes the chapter on I.V. calculation.

Points to Remember:

✔ Calculation of gtt/min can be done using $\dfrac{V_1}{T_1} \times \dfrac{V_2}{T_2} = $ gtt/min

✔ For the nurse to calculate I.V. flow rate she must have the volume of solution, the time factor, and the drop factor of the tubing.

✔ Microdrops always deliver 60 gtt/mL.

✔ Macrodrops differ according to manufacturer. They can deliver 10, 15, or 20 gtt/mL.

✔ I.V. flow rates must be monitored by the nurse. When I.V. solutions are behind or ahead of schedule, the flow rate must be recalculated.

✔ Never increase an I.V. flow rate without recalculating or assessing a client to determine if they can tolerate a rate increase.

✔ Read I.V. labels carefully to determine whether the correct solution is being administered.

Chapter Review

Calculate the I.V. flow rate in gtt/min for the following I.V. administrations, unless another unit of measure is stated.

1. 1000 mL D5 Ringers Lactate to infuse in 8 hours. The administration set is 20 gtt/mL.

2. 2500 mL D5 0.9% Normal Saline to infuse in 24 hours. The administration set is 10 gtt/mL.

3. 500 mL D5W to infuse in 4 hours. The administration set is 15 gtt/mL.

4. 300 mL 0.9% Normal Saline to infuse in 6 hours. The administration set is 60 gtt/mL.

5. 1000 mL D5W for 24 hours KVO (keep vein open). The administration set is 60 gtt/mL.

6. 1000 mL D5 0.45% Normal Saline with 20 mEq KCl over 12 hours. The administration set is 10 gtt/mL.

7. 1000 mL Ringers Lactate to infuse in 10 hours. The administration set is 20 gtt/mL.

8. 1500 mL Normal Saline to infuse in 12 hours. The administration set is 10 gtt/mL.

9. A unit of whole blood (500 mL) to infuse in 4 hours. The administration set is 10 gtt/mL.

10. A unit of packed cells (250 mL) to infuse in 3 hours. The administration set is 10 gtt/mL.

11. 1500 mL D5W in 8 hours. The administration set is 20 gtt/mL.

12. 3000 mL Ringers Lactate in 24 hours. The administration set is 15 gtt/mL.

13. Infuse 2 L of Ringers Lactate in 24 hours. The administration set is 15 gtt/mL.

14. 1000 mL D5W with 10 mEq KCl to infuse in 7 hours. The administration set is 10 gtt/mL.

15. 500 mL D5W in 4 hours. The administration set is 60 gtt/mL.

16. 1000 mL D5 0.45% Normal Saline in 6 hours. The administration set delivers 20 gtt/mL.

17. 250 mL D5W in 8 hours. The administration set delivers 60 gtt/mL.

18. 1 L of 5% Dextrose in water to infuse at 50 mL/hr. The administration set is 60 gtt/mL.

19. 2 L of D5 Ringers Lactate at 150 mL/hr. The administration set is 15 gtt/mL.

20. 500 mL D5W in 6 hours. The administration set is 12 gtt/mL.

21. 1500 mL 0.9% Normal Saline in 12 hours. The administration set is 10 gtt/mL.

22. 1500 mL D5W in 24 hours. The administration set is 12 gtt/mL.

23. 2000 mL D5W in 16 hours. The administration set is 20 gtt/mL.

24. 500 mL D5W in 8 hours. The administration set is 15 gtt/mL.

25. 250 mL D5W in 10 hours. The administration set is 60 gtt/mL.

26. Infuse 300 mL of 5% D/W at 75 mL/hr. The administration set is 60 gtt/mL.

27. Infuse 125 mL/hr of D5 Ringers Lactate. The administration set is 20 gtt/mL.

28. Infuse 40 mL/hr of D5W. The administration set is 60 gtt/mL.

29. Infuse an I.V. medication with a volume of 50 mL in 45 minutes. The administration set is a microdrip.

30. Infuse 90 mL/hr of 0.9% Normal Saline. The administration set delivers 15 gtt/mL.

31. Infuse 150 mL/hr of D5 Ringers Lactate. The administration set delivers 10 gtt/mL.

32. Infuse 3000 mL of D5W in 24 hours. The administration set delivers 15 gtt/mL.

33. Infuse an I.V. medication with a volume of 50 mL in 40 minutes. The administration set delivers 10gtt/mL.

34. Infuse 100mL of an I.V. with medication in 30 minutes. The administration set delivers 20 gtt/mL.

35. Infuse 250 mL of 0.45% Normal Saline in 5 hours. The administration set delivers 20 gtt/mL.

36. Infuse 1000 mL of D5W at 80 mL/hr. The administration set delivers 20 gtt/mL.

37. Infuse 150 mL of D5 Ringers Lactate in 30 minutes. The administration set delivers 12 gtt/mL.

38. Infuse Kefzol 0.5 g in 50 mL D5W in 30 minutes. The administration set is a microdrip.

39. Infuse Plasmanate 500 mL over 3 hours. The administration set delivers 10 gtt/mL.

40. Infuse Albumin 250 mL over 2 hours. The administration set delivers 15gtt/mL.

41. The doctor orders the following I.V.s for 24 hours.
    The administration set delivers 10 gtt/mL.
    1000 cc D5W with 1 ampule MVI (multivitamin).
    500 cc D5W.
    250 cc D5W.

42. Infuse Vancomycin 1 g IVPB in 150 mL D5W in 1.5 hours. The administration set is a microdrip.

43. If 2 L of D5W is to infuse in 16 hours, how many mL are to be administered per hour?

44. If 500 mL of Ringers Lactate is to infuse in 4 hours, how many mL are to be administered per hour?

45. If 200 mL of 0.9% Normal Saline is to infuse in 2 hours, how many mL are to be administered per hour?

46. If 500 mL of 5% D/W is to infuse in 8 hours, how many mL are to be administered per hour?

47. Infuse 500 mL Intralipids I.V. in 6 hours. The administration set delivers 10 gtt/mL.

48. Infuse a Hyperalimentation solution of 1100 mL in 12 hours. The administration set delivers 20 gtt/mL.

49. Infuse 3000 mL D5W in 20 hours. The administration set delivers 20 gtt/mL.

50. An I.V. of 500 mL D5W with 200 mg of Minocycline is to infuse in 6 hours. The administration set delivers 10 gtt/mL.

51. An I.V. of D5W 500 mL was ordered to infuse over 10 hours at a rate of 13 gtt/min. The administration set delivers 15 gtt/mL. After 3 hours you notice that 300 mL of I.V. solution is left. Recalculate the gtt/min for the remaining solution.

52. An I.V. of D5W 1000 mL was ordered to infuse over 8 hours at a rate of 42 gtt/min. The administration set delivers 20 gtt/mL. After 4 hours you notice only 400 mL has infused. Recalculate the gtt/min for the remaining solution.

53. An I.V. of 1000 mL D5 0.45% Normal Saline has been ordered to infuse at 125 mL/hr. The administration set delivers 15 gtt/mL. The I.V. was hung at 7 AM. At 11 AM you check the I.V. and there is 400 mL left. Recalculate the gtt/min for the remaining solution.

54. An I.V. of 500 mL of Normal Saline is to infuse in 6 hours at a rate of 14 gtt/min. The administration set delivers 10 gtt/mL. The I.V. was started at 7 AM. You check the I.V. at 8 AM and 250 mL has infused. Recalculate the gtt/min for the remaining solution.

55. An I.V. of 1000 cc D5W is to infuse in 10 hours. The administration set delivers 15 gtt/mL. The I.V. was started at 4 AM. At 10 AM 600 mL remain in the bag. Is the I.V. on time? If not recalculate the gtt/min for the remaining solution.

56. 900 mL of Ringers Lactate is infusing at a rate of 80 gtt/min. The administration set delivers 15 gtt/mL. How long will it take for the I.V. to infuse?

57. A client is receiving 1000 mL of D5W at 100 cc/hr. How many hours will it take for the I.V. to infuse?

58. 1000 mL of D5W is infusing at 20 gtt/min. The administration set delivers 10 gtt/mL. How long will it take for the I.V. to infuse? (Express time in hours and minutes.)

59. 450 mL of 0.9% Normal Saline is infusing at 25 gtt/min. The administration set delivers 20 gtt/mL. How long will it take for the I.V. to infuse?

60. 100 mL of D5W is infusing at 10 gtt/min. The administration set delivers 15 gtt/cc. How many hours will it take for the I.V. to infuse?

61. An I.V. is regulated at 25 gtt/min. The administration set delivers 15 gtt/mL. How many mL of fluid will the client receive in 8 hours?

62. An I.V. is regulated at 40 gtt/min. The administration set delivers 60 gtt/mL. How many mL of fluid will the client receive in 10 hours?

63. An I.V. is regulated at 30 gtt/min. The administration set delivers 15 gtt/mL. How many mL of fluid will the client receive in 5 hours?

64. 10 mEq of Potassium chloride is placed in 500 mL of D5W to be administered at the rate of 2 mEq per hour.
    a) How many mL of solution is needed to administer 2 mEq?
    b) Calculate the gtt/min to deliver 2 mEq per hour. The administration set delivers 20 gtt/mL.

65. 30 mEq of Potassium chloride is added to 1000 mL of D5W to be administered at the rate of 4 mEq per hour.
    a) How many mL of solution is needed to administer 4 mEq?
    b) Calculate the gtt/min to deliver 4 mEq per hour. The administration set delivers 15 gtt/mL.

66. Doctor's order: Regular insulin 7 U. per hour. The I.V. solution contains 50 U. of Regular insulin in 250 mL of 0.9% Normal Saline. How many mL/hr should the I.V. infuse at?

67. Doctor's order: Regular insulin 18 U. per hour. The I.V. solution contains 100 U. of Regular insulin in 250 mL of 0.9% Normal Saline. How many mL/hr should the I.V. infuse at?

68. Doctor's order: 11 U. per hour of Regular insulin. The I.V. solution contains 100 U. of Regular insulin in 100 mL of Normal Saline. How many mL/hr should the I.V. infuse at?

69. Infuse 150 mL Gentamicin IVPB over 1 hour. The administration set delivers 10 gtt/mL. How many gtt/min should the I.V. infuse at?

70. Infuse Ampicillin 1g that has been diluted in 40 mL D5W in 40 minutes using a microdrip set. How many gtt/min should the I.V. infuse at?

71. Administer I.V. medication with a volume of 35 mL in 30 minutes using a microdrip set. How many gtt/min should the I.V. infuse at?

72. Administer I.V. medication with a volume of 80 mL in 40 minutes using an administration set that delivers 15 gtt/mL. How many gtt/min would you infuse?

73. Administer 50 mL of an antibiotic in 25 minutes. The administration set delivers 10 gtt/mL. How many gtt/min would you regulate the I.V. at?

74. An I.V. is to infuse at 65 mL/hr. The administration set delivers 15 gtt/mL. How many gtt/min should infuse?

21 Heparin Calculations

Objectives

After reviewing this chapter the student will be able to do the following:

1. State the importance of calculating Heparin dosages
2. Calculate Heparin dosages being administered I.V.
3. Calculate s.c. doses of Heparin

Heparin is a potent anticoagulant that prevents clot formation and blood coagulation. The therapeutic range for Heparin is determined individually by monitoring the client's PTT (Partial Thromboplastin Time).

Heparin is always measured in Units and can be administered intravenously or subcutaneously. When given I.V. Heparin is ordered in units per hour. Heparin comes in different strengths, therefore it is important to read labels carefully when administering it (Figure 21.1).

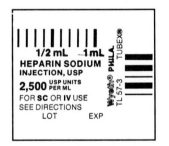 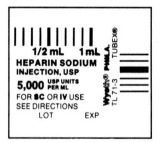

Figure 21.1 Heparin labels **A,** Heparin Sodium 2500 Units/mL (From Smith: *Dosages and solutions calculations,* St Louis, 1989, Mosby.) **B,** Heparin Sodium 5000 Units/mL (From Smith: *Dosages and solutions calculations,* St Louis, 1989, Mosby.)

Calculation of s.c. Dosages

Heparin is administered s.c. using a Tuberculin syringe to ensure accurate dosage. The same methods of calculating that were presented earlier are used to calculate s.c. Heparin, except that the dosage is never rounded off.

Example 1:   Doctor's order: Heparin 7500 U. s.c.
Available: Heparin labeled 10,000 U/mL.
What will you administer to the client?

Set-up:

1. No conversion is necessary. There is no conversion for Units.

2. Think – what would a logical dose be?

3. Set up in ratio-proportion or formula and solve.

Solution Using Ratio-Proportion:

$$10,000 \text{ U. : } 1\text{mL} = 7500 \text{ U. : } x \text{ mL}$$

$$10,000x = 7500$$

$$x = \frac{7500}{10,000}$$

$$x = 0.75 \text{ mL}$$

Solution Using Formula:

$$\frac{7500 \text{ U.}}{10,000 \text{ U.}} \times 1 \text{ mL} = x$$

$$x = 0.75 \text{ mL}$$

The dosage of 0.75 mL is reasonable since the available dosage is less than what is available. Therefore less than 1 cc would be needed to administer the dose. This dose can only be measured accurately using a Tuberculin syringe. This dosage would not be rounded to the nearest tenth of a mL. A Tuberculin syringe is shown below illustrating the dosage to be administered (Figure 21.2).

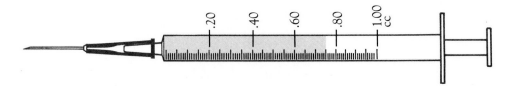

Figure 21.2 Tuberculin syringe illutstrating 0.75 mL drawn up (From Dison: *Simplified drugs and solutions for nurses*, ed 10, St Louis, 1992, Mosby.)

Calculation of I.V. Heparin Solutions

1. Calculating mL/hr of Heparin – This can be done by using a ratio-proportion.

> **Example:** An I.V. solution of Heparin is ordered for a client. D₅W 1000 mL containing 20,000 U. of Heparin is to infuse at 30 mL/hr. Calculate the dosage of Heparin the client is to receive per hour.

Set up a proportion:

$$20{,}000 \text{ U.} : 1000 \text{ mL} = x \text{ U.} : 30 \text{ mL}$$

$$1000 \, x = 20{,}000 \times 30$$

$$\frac{1000 \, x}{1000} = \frac{600{,}000}{1000} = 600 \text{ U/hr}$$

2. Calculating hourly dosages when given the set calibration and flow rate.

> **Example:** A client is receiving 12,500 U. of Heparin in 250 mL of D₅W. The set calibration is 15 gtt/mL, and the flow rate is 30 gtt/min. Calculate the hourly dosage the client is receiving. This is solved using a series of steps.

First – Convert the drops per minute to mL/min.

$$15 \text{ gtt} : 1\text{mL} = 30 \text{ gtt} : x \text{ mL}$$

$$\frac{15 \, x}{15} = \frac{30}{15}$$

$$x = 2 \text{ mL/min}$$

Then – Convert mL/min to mL/hr

$$2 \text{ mL/min} \times 60 \text{ min} = 120 \text{ mL/hr}$$

After doing these steps the proportion can be set up to calculate the units per hour that were illustrated.

$$12{,}500 \text{ U.} : 250 \text{ mL} = x \text{ U.} : 120 \text{ mL}$$

$$250 \, x = 1{,}500{,}000$$

$$x = 6000 \text{ U/hr}$$

The client is receiving 6000 U. of Heparin per hour.

Since I.V. Heparin is ordered in Units per hour, after calculating the mL/hr another calculation must be done to determine the flow rate.

Example 1:   Infuse 8000 U/hr of Heparin from a solution containing 20,000 U. in 250 cc D5W. The administration set delivers 10 gtt/mL.

First calculate mL/hr to be administered:

$$20{,}000 \text{ U.} \; : \; 250 \text{ mL} \; = \; 8000 \text{ U.} \; : \; x \text{ mL}$$

$$20{,}000 \, x \; = \; 8000 \times 250$$

$$\frac{20{,}000}{20{,}000} x \; = \; \frac{2{,}000{,}000}{20{,}000} \; = \; 100 \text{ mL/hr}$$

Then calculate the flow rate in gtt/min:

$$\frac{100 \text{ mL}}{1 \text{ hr}} \times \frac{10 \text{ gtt/mL}}{60 \text{ min}} \; = \; 16.6$$

Answer: 17 gtt/min

This concludes the chapter on Heparin.

Points to Remember:

✔ Dosages of Heparin must be accurately calculated.

✔ Heparin dosages are administered s.c. and I.V.

✔ When being administered I.V., calculations involving Heparin may involve a series of steps.

✔ The method of calculating I.V. Heparin dosages can also be used to calculate I.V. doses of other medications.

Chapter Review

For questions 1 through 12 calculate the dose of Heparin you will administer, and shade the dosage in on the syringes provided. Questions 13 through 40 calculate the units as indicated by the problem. Use labels where provided to calculate dosages.

1. Doctor's order: Heparin 3500 U. s.c. o.d.
   Available:

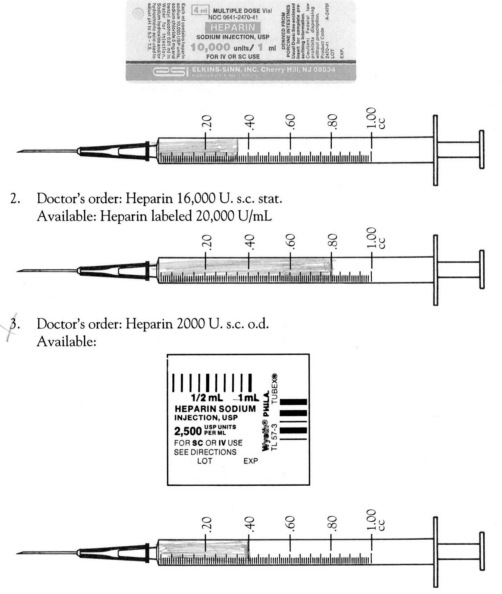

2. Doctor's order: Heparin 16,000 U. s.c. stat.
   Available: Heparin labeled 20,000 U/mL

3. Doctor's order: Heparin 2000 U. s.c. o.d.
   Available:

4. Doctor's order: Heparin 2000 U. s.c. o.d.
    Available

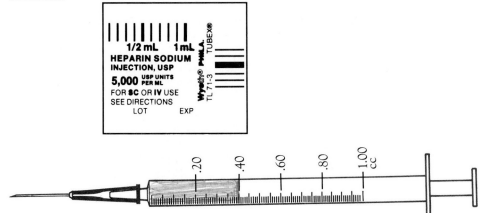

5. Prepare a dosage of 500 U. of Heparin
    Available:

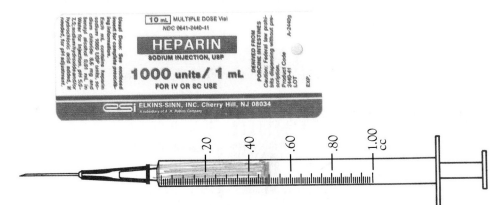

6. Doctor's order: Heparin flush 10 U. q shift to flush a Heparin lock.
    Available:

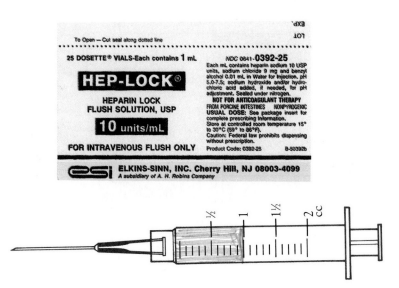

7. Doctor's order: Heparin 50,000 U. in D5W 500 mL.
    Available:

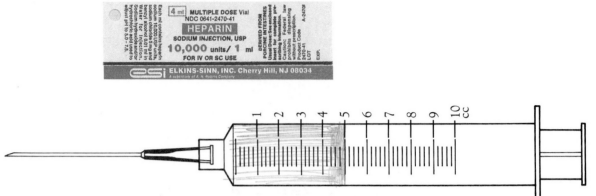

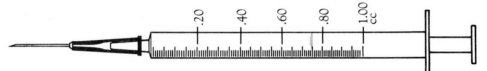

8. Doctor's order: Heparin 15,000 U. s.c. o.d.
    Available: Heparin labeled 20,000 U/mL

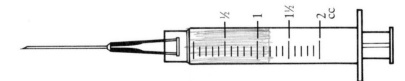

9. Doctor's order: 3000 U. of Heparin to a liter of I.V. solution.
    Available:

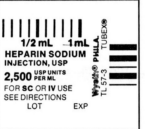

10. Doctor's order: Heparin 17,000 U. s.c. o.d.
    Available: Heparin labeled 20,000 U/mL.

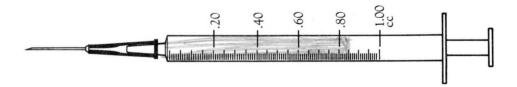

11.   Doctor's order: Heparin bolus of 8500 U. I.V. stat.
       Available:

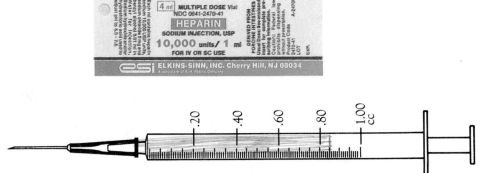

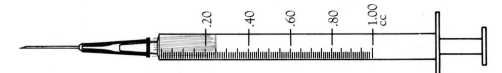

12.   Doctor's order: Heparin 2500 U. s.c. q6h.
       Available: Heparin labeled 10,000 U/mL.

13.   Doctor's order: Heparin 2000 U/hr I.V. You have 25,000 U. per 1000 mL of 0.9%
       Normal Saline. How many mL per hour will deliver 2000 U/hr?

14.   Doctor's order: Heparin 1500 U/hr I.V. Available 25,000 U. per 500 mL of D5W.
       How many mL per hour will deliver 1500 U/hr?

15.   Doctor's order: Heparin 1800 U/hr I.V. Available 25,000 U. per 250 mL of D5W.
       How many mL/hr will deliver 1800 U/hr?

16.   Doctor's order: Add 40,000 U. Heparin to 1 L Normal Saline and infuse at 25 mL/hr.
       Calculate the hourly Heparin dosage.

17.   Doctor's order : Add Heparin 25,000 U. to 250 cc D5W and infuse at 11 mL/hr.
       Calculate the hourly Heparin dosage.

18.   Doctor's order: Add 40,000 U. Heparin to 500 mL D5W and infuse at 30 mL/hr.
       Calculate the hourly Heparin dosage.

19.   Doctor's order: Add 20,000 U. to 500 mL D5W to infuse at 12 mL/hr. Calculate the
       hourly Heparin dosage.

20.   Doctor's order: Add Heparin 25,000 U. to 500 cc D5W to infuse at 15 mL/hr.
       Calculate the hourly Heparin dosage.

21.   Doctor's order: Infuse 1 L of Normal Saline with 40,000 U. Heparin over 24 hours.
       The administration set delivers 15 gtt/mL. Calculate the hourly dose of Heparin.
       Calculate the gtt/min.

22.   Doctor's order: Infuse 1 L of D5W with 15,000 U. Heparin over 10 hours.
       Calculate mL/hr and U/hr being administered.

23. Doctor's order: Infuse 20 mL/hr of 1 Liter of D_5W with 35,000 U. of Heparin. Calculate the hourly dosage and gtt/min using a microdrop administration set.

24. Doctor's order: Infuse 500 mL of Normal Saline with 10,000 U. Heparin at 20 gtt/min. The administration set delivers 10 gtt/mL. Calculate the mL/hr and the hourly unit dose the client is receiving.

25. Doctor's order: Infuse 500 mL of D_5W with 25,000 U. Heparin at 25 mL/hr. Calculate the hourly unit dose of Heparin.

26. Doctor's order: Infuse 500 mL of D_5W with 20,000 U. Heparin at 40 mL/hr. Calculate the hourly unit dosage.

27. Doctor's order: Infuse 1400 U/hr of Heparin I.V. Heparin 40,000 U. is in 1000 mL of D_5W. The administration set delivers 15 gtt/mL. Calculate the mL/hr and gtt/min.

28. Doctor's order: Infuse 1000 U/hr of Heparin I.V. Heparin 40,000 U. is in 1 L of Normal Saline. The administration set delivers 15 gtt/mL. Calculate mL/hr and gtt/min.

29. Doctor's order: Administer 1000 U. Heparin I.V. every hour. Solution available is 25,000 U. of Heparin in 500 mL D_5W. The administration set is a microdrip. Calculate the gtt/min.

30. Doctor's order: Administer 2000 U. Heparin I.V. every hour. The solution available is 25,000 U. of Heparin in 1 L Normal Saline. The administration set delivers 15 gtt/mL. Calculate the gtt/min.

31. A client is receiving an I.V. of 1000 mL of D_5W with 50,000 U. Heparin infusing at 15 gtt/min. The administration set delivers 15 gtt/mL. Calculate the hourly dose of Heparin the client is receiving.

32. A client is receiving an I.V. of 250 mL Normal Saline with 25,000 U. Heparin at 20 gtt/min. The administration set delivers 10 gtt/mL. Calculate the hourly dose of Heparin.

33. A client is receiving 500 mL of D_5W with 20,000 U. of Heparin at 20 gtt/min. The administration set is a microdrip. Calculate the hourly dose of Heparin.

34. A client is receiving an I.V. of 25,000 U. Heparin in 1 L of D_5W infusing at 14 gtt/min. The administration set delivers 15 gtt/mL. Calculate the hourly dose of Heparin.

35. A client is receiving an I.V. at 1000 mL D_5W with 20,000 U. Heparin infusing at 24 gtt/min. The administration set delivers 10 gtt/mL. Calculate the hourly dosage of Heparin.

Directions: Calculate the following hourly dosages of Heparin.

36.   Order: 30,000 U. of Heparin in 500 mL of D₅W to infuse at 25 mL/hr.

37.   Order: 20,000 U. of Heparin in 1 L of D₅W to infuse at 40 mL/hr.

38.   Order: 40,000 U. of Heparin in 500 mL Normal Saline to infuse at 25 mL/hr.

39.   Order: 35,000 U. of Heparin in 1 L of D₅W to infuse at 20 mL/hr.

40.   Order: 25,000 U. of Heparin in 1 L of D₅W to infuse at 30 mL/hr.

22 Critical Care Calculations

Objectives

After reviewing this chapter the student will be able to do the following:

1. Calculate dosage in mcg/min, mcg/hour, and mg/min
2. Calculate dosage in mg/kg/hr, mg/kg/min, and mcg/kg/min

This chapter will provide the basic information on medicated intravenous drips and titration. Critically ill clients receive medications that are potent and require close monitoring. Because of the potency of the medications and their tendency to induce changes in blood pressure and heart rate, accurate calculation of dosages is essential. Medications in the critical care area can be ordered by mL/hr, gtt/min, mcg/kg/min, or mg/hr. Infusion pumps and volume control devices are usually used to administer these medications. The process of administering calculated doses of potent drugs is referred to as *titration*. Examples of medicated I.V. drips that require titration are Aramine, Nitroprusside, Levophed, and Epinephrine.

Points to Remember:

✔ When calculating dosages to be administered without any type of electronic infusion pumps always use microgtt tubing (60 gtt = 1cc). This is preferred because the drops are smaller, so more accurate titration is possible.

✔ Calculate dosages accurately. Double-checking math calculations helps to ensure a proper dosage.

✔ Obtain an accurate weight of your client.

✔ Before determining mL/hr or gtt/min calculate the dosage first.

Calculating Critical Care Dosages per Hour or per Minute

Example 1:   Infuse Dopamine 400 mg in 500 mL D5W at 30 mL/hr.
Calculate the dosage in mcg/min and mcg/hr.

Solution:

A. Use ratio-proportion to determine the dosage per hour first.

$$400 \text{ mg} : 500 \text{ mL} = x \text{ mg} : 30 \text{ mL}$$
$$\text{known} \qquad\qquad \text{unknown}$$

$$500\,x = 400 \times 30$$

$$500\,x = 12000$$

$$x = \frac{12000}{500}$$

$$x = 24 \text{ mg/hr}$$

B. The next step is to convert 24 mg to mcg since the question asked for mcg/min and mcg/hr. Change mg to mcg by using the equivalent 1000 mcg = 1 mg. To change mg to mcg multiply by 1000 or move the decimals three places to the right, since it's a metric measure.

$$24 \text{ mg} = 24000 \text{ mcg/hr.}$$

C. Now that you have the mcg per hour, the next step is to change mcg/hr to mcg/min. This is done by dividing the number of mcg/hr by 60 (60 minutes = 1 hour).

$$24,000 \text{ mcg/hr} \div 60 = 400 \text{ mcg/min.}$$

Remember accurate math is essential since these medications are extremely potent.

Drugs Ordered in Milligrams per Minute

Drugs such as Lidocaine and Pronestyl are ordered in mg/min.

Example 2:   A client is receiving Pronestyl at 60 mL/hr. The solution available is Pronestyl 2 g in 500 mL D5W. Calculate the mg/hr and the mg/min the client will receive.

A. A conversion is necessary; g has to be converted to mg. This is what you are being asked for (mg/min, mg/hr).

To convert g to mg use the equivalent 1 g = 1000 mg.

Therefore 2 g = 2000 mg (1000 × 2).

   B. Now determine the mg/hr by setting up a proportion.

$$2000 \text{ mg} : 500 \text{ mL} = x \text{ mg} : 60 \text{ mL}$$

$$500 \, x = 2000 \times 60$$

$$500 \, x = 120,000$$

$$x = 240 \text{ mg/hr}$$

   C. Convert mg/hr to mg/min.

$$240 \text{ mg/hr} \div 60 = 4 \text{ mg/min}.$$

Calculating Dosages Based on mcg/kg/min

Drugs are also ordered for clients based on dosage per kg per minute. These drugs include Nipride, Dopamine, and Dobutamine for example.

   Example 3:   Doctor's order: Dopamine 2 mcg/kg/min. The solution available is 400 mg in 250 cc D5W. The client weighs 150 pounds.

   A. Convert the client's weight in lb to kg.

$$2.2 \text{ lb} = 1 \text{ kg}.$$

To convert the client's weight divide 150 pounds by 2.2.

$$150 \text{ lb} \div 2.2 = 68.18 \text{ kg} = 68 \text{ kg}.$$

   B. Now that you have the client's weight in kg, determine the dosage per minute.

$$68 \text{ kg} \times 2 \text{ mcg} = 136 \text{ mcg/min}.$$

Points to Remember:

✔ Always calculate dosages first, and check your answers for accuracy.

✔ The safest way to administer medications is by an infusion device, however when not available use microgtt tubing (60 gtt = 1 mL).

Practice Problems

1. Doctor orders Epinephrine at 30 mL/hr. Solution available is 2 mg in 250 cc D5W. Calculate the mg/hr, mcg/hr, and mcg/min.

2. Aminophylline 0.25 g is added to 500 cc D5W to infuse in 8 hours. Calculate mg/hr and mg/min that the client will receive.

3. The doctor orders Pitocin at 15 microdrops per minute. The solution contains 10 U. Pitocin in 1000 cc D5W. Calculate the number of Units per hour the client is receiving.

4. Doctor's order: 3 mcg/kg/min of Nipride.
   Solution available: 50 mg of Nipride in 250 mL D5W. Client's weight 60 kg. Calculate the flow rate in mL/hr that will deliver this dosage.

5. A Nitroglycerine drip is infusing at 3 mL/hr. Available solution is 50 mg in 250 cc D5W. How many mcg/hr and mcg/min is the client receiving?

Chapter Review

Calculate the dosages as indicated. Use the labels where provided.

1. Client is receiving Isuprel at 30 mL/hr. Solution is available in 2 mg of Isuprel in 250 mL D5W. Calculate mg/hr, mcg/hr, and mcg/min.

2. Client is receiving Epinephrine at 40 mL/hr. Solution is available in 4 mg of Epinephrine in 500 mL D5W. Calculate mg/hr, mcg/hr, and mcg/min.

3. Infuse Dopamine 800 mg in 500 mL D5W at 30 mL/hr. Calculate the dosage in mcg/min and mcg/hr. Calculate the number of mL you will add to the I.V. for this dose.

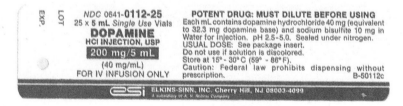

4. Infuse Nipride at 30 mL/hr. The solution available is 50 mg Nipride in D5W 250 mL. Calculate mcg/hr and mcg/min.

5.   Doctor's Order: 100 mg Aramine in 250 mL D5W to infuse at 25 mL/hr. Calculate the dosage in mcg/min and mcg/hr.

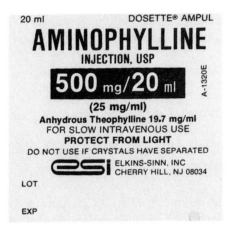

6.   Doctor's Order: Lidocaine 2 g in 250 mL D5W to infuse at 60 mL/hr. Calculate the mg/hr and mg/min the client will receive.

7.   Doctor orders: Aminophylline 0.25 g to be added to 250 mL of D5W. The order is to infuse over 6 hours. Calculate the mg/hr the client will receive.

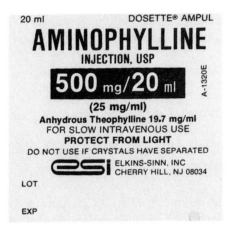

8.   A client is receiving Pronestyl at 30 mL/hr. The solution available is 2 g Pronestyl in 250 mL D5W. Calculate mg/hr and mg/min the client is receiving.

9.   Doctor orders a Pitocin (Oxytocin) drip at 45 microdrops/minute. The solution contains 20 U. Pitocin in 1000 mL D5W. Calculate the U/min and U/hr the client is receiving.

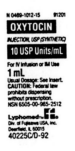

10. Doctor's Order: 30 U. Pitocin in 1000 mL D5W. Client is receiving 40 mL/hr. How many U/hr of Pitocin is the client receiving?

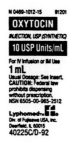

11. 30 units of Pitocin are added to 500 mL D5 R/L for an induction. The client is receiving 45 mL/hr. How many U/hr of Pitocin is the client receiving?

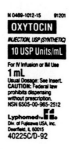

12. A client is receiving Bretylium at 30 microdrops/min. The solution available is 2 g Bretylium in 500 mL D5W. Calculate the mg/hr and mg/min the client is receiving.

13. A client is receiving Bretylium at 45 microdrops/min. The solution available is 2 g Bretylium in 500 mL D5W. Calculate mg/hr the client is receiving and mg/min.

14. A client is receiving Niroglycerine 50 mg in 250 mL D5W. The order is to infuse 400 mcg/min. How many mL/hr would be needed to deliver this amount?

15. Dopamine has been ordered to maintain a client's B/P. 400 mg Dopamine has been placed in 500 mL D5W to infuse at 35 mL/hr. How many mg are being administered per hour?

16. Doctor orders Isuprel at 30 mL/hr. The solution available is 2 mg Isuprel in 250 mL D5W. Calculate mg/hr, mcg/hr, and mcg/min the client will be receiving.

17. Doctor's Order: 1 g of Aminophylline in 1000 mL D5W to infuse over 10 hours. Calculate the mg/hr the client will receive.

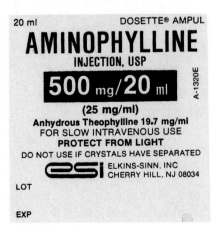

18. Ritodrine (Yutopar) 150 mg is placed in 500 cc D5W to infuse at 30 mL/hr. Calculate mg/hr the client is receiving.

19. A Lidocaine drip is infusing at 22 mL/hr. The solution available is 2 g Lidocaine in 250 mL D5W. How many mg/hr and mg/min is the client receiving?

20. Doctor's Order: Epinephrine 8 mL/hr. Available solution is Epinephrine 4 mg in 250 mL D5W. Calculate the mcg/min and mcg/hr the client is receiving.

21. Doctor's Order: Infuse Afronad at 30 mL/hr. Solution available: 500 mg Afronad in 250 mL Normal Saline. Calculate the mg/hr and mg/min that the client is receiving.

22. Infuse Dobutamine at 30 mL/hr. Dobutamine 500 mg is placed in 500 mL of D5W. Calculate the dosage in mcg/min and mcg/hr.

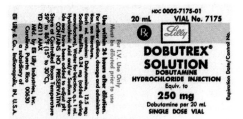

23. Doctor's Order: 2 g/hr of Magnesium Sulfate.
Solution available: 25 g, 50% Magnesium Sulfate in 300 mL D5W. How many mL/hr would be needed to administer the required dose?

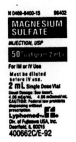

Answers

24. Doctor's Order: Infuse 200 mcg/min of Dopamine I.V. The solution available is 400 mg Dopamine in 500 mL Normal Saline. Using a volumetric pump calculate the mL/hr.

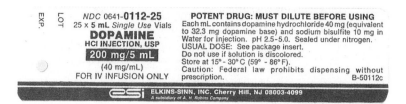

25. Doctor's Order: 3 g/hr of Magnesium Sulfate. Solution available: 25 g of 50% Magnesium Sulfate in 300 mL D5W. How many mL/hr would be needed to administer the required dose?

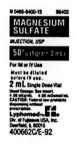

26. A client with chest pain has an order for Nitroglycerine 10 mcg/min. Solution available is 50 mg Nitroglycerine in 250 mL D5W. Calculate the I.V. rate in gtt/min using a microdrip administration set.

27. Doctor's Order: 2 mcg/kg/min of Nipride.
     Solution available: 50 mg Nipride in 250 mL D5W.
     Client's weight = 120 lb.
     Calculate the dosage per minute.

28. Doctor's Order: Infuse 500 mL of D5W with Dobutrex 250 mg at 3 mcg/kg/min. The client weighs 80 kg. How many mcg/min should the client receive?

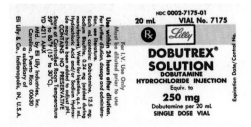

29.   Doctor's Order: Infuse 500 mL D5W with 800 mg Theophylline at 0.7 mg/kg/hr. The client weighs 73.5 kg. How many mg should this patient receive per hour?

30.   Doctor's Order: Infuse 1 g of Aminophylline in 1000 mL of D5W at 0.7 mg/kg/hr. The patient weighs 110 lb. Calculate the dosage in mg/hr and mg/min. Reference states no more than 20 mg/min. Is the order safe?

Pre-Test

1. ix, īx, IX
2. xvi, x̄vi, XVI
3. xxiii, x̄xiii, XXIII
4. xss, x̄ss
5. xxii, x̄xii, XXII
6. 11 1/2
7. 12
8. 18
9. 24
10. 6
11. 2/3
12. 1/4
13. 1/75
14. 4/5
15. 4/6 = 2/3
16. 2
17. 5 1/3
18. 23/45
19. 4 13/42
20. 18 2/3
21. 0.9
22. 0.3
23. 0.7
24. 0.9
25. 7/8
26. 11/12
27. 87.45
28. 5. 008
29. 40.112
30. 47.77
31. 1875
32. 23.7
33. 36.8
34. 0.674
35. 0.375
36. 0.6
37. x = 12
38. x = 2
39. x = 3
40. x = 0.5 or 1/2
41. 0.4
42. 0.7
43. 1.5
44. 0.74
45. 0.83
46. 1.23

	Percent	Decimal	Ratio	Fraction
47.	6%	0.06	3:50	3/50
48.	35%	0.35	7:20	7/20
49.	525%	5.25	21:4	5 1/4
50.	1.5%	0.015	3:200	3/200

Chapter 1

Answers to Practice Problems

1. xv, x̄v, XV
2. xiii, x̄iii, XIII
3. xxx, x̄xx, XXX
4. xi, x̄i, XI
5. xiv, x̄iv, XIV
6. xxix, x̄xix, XXIX
7. iv, īv, IV
8. xix, x̄ix, XIX

Answers to Chapter Review

1. vi, v̄i, VI
2. xxx, x̄xx, XXX
3. iss, īss
4. xxvii, x̄xvii, XXVII
5. xii, x̄ii, XII
6. xviii, x̄viii, XVIII
7. xx, x̄x, XX
8. iii, īii, III
9. xxi, x̄xi, XXI
10. xxvi, x̄xvi, XXVI
11. 7 1/2
12. 19
13. 15
14. 30
15. 1/2
16. 3
17. 22
18. 16
19. 5
20. 27

Chapter 2

Answers to Practice Problems

1. LCD = 30, therefore 6/30 lesser value.
2. LCD = 8, therefore 6/8 lesser value.
3. 1/150 lesser value, the denominator (150) is larger.

4. 6/18 lesser value, the numerator (6) is smaller.
5. 3/5 lesser value, the numerator (3) is smaller.
6. 1/8 lesser value, the numerator (1) is smaller.
7. 1/40 lesser value, the denominator (40) is larger.
8. 1/300 lesser value, the denominator (300) is larger.
9. 4/24 lesser value, the numerator (4) is smaller.
10. LCD = 6, therefore 1/6 lesser value.
11. LCD = 72, therefore 6/8 has the higher value.
12. LCD = 6, therefore 7/6 higher value.
13. LCD = 72, therefore 6/12 has the higher value.
14. LCD = 120, therefore 1/6 has the higher value.
15. 1/75 higher value, the denominator (75) is smaller.
16. 6/5 higher value, the numerator (6) is larger.
17. LCD = 24, therefore 4/6 has the higher value.
18. 8/9 higher value, the numerator (8) is larger.
19. LCD = 150, therefore 1/10 has the higher value.
20. 6/15 higher value, the denominator (6) is larger.

Answers

21. $\dfrac{10 \div 5}{15 \div 5} = \dfrac{2}{3}$

22. $\dfrac{7 \div 7}{49 \div 7} = \dfrac{1}{7}$

23. $\dfrac{64 \div 2}{128 \div 2} = \dfrac{32}{64} = \dfrac{1}{2}$

24. $\dfrac{100 \div 2}{150 \div 2} = \dfrac{50}{75} = \dfrac{2}{3}$

25. $\dfrac{20 \div 4}{28 \div 4} = \dfrac{5}{7}$

26. $\dfrac{14 \div 2}{98 \div 2} = \dfrac{7}{49} = \dfrac{1}{7}$

27. $\dfrac{10 \div 2}{18 \div 2} = \dfrac{5}{9}$

28. $\dfrac{24 \div 12}{36 \div 12} = \dfrac{2}{3}$

29. $\dfrac{10 \div 10}{50 \div 10} = \dfrac{1}{5}$

30. $\dfrac{9 \div 9}{27 \div 9} = \dfrac{1}{3}$

31. $\dfrac{9 \div 9}{9 \div 9} = \dfrac{1}{1} = 1$

32. $\dfrac{15 \div 15}{45 \div 15} = \dfrac{1}{3}$

33. $\dfrac{124 \div 31}{155 \div 31} = \dfrac{4}{5}$

34. $\dfrac{12 \div 6}{18 \div 6} = \dfrac{2}{3}$

35. $\dfrac{36 \div 4}{64 \div 4} = \dfrac{9}{16}$

Answers to Chapter Review

1. 1 2/8 = 1 1/4
2. 7 2/4 = 7 1/2
3. 3 4/6 = 3 2/3
4. 2 3/4
5. 4 3/14
6. 6 7/10
7. 4 1/2
8. 2 1/5
9. 4 4/15
10. 7 9/13
11. 5/2
12. 59/8
13. 43/5
14. 65/4
15. 16/5
16. 13/5
17. 84/10
18. 37/4
19. 51/4
20. 47/7
21. LCD = 30.   1 13/30
22. LCD = 24.   13/24
23. LCD = 4.   88/4 = 22
24. LCD = 10.   7/10
25. LCD = 36.   234/36 = 6 18/36
             = 6 1/2
26. LCD = 4.   1
27. LCD = 4.   3/4
28. LCD = 4.   2 2/4 = 2 1/2
29. LCD = 30.   19/30
30. 1/9

31. LCD = 20.   11/20
32. LCD = 24.   7/24
33. LCD = 6. 17/6 = 2 5/6
34. LCD = 15.   19/15 = 1 4/15
35. LCD = 21.   5/21
36. 4/36 = 1/9
37. 9 11/32
38. 14
39. 10
40. 27
41. 10/16 = 5/8
42. 2/30 = 1/15
43. 12/120 = 1/10
44. 7/27
45. 50/75 = 2/3
46. 42/75 = 14/25
47. 2/3
48. 2
49. 28/72 = 7/18
50. 24/6 = 4
51. 8/6 = 4/3 = 1 1/3
52. 1 25/50 = 1 1/2
53. 7 1/2
54. 15/300 = 1/20
55. 1

Chapter 3

Answers to Practice Problems

1. eight and thirty-five hundredths.
2. eleven and one thousandths
3. four and fifty-seven hundredths
4. five and seven ten thousandths
5. ten and five tenths
6. one hundred sixty-three thousandths
7. 0.4
8. 84.07
9. 0.07
10. 2.23
11. 0.05
12. 0.009
13. 0.5
14. 2.87
15. 0.375
16. 0.175
17. 7.35
18. 0.087
19. 18.4
20. 40.449
21. 3.95

22. 3.87
23. 2.92
24. 43.1
25. 0.035
26. 5.88
27. 0.04725
28. 0.9125
29. 9,650
30. 1.78
31. 100.8072
32. 4
33. 1.16
34. 70.88
35. 30.46
36. 0.6
37. 3.6
38. 1
39. 2
40. 3.55
41. 0.61
42. 0.74
43. 0.0005
44. 0.00004
45. 584
46. 500
47. 0.75
48. 0.555
49. 0.5
50. 3/4
51. 1/2000
52. 1/25

Answers to Chapter Review

1. 0.444
2. 0.8
3. 1.5
4. 0.2
5. 0.725
6. 9.783
7. 28.9
8. 2.743
9. 5.12
10. 2.5
11. 6.33
12. 1.5
13. 1.5
14. 15
15. 31.2
16. 0.9448
17. 1.8
18. 0.1

19. 1.43
20. 0.15
21. 0.125
22. 0.06
23. 6.5
24. 1 1/100
25. 13/200

Chapter 4

Answers to Chapter Review

1. 2 : 3
2. 1 : 9
3. 3 : 4
4. 1 : 5
5. 1 : 2
6. 1 : 5
7. 3/7
8. 2/3
9. 1/7
10. 4/3
11. 3/4
12. x = 5
13. x = 2
14. x = 4
15. x = 3.33
16. x = 4.5
17. x = 0.8
18. x = 1.33
19. x = 0.16
20. x = 0.1

Chapter 5

Answers to Practice Problems

1. 1/100
2. 1/50
3. 1/2
4. 4/5
5. 3/100
6. 0.1
7. 0.35
8. 0.5
9. 0.142
10. 0.0025
11. 1:4
12. 11:100
13. 3:4
14. 9:200

15. 1:250
16. 40%
17. 125%
18. 50%
19. 25%
20. 70%
21. 4%
22. 75%
23. 10%
24. 1%
25. 50%

Answers to Chapter Review

	Percent	Ratio	Fraction	Decimal
1.	0.25%	1:400	1/400	0.0025
2.	71%	71:100	71/100	0.71
3.	7%	7:100	7/100	0.07
4.	2%	1:50	1/50	0.02
5.	6%	3:50	3/50	0.06
6.	3.3%	1:30	1/30	0.0333
7.	61%	61:100	61/100	0.61
8.	0.7%	7:1000	7/1000	0.007
9.	5%	1:20	1/20	0.05
10.	2.5%	1:40	1/40	0.025

Post-Test

1. v, $\overline{v}$, V
2. xvii, $\overline{xvii}$, XVII
3. xxvii, $\overline{xxvii}$, XXVII
4. xxix, $\overline{xxix}$, XXIX
5. xxx, $\overline{xxx}$, XXX
6. 6 1/2
7. 24
8. 19
9. 25
10. 15
11. 1 1/3
12. 2/3
13. 3/7
14. 2/3
15. 1 3/5
16. 1 4/21
17. 1 2/9
18. 25 1/3
19. 1 22/35
20. 1 17/36
21. 1.1
22. 0.1
23. 0.1

24. 0.9
25. 2/3
26. 3/4
27. 37.70
28. 17.407
29. 105.7
30. 32.94
31. 84.8
32. 22.5
33. 0.5
34. 0.850
35. 3.002
36. 0.493
37. $x = 4$
38. $x = 2.5$
39. $x = 0.1$
40. $x = 4$
41. 0.6
42. 1
43. 1.4
44. 0.68
45. 0.83
46. 1.22

	Percent	Decimal	Ratio	Fraction
47.	10%	0.1	1:10	1/10
48.	60%	0.6	3:5	3/5
49.	66 2/3%	0.67	2:3	2/3
50.	25%	0.25	1:4	1/4

Chapter 6

Answers to Chapter Review

1. gram (g), liter (L), meter (m).
2. kilogram (kg).
3. 0.001 L.
4. a) L (liter), mL (milliliter),
    cc (cubic centimeter)
   b) g (gram), mg (milligram),
    mcg (microgram), kg (kilogram)
5. 1 g.
6. 1 cc.
7. 1 mg.
8. 1 L.
9. 10 mL.
10. mcg.
11. mL.
12. g.
13. cc.
14. 1,000 times.

15. the thousandth part of.
16. 0.6 g
17. 50 kg
18. 0.4 mg
19. 0.04 L
20. 4.2 mcg
21. 0.005 g
22. 0.06 g
23. 2.6 mL
24. 100 mL
25. 0.03 mL

Chapter 7

Answers to Chapter Review

1. gr 8 1/2, gr viiiss
2. m 3, miii
3. dr 5,ʒv
4. oz 8,ʒviii
5. qt
6. pt
7. gr 1/125
8. fʒviss, fʒv̄īss
9. fʒii, fʒīī
10. oz 5,ʒv
11. m i, m 1
12. m 60
13. fʒv̄īīī
14. fʒx̄v̄ī, fʒ16
15. fʒx̄x̄x̄īī, fʒ32
16. fʒ1/2
17. gtt
18. tablespoon
19. teaspoon

Chapter 8

Answers to Practice Problems

1. 0.6 L
2. 16 mg
3. 4000 g
4. 0.003 mg
5. 0.0003 g
6. 10 g
7. 1900 mL
8. 0.0005 kg
9. 70 mcg
10. 0.65 L
11. 40 mg

12. 0.00012 kg
13. 0.18 g
14. 1.7 L
15. 15000 g
16. 0.5 L
17. 4000 g
18. 1400 cc
19. ʒ3/4
20. ʒii, ʒ2
21. ʒiv, ʒ4
22. 1/6 tsp
23. 0.06 kg
24. 0.6 g
25. 736 mcg
26. 1.6 L
27. 15 mL
28. 180 mg
29. 0.025 mg
30. 0.0052 kg
31. 27.27 kg
32. gr 1/4
33. 20 cc (25 cc if conversion is 5 cc)
34. 300 mg
35. 210 cc
36. 1/4 qt
37. 3 tbs
38. 3 g
39. 90 mg
40. 3 mL
41. 1000 mg (900 mg if gr 1 = 60 mg)
42. 4,000 mL
43. 158.4 lbs or 158 2/5
44. 0.48 mg
45. 2400 cc

Answers to Chapter Review

1. 7 mg
2. 0.001 g
3. 6 kg
4. 0.005 L
5. 450 cc
6. ʒii, or ℥2
7. 0.2 mg
8. gr 1/60
9. ʒ3, ʒiii
10. 120 mg
11. 1500 mL
12. gr ss, or gr 1/2
13. 1600 mL
14. 103.4 or 103 2/5
15. m 15 or m 16

16. 34.09 kg
17. 8 mg
18. m 45 or m 48
19. 30 mg
20. 0.4 mg
21. 6.17 kg
22. 40 tsp (50 tsp if conversion is 4 cc)
23. 46.36 kg
24. 0.204 kg
25. 1500 cc
26. 0.2 mg
27. 48,600 cc
28. 700 cc
29. 165 mL
30. 20 cc
31. 240 mg
32. 30 mL
33. 8 mL
34. gr 3/4
35. 3 g
36. 600 mL
37. 150 mg
38. 22.5 mg
39. 600 mg
40. 8.8 lbs or 8 2/5 lbs
41. 3,250 mcg
42. ℥iiss, or ℥2 1/2
43. 0.5 mg
44. 6,653 mg
45. 4000 mg
46. 0.036 g
47. 800 mg
48. gr 135, or gr cxxxv
49. gr 1/120
50. 2 L

Chapter 9

Answers to Chapter Review

1. drug, dose, client, route, time
2. identification band, asking the name, getting a staff member to help identify the client.
3. three
4. after
5. parenteral

Chapter 10

Answers to Chapter Review

1. the name of the client.
2. the date and time the order was written.
3. name of the medication.
4. dosage of medication.
5. route by which medication is to be administered.
6. time/and or frequency of administration.
7. signature of person writing the order.
8. twice a day.
9. both eyes.
10. as desired.
11. subcutaneous.
12. with.
13. before meals.
14. four times a day.
15. twice a week.
16. hours of sleep (bedtime).
17. once a day.
18. elixir.
19. left eye.
20. syrup.
21. nothing by mouth.
22. sublingual.
23. p.c., $\overline{pc}$
24. t.i.d., tid
25. I.M., IM
26. q.8.h., q8h
27. supp
28. I.V., IV
29. s.o.s., sos
30. s, $\overline{s}$
31. stat, STAT
32. O.D.
33. ung, oint
34. ss, $\overline{ss}$
35. mEq
36. q.h.s., qhs
37. p.r., pr
38. Give 0.2 milligrams of Methergine orally (by mouth) every four hours for six doses.
39. Give 0.125 milligrams of Digoxin orally (by mouth) once a day.
40. Give Regular Humulin Insulin 14 Units by subcutaneous injection every day at 7:30 a.m.
41. Give Demerol 50 milligrams by intramuscular injection and Atropine grains 1/150 by intramuscular injection on call to the operating room.
42. Give Ampicillin 500 milligrams orally (by mouth) immediately and then 250 milligrams four times a day thereafter.
43. Give Lasix 40 milligrams by intramuscular injection immediately.
44. Give Librium 50 milligrams orally (by mouth) every four hours when necessary for agitation.
45. Give two 20 milliequivalent doses of Potassium Chloride intravenously x 2L. (20 mEq per 2000 cc)
46. Give Tylenol 10 grains orally (by mouth) every four hours whenever necessary for pain.
47. Give Mylicon 80 milligrams orally (by mouth) after meals and at bedtime.
48. Give Folic Acid 1 milligram orally (by mouth) once a day (every day).
49. Give Nembutal 100 milligrams orally (by mouth) at bedtime when necessary/required.
50. Give Aspirin ten grains orally (by mouth) every four hours when necessary/required for temperature greater than 101.
51. Give Dilantin 100 milligrams orally (by mouth) three times a day.
52. Give Minipress orally (by mouth) two times a day. Hold for systolic blood pressure less than 120.
53. Give Compazine 10 milligrams by intramuscular injection every four hours as needed/required for nausea and vomiting.
54. Give four one gram doses of Ampicillin intravenous piggyback every six hours.
55. Give Heparin 5,000 Units by subcutaneous injection every twelve hours.
56. Give Dilantin suspension 200 milligrams every morning and 300 milligrams at bedtime through a nasogastric tube.
57. Give Benadryl 50 milligrams orally (by mouth) immediately.
58. route of administration.
59. fequency/time interval of administration.
60. dosage of medication (drug).
61. name of medication (drug).
62. dosage of medication (drug), and route of administration.

Chapter 11

Answer to Exercise in Transcribing (Fig. 11-11)

MONTEFIORE MEDICAL CENTER
JACK D. WEILER HOSPITAL OF THE ALBERT EINSTEIN COLLEGE OF MEDICINE DIVISION
STANDING ORDERS MEDICATION RECORD

INIT.	SIGNATURE	INIT.	SIGNATURE	INIT.	SIGNATURE
D.G.	Deborah C. Gray				

A D D R E S S O G R A P H

DRUG SENSITIVITIES	☒ NONE KNOWN	DATE 4-9-92	DATE	DATE	DATE	DATE	DATE	DATE	☐ PATIENT DISCHARGED
MEDICATIONS		TIME AND INITIALS	TIME AND INITIALS	TIME AND INITIALS	TIME AND INITIALS	TIME AND INITIALS	TIME AND INITIALS	TIME AND INITIALS	

1
DRUG Potassium chloride DOSE 20 mEq
FREQUENCY Qd x LOS ADMINISTRATIVE TIMES 9A ROUTE P.O.
DATE ORDERED 4-9-92
Time: 9A

2
DRUG Digoxin DOSE 0.125 mg.
FREQUENCY Qd x LOS ADMINISTRATIVE TIMES 9A ROUTE P.O.
DATE ORDERED 4-9-92
Time: 9A

3
DRUG Lasix DOSE 30 mg
FREQUENCY bid x LOS ADMINISTRATIVE TIMES 9A-5P ROUTE P.O.
DATE ORDERED 4-9-92
Time: 9A 5P

4
DRUG Aldomet DOSE 500 mg
FREQUENCY bid x LOS ADMINISTRATIVE TIMES 9A-5P ROUTE P.O.
DATE ORDERED 4-9-92
Time: 9A 5P

5
DRUG DOSE
FREQUENCY ADMINISTRATIVE TIMES ROUTE
DATE ORDERED

6
DRUG DOSE
FREQUENCY ADMINISTRATIVE TIMES ROUTE
DATE ORDERED

7
DRUG DOSE
FREQUENCY ADMINISTRATIVE TIMES ROUTE
DATE ORDERED

S T A N D I N G O R D E R S

DATE	TIME	DRUG	REASON NOT GIVEN	DATE	TIME	DRUG	REASON NOT GIVEN

NR 1586E 1/89   **CHART COPY**

Chapter 11

Answer to Exercise in Transcribing (Fig. 11-12)

MONTEFIORE MEDICAL CENTER
HOSPITAL OF THE ALBERT EINSTEIN COLLEGE OF MEDICINE DIVISION

PRE-OP, STAT AND PRN MEDICATION RECORD

INIT.	SIGNATURE	INIT.	SIGNATURE	INIT.	SIGNATURE
DG	Deborah C. Gray				

DRUG SENSITIVITIES ☐ NONE KNOWN	DATE 4·9·92	DATE	DATE	DATE	DATE	DATE	DATE	☐ PATIENT DISCHARGED
MEDICATIONS	TIME AND INITIALS	TIME AND INITIALS	TIME AND INITIALS	TIME AND INITIALS	TIME AND INITIALS	TIME AND INITIALS	TIME AND INITIALS	SEND 2ND COPY TO PHARMACY WHEN COMPLETED

PRE-OP AND STAT

#	DRUG / DOSE / FREQUENCY / ADMINISTRATIVE TIMES / ROUTE / DATE ORDERED								
1	DRUG: Tylenol DOSE: 650 mg. FREQUENCY: q4h×LOS ADMINISTRATIVE TIMES: prn T>38² ROUTE: P.O. DATE ORDERED: 4·9·92								
2	DRUG: Percocet DOSE: 2 tabs FREQUENCY: q3-4h × 2days prn pain ROUTE: P.O. DATE ORDERED: 4·9·92	2p D.G.							
3	DRUG: DOSE: FREQUENCY: ADMINISTRATIVE TIMES: ROUTE: DATE ORDERED:								
4	DRUG: DOSE: FREQUENCY: ADMINISTRATIVE TIMES: ROUTE: DATE ORDERED:								
5	DRUG: DOSE: FREQUENCY: ADMINISTRATIVE TIMES: ROUTE: DATE ORDERED:								
6	DRUG: DOSE: FREQUENCY: ADMINISTRATIVE TIMES: ROUTE: DATE ORDERED:								

PRN

Chapter 11

Answers to Practice Reading of Medication
Record (Fig. 11-10)

1. 4/6/92-Procardia 10 mg sublingual 5 p.m.
2. 4/8/92-Digoxin 0.25 mg p.o. 9 a.m.
3. Lasix 20 mg p.o. 9 a.m. and 5 p.m.
4. Procardia 10 mg sublingual 9 a.m.,
   1p.m., and 5 p.m.
5. Colace 100 mg p.o. 9 a.m. and 5 p.m.
6. Heparin 5,000 Units subcutaneous 9 a.m.

Chapter 12

Answers to Chapter Review

1. Generic name-prazosin hydrochloride
   Trade name-Minipress
   Form-Capsules
   Dosage strength-1 mg per capsule
2. Generic name-Digoxin
   Trade name-Lanoxin
   Total Volume-2 mL
   Dosage strength-0.25 mg per mL
   Form-Injectable
3. Generic name-Dexamethasone, MSD
   Trade name-Decadron
   Drug Form-Tablets
   Dosage Strength-0.25 mg per tablet
4. Generic name-Gentamicin sulfate
   Trade name-Garamycin
   Total Volume-20 mL
   Dosage Strength-40 mg per mL
   Form-injectable
   Instructions-should not be physically
   premixed with other drugs
5. Generic name-Digitoxin
   Trade name-Crystodigin
   Form-Tablets
   Dosage strength-0.1 mg per tablet
6. Generic name-Levothyroxine sodium
   Trade name-Synthroid
   Form-tablets
   Dosage strength-50 mcg per tablet,
   0.05 mg per tablet
7. Generic name-Penicillin V potassium
   Trade name-V-Cillin K
   Total volume-100 mL
   Dosage strength-125 mg per 5 mL,
   200,000 units per 5 mL

Directions for storage-15° to 86° F
(15° to 30° C). Store in refrigerator
after mixing.
8. Generic name-Potassium Chloride
   Trade name-None stated
   Form-Injectable
   Dosage strength-2 mEq per mL
9. Generic name-docusate calcium
   Trade name-Surfak
   Form-Capsules
   Dosage Strength-50 mg per capsule
10. Generic name-Streptomycin Sulfate
    Trade name-None
    Form-Injectable
    Directions for mixing-The dry powder
    is dissolved by adding 9 mL water,
    USP or Sodium Chloride for injection.
    Dosage strength after reconstitution -
    400 mg per mL.
    Storage Instructions-In dry form store
    below 86° F (30° C). Protect reconsti-
    tuted solution from light, may be stored
    at room temperature for four weeks.

Chapter 13

Answers to Practice Problems

1. Less than one tablet.
2. More than one tablet.
3. Less than one tablet.
4. More than one tablet.
5. More than one tablet.

Answers to Problems Using Ratio-Proportion

6. 5 mg : 1 tab = 7.5 mg : x tab

$$\frac{5\,x}{5} = \frac{7.5}{5}$$

$$x = \frac{7.5}{5}$$

OR

$$\frac{5\text{ mg}}{1\text{ tab}} = \frac{7.5\text{ mg}}{x\text{ tab}}$$

$$\frac{5x}{5} = \frac{7.5}{5}$$

x = 1.5 tab, or 1 1/2 tab. (5 mg is smaller than 7.5 mg, therefore you will need more than 1 tablet to administer the dosage.)

7. equivalent 60 mg = gr 1. (gr 1/4 = 15 mg)

    15 mg : 1 tab = 15 mg : x tab

    $$\frac{15x}{15} = \frac{15}{15}$$

    $$x = \frac{15}{15}$$

    OR

    $$\frac{15 \text{ mg}}{1 \text{ tab}} = \frac{15 \text{ mg}}{x \text{ tab}}$$

    $$\frac{15x}{15} = \frac{15}{15}$$

    $$x = \frac{15}{15}$$

    x = 1 tab. (15 mg is equal to one tablet.)

8. equivalent 60 mg = gr 1.
    (gr 1 1/2 = 90 mg)

    100 mg : 1 caps = 90 mg : x caps

    $$\frac{100x}{100} = \frac{90}{100}$$

    $$x = \frac{90}{100}$$

    OR

    $$\frac{100 \text{ mg}}{1 \text{ caps}} = \frac{90 \text{ mg}}{x \text{ caps}}$$

    $$\frac{100x}{100} = \frac{90}{100}$$

    $$x = \frac{90}{100}$$

x = 1 caps. It would be impossible to administer 0.9 of a capsule. There is a 10% margin of difference allowed between what is ordered and what is administered. Using this 10% safety margin, no more than 110 mg and no less than 90 mg may be given. The doctor ordered gr iss (90 mg). The capsules available are 100 mg. Capsules are not dividable, administering 1 capsule is within the 10% margin of difference allowed.

9. 0.5 mg : 1 cc = 0.25 mg : x cc

    $$\frac{0.5x}{0.5} = \frac{0.25}{0.5}$$

    $$x = \frac{0.25}{0.5}$$

    OR

    $$\frac{0.5 \text{ mg}}{1 \text{ cc}} = \frac{0.25 \text{ mg}}{x \text{ cc}}$$

    $$\frac{0.5x}{0.5} = \frac{0.25}{0.5}$$

    $$x = \frac{0.25}{0.5}$$

x = 0.5 cc, 0.5 mL, or 1/2 mL. (0.25 mg is less than 0.5 mg, you would need less than a cc to administer the dose.)

10. gr 3/4 : 1 cc = gr 1/4 : x cc

    $$\frac{\frac{3}{4}x}{\frac{3}{4}} = \frac{\frac{1}{4}}{\frac{3}{4}}$$

    x = 1/4 ÷ 3/4 = 1/4 × 4/3 =

    4/12 = 1/3

    OR

    $$\frac{\text{gr } \frac{3}{4}}{1 \text{ cc}} = \frac{\text{gr } \frac{1}{4}}{x \text{ cc}}$$

$$\frac{\frac{3}{4}x}{\frac{3}{4}} = \frac{\frac{1}{4}}{\frac{3}{4}}$$

$$x = \frac{\frac{1}{4}}{\frac{3}{4}}$$

$x = 1/4 \div 3/4 = 1/4 \times 4/3 =$

$$4/12 = 1/3$$

$x = 0.33 = 0.3$ cc, or 0.3 mL. (gr 1/4 is less than gr 3/4, therefore you will need less than a cc to administer the dose.)

11. 40 mEq : 10 cc = 20 mEq : x cc

$$\frac{40\,x}{40} = \frac{200}{40}$$

$$x = \frac{200}{40}$$

OR

$$\frac{40\ \text{mEq}}{10\ \text{cc}} = \frac{20\ \text{mEq}}{x\ \text{cc}}$$

$$\frac{40\,x}{40} = \frac{200}{40}$$

$x = 5$ mL, 5 cc. (20 mEq is less than 40 mEq, you would need less than 10 cc to administer the dose.)

12. 10,000 U. : 1 cc = 5,000 U. : x cc

$$\frac{10,000\,x}{10,000} = \frac{5,000}{10,000}$$

$$x = \frac{5,000}{10,000}$$

OR

$$\frac{10,000\ \text{U.}}{1\ \text{cc}} = \frac{5,000\ \text{U.}}{x\ \text{cc}}$$

$$\frac{10,000\,x}{10,000} = \frac{5,000}{10,000}$$

$$x = \frac{5,000}{10,000}$$

$x = 0.5$ mL, 0.5 cc, or 1/2 mL, 1/2 cc. (10,000 U. is more than 5,000 U., therefore you will need less than a cc to administer the dose.)

13. 80 mg : 2 cc = 50 mg : x cc

$$\frac{80\,x}{80} = \frac{100}{80}$$

$$x = \frac{100}{80}$$

OR

$$\frac{80\ \text{mg}}{2\ \text{cc}} = \frac{50\ \text{mg}}{x\ \text{cc}}$$

$$\frac{80\,x}{80} = \frac{100}{80}$$

$$x = \frac{100}{80}$$

$x = 1.25 = 1.3$ cc, or 1.3 mL. (50 mg is less than 80 mg, therefore you will need less than 2 cc to administer the dose.)

14. equivalent 1000 mg = 1 g.
(0.5 g = 500 mg)

250 mg : 1 caps = 500 mg : x caps

$$\frac{250\,x}{250} = \frac{500}{250}$$

$$x = \frac{500}{250}$$

OR

$$\frac{250\ \text{mg}}{1\ \text{caps}} = \frac{500\ \text{mg}}{x\ \text{caps}}$$

$$\frac{250\,x}{250} = \frac{500}{250}$$

$x = 2$ caps. (500 mg is more than 250 mg, therefore you would need more than 1 capsule to administer the dose.)

15. 125 mg : 5 cc = 400 mg : x cc

$$\frac{125\,x}{125} = \frac{2,000}{125}$$

$$x = \frac{2,000}{125}$$

OR

$$\frac{125\text{ mg}}{5\text{ cc}} = \frac{400\text{ mg}}{x\text{ cc}}$$

$$\frac{125\,x}{125} = \frac{2,000}{125}$$

$$x = \frac{2,000}{125}$$

$x = 16$ cc, 16 mL. (400 mg is larger than 125 mg, therefore you will need more than 5cc to administer the dose.)

Answers to Review Questions

1. 1 tab.
2. 1 caps
3. 2 caps
4. 2 tabs
5. 2 tabs
6. 1/2 tab
7. 1 tab
8. 1 tab
9. 1 tab
10. 1 tab
11. 2 caps
12. 1 tab
13. 2 caps
14. 2 caps

Part II

15. 4 mL
16. 20 mL

17. 1.3 mL
18. 10 mL
19. 0.7 mL
20. 2.3 mL
21. 1 mL
22. 1 mL
23. 0.66 mL
24. 7.5 mL
25. 1 mL
26. 0.5 mL
27. 0.5 mL
28. 10 mL
29. 0.75 mL
30. 1.1 mL
31. 0.5 mL
32. 0.5 mL
33. 0.8 mL
34. 4 mL

Chapter 14

Answers to Chapter Review

1.
$$\frac{\text{gr}\,\dfrac{1}{150} \times (1\text{ tab})}{\text{gr}\,\dfrac{1}{300}} = x\text{ tab}$$

$$\frac{1}{150} \div \frac{1}{300} = \frac{1}{150} \times \frac{300}{1} = \frac{300}{150} = 2$$

$x = 2$ tabs. (gr 1/300 is smaller than gr 1/150, therfore you will need more than one tablet to administer the dose.)

2. equivalent 1000 mg = 1 g.
(0.75 g=750 mg)

$$\frac{750\text{ mg}}{250\text{ mg}} \times (1\text{caps}) = x\text{ caps}$$

$x = 3$ caps. (750 mg is larger than 250 mg, therefore more than one capsule is needed to administer the dose.)

3. $\dfrac{90\text{ mg}}{60\text{ mg}} \times (1\text{ tab}) = x\text{ tabs}$

$x = 1.5$ or 1 1/2 tabs. (90 mg is larger than 60 mg therefore you will need more than one tablet to administer the dose.)

4. $\dfrac{7.5 \text{ mg}}{2.5 \text{ mg}} \times 1 \text{ tab} = x \text{ tabs}$

   $x = 3$ tabs. (7.5 mg is larger than 2.5 mg, therefore you will need more than one tablet to administer the dosage.)

5. equivalent 1000 mcg = 1 mg.
   (0.05 mg = 50 mcg)

   $\dfrac{50 \text{ mcg}}{25 \text{ mcg}} \times 1 \text{ tab} = x \text{ tabs}$

   $x = 2$ tabs. (50 mcg is larger than 25 mcg, therefore you will need more than one tablet to administer the dosage.)

6. $\dfrac{40 \text{ mg}}{80 \text{ mg}} \times 2 \text{ ml} = x$

   $x = 1$ mL. (40 mg is 1/2 of the dose available, you would need less than 2 mL to administer the dose.)

7. $\dfrac{4,500 \text{ U.}}{5,000 \text{ U.}} \times 1 \text{ mL} = x \text{ mL}$

   $\dfrac{4,500}{5,000} = x$

   $x = 0.9$ mL. (4,500 U. is less than 5,000 U., you need less than 1 mL to administer the dose.)

8. equivalent is 60 mg = gr 1.
   (gr 1/200=0.3 mg)

   $\dfrac{0.3 \text{ mg}}{0.3 \text{ mg}} \times 1 \text{ mL} = x \text{ mL}$

   $x = 1$ mL. (0.3 mg is equal to 1 mL, therefore you would need 1 mL to administer the dose.)

9. $\dfrac{0.75 \text{ mg}}{0.25 \text{ mg}} \times 1 \text{ mL} = x \text{ mL}$

   $x = 3$ mL. (0.75 mg is larger than 0.25 mg, you would need more than 1 mL to administer the dose.)

10. equivalent 60 mg = gr 1.
    (gr 1/6 = 10 mg)

    $\dfrac{10 \text{ mg}}{15 \text{ mg}} \times 1 \text{ mL} = x \text{ mL}$

    $x = 0.66 = 0.7$ mL. (10 mg is less than 15 mg, you will need less than 1 mL to administer the dose.)

11. 1 tab
12. 1 tab
13. 2 caps
14. 1 tab
15. 2 tabs
16. 1 1/2 tabs
17. 1 caps
18. 1 caps
19. 2 caps
20. 2 tabs
21. 1 1/2 tabs
22. 2 caps
23. 1 tab
24. 3 tab
25. 2 caps
26. 0.7 mL
27. 1 mL
28. 0.4 mL
29. 12 mL
30. 7.5 mL
31. 11.3 mL
32. 0.6 mL
33. 2 mL
34. 1.8 mL
35. 10 mL
36. 0.8 mL
37. 2 mL
38. 0.6 mL
39. 0.8 mL
40. 0.5 mL
41. 0.3 mL
42. 1 mL
43. 2 mL
44. 3.2 mL
45. 5 mL

Chapter 15

Answers to Practice Problems

The answers to the practice problems are included below with the rationale for the answer where indicated. In problems where necessary, the methods for calculation of the dosage are shown as well. (Note) In problems that required a conversion before calculating the dosage, the problem set-up shown illustrates the problem after appropriate conversions have been made.

1. 50 mcg : 1 tab = 25 mcg : x tab

    OR

    $$\frac{25 \text{ mcg}}{50 \text{ mcg}} = \frac{1}{2}\text{tab}$$

    Answer: 0.5 or 1/2 tab. This is an acceptable answer since the tabs are scored.

2. 25 mg : 1 tab = 6.25 mg : x tab

    OR

    $$\frac{6.25 \text{ mg}}{25 \text{ mg}} = \frac{1}{4}\text{ tab}$$

    Answer: 1/4 of a tab, this is logical since the tablets are scored in quarters, therefore you could accurately administer the dosage.

3. Conversion is necessary: 1000 mg = 1g. Therefore 1.2g = 1200 mg.

    400 mg : 1 tab = 1200 mg : x tab

    $$\frac{400 \, x}{400} = \frac{1200}{400}$$

    OR

    $$\frac{1200 \text{ mg}}{400 \text{ mg}} = 3 \text{ tablets}$$

    x = 3 tabs
    The dose ordered is greater than what's available. You would need more than one

tablet to administer the dose.

4. It would be best to administer 1 of the 5 mg tablets and 1 of the 2.5 mg tablets. (5mg + 2.5 mg = 7.5 mg).

5. a)125 mcg tablet is the appropriate strength to use. (0.125 mg=125 mcg)
    b) 1 tab. Even though the tablets are scored 1/2 of 500 mcg would still be twice the dosage desired.

    125 mcg : 1 tab = 125 mcg : x tab

    OR

    $$\frac{125 \text{ mcg}}{125 \text{ mcg}} = 1 \text{ tab}$$

6. a) 500 mg caps would be appropriate to use.
    b) 2 caps. (500 mg each) 1000 mg = 1g. Therefore two capsules 500 mg each would be the least number of capsules. Using the 250 mg strength capsules would require 4 caps.
    c) 2 caps q6h = 8 caps. When the number of caps needed is multiplied by the number of days it gives you the number of capsules required.

    8 (# of caps per day) × 7 (# of days) = 56 (total number of caps needed)

    500 mg : 1 caps = 1000 mg : x caps

    $$\frac{1000 \text{ mg}}{500 \text{ mg}} = 2 \text{ caps}$$

7. 5 mg : 1 tab = 10 mg : x tab

    $$\frac{10 \text{ mg}}{5 \text{ mg}} = 2 \text{ tabs}$$

    Answer: 2 tabs. The dosage ordered is larger than what's available, therefore more than one tablet would be needed to administer the dosage.

8. a) 1 1/2 tabs, the tablets are scored

    10 mg : 1 tab = 15 mg : x tab

OR

$$\frac{15 \text{ mg}}{10 \text{ mg}} = 1.5 \text{ tab}$$

b) 15 mg × 3 (tid) = 45 mg per day. The total number of mg received for three days = 135 mg. 45 mg × 3 = 135 mg.

9.   0.075 mg = 75 mcg.

50 mcg : 1 tab = 75 mcg : x tab

OR

$$\frac{75 \text{ mg}}{50 \text{ mg}} = 1\frac{1}{2} \text{ tab}$$

Answer: 1.5 or 1 1/2 tablets, since the tabs are scored.

10.   1.3 g = 1300 mg

650 mg : 1 tab = 1300 mg : x tab

OR

$$\frac{1300 \text{ mg}}{650 \text{ mg}} = 2 \text{ tabs}$$

Answer: 2 tabs. The dosage ordered is more than what's available, therefore more than one tab would be needed to administer the dosage.

11.   No conversion necessary.

30 mg : 1 caps = 90 mg : x caps

$$\frac{30\,x}{30} = \frac{90}{30}$$

OR

$$\frac{90 \text{ mg}}{30 \text{ mg}} = 3 \text{ caps}$$

x = 3 caps.
The dosage ordered is greater than what's available. You would need more than one

capsule to administer the dosage.

12.   No conversion necessary.

100 mg : 1 tab = 200 mg : x tab

$$\frac{100\,x}{100} = \frac{200}{100}$$

OR

$$\frac{200 \text{ mg}}{100 \text{ mg}} = 2 \text{ tabs}$$

x = 2 tabs.

The dosage ordered is greater than what's available. More than one tablet would be needed to administer the dose.

13.   a) 2 caps. (1 g = 1000 mg)
         500 mg × 2 = 1000 mg.
      b) 1 caps. (500 mg = 0.5 g)
         (1) capsule of 500 mg.

Initial dose:
500 mg : 1 caps = 1000 mg : x caps

OR

$$\frac{1000 \text{ mg}}{500 \text{ mg}} = 2 \text{ cap}$$

Daily dose:
500 mg : 1 caps = 500 mg : x caps

OR

$$\frac{500 \text{ mg}}{500 \text{ mg}} = 1 \text{ cap}$$

14.   No conversion necessary.

125 mg : 1 tab = 250 mg : x tab

$$\frac{125\,x}{125} = \frac{250}{125}$$

x = 2 tabs.

OR

$$\frac{250 \text{ mg}}{125 \text{ mg}} = x \text{ tab}$$

$$\frac{250}{125} = x$$

$$2 = x$$

$$x = 2 \text{ tabs.}$$

The dosage ordered is more than what's available or 1/2 the dose ordered. Therefore you would need more than one tablet to administer the dose.

15. gr iss = 90 mg.
a) 30 mg tablets.
b) (3) 30 mg tablets. This strength would allow the client to take 3 tabs to achieve the desired dose, as opposed to (6) 15 mg tabs. This dose is logical since the maximum number of tablets administered is three.

$$30 \text{ mg} : 1 \text{ tab} = 90 \text{ mg} : x \text{ tab}$$

OR

$$\frac{90 \text{ mg}}{30 \text{ mg}} = 3 \text{ tablets}$$

16. No conversion needed.
The best strength to use is 1.5 mg. This would allow the client to swallow the least amount.

$$1.5 \text{ mg} : 1 \text{ tab} = 3 \text{ mg} : x \text{ tab}$$

$$\frac{1.5 \, x}{1.5} = \frac{3}{1.5}$$

$$x = 2 \text{ tabs}$$

OR

$$\frac{3 \text{ mg}}{1.5 \text{ mg}} = 2 \text{ tab}$$

Two tablets would be the least number of tablets. 0.75 mg would require the client to swallow 4 tabs to receive the dose

$$(0.75 \times 4 = 3.0)$$

17. $50 \text{ mg} : 1 \text{ tab} = 100 \text{ mg} : x \text{ tab}$

OR

$$\frac{100 \text{ mg}}{50 \text{ mg}} = 2 \text{ tabs}$$

Answer: a) you need (2) tabs to administer 100 mg.
(2) tabs tid (three times a day) =
6 tabs × (3) days = 18 tabs.

18. It would be best to administer 1 of the 80 mg tablets and 1 of the 40 mg tablets (80 + 40 = 120 mg).

19. The conversion to use here would be 65 mg = gr 1.

$$\text{gr } x = 650 \text{ mg}$$

$$325 \text{ mg} : 1 \text{ tab} = 650 \text{ mg} : x \text{ tab}$$

OR

$$\frac{650 \text{ mg}}{325 \text{ mg}} = 2 \text{ tabs}$$

Answer: 2 tabs. The dosage ordered is larger than the required dose, therefore more than 1 tab. would be required.

20. $0.5 \text{ mg} : 1 \text{ tab} = 1 \text{ mg} : x \text{ tab}$

OR

$$\frac{1 \text{ mg}}{0.5 \text{ mg}} = 2 \text{ tabs}$$

Answer: 2 tabs. (0.5 × 2 = 1)

21. $1 \text{ mg} : 1 \text{ caps} = 3 \text{ mg} : x \text{ caps}$

OR

$$\frac{3 \text{ mg}}{1 \text{ mg}} = 3 \text{ caps}$$

Answer: 3 caps. They are administered in

whole numbers. The answer is logical. The maximum number of tablets or capsules administered is 3.

22. 60 mg = gr 1. Therefore,
gr 1/150 = 0.4 mg

0.4 mg : 1 tab = 0.4 mg : x tab

$$\frac{0.4\,x}{0.4} = \frac{0.4}{0.4}$$

OR

$$\frac{0.4\,mg}{0.4\,mg} = 1\ tab$$

x = 1 tab.

The label indicates gr 1/150 = 0.4 mg. Therefore only one tablet is needed to administer the dose.

23. Choose the 6 mg tablets and give 1 tablet.

6 mg : 1 tab = 6 mg : x

OR

$$\frac{D}{H} = \frac{6\,mg}{6\,mg} = 1\ tablet$$

24. 0.2 g = 200 mg.

100 mg : 1 tab = 200 mg : x tab

OR

$$\frac{200\,mg}{100\,mg} = 2\ tabs$$

Answer: 2 tabs. The dosage ordered is larger than what's available, therefore more than one tab is needed.

25. 40 mg : 1 tab = 60 mg : x tab

OR

$$\frac{60\,mg}{40\,mg} = 1\frac{1}{2}\ tabs$$

Answer: 1 1/2 tabs or 1.5 tabs. The tabs are scored so a half of a tablet can be administered.

26. No conversion needed.

5 mg : 1 tab = 2.5 mg : x tab

$$\frac{5\,x}{5} = \frac{2.5}{5}$$

OR

$$\frac{2.5\,mg}{5\,mg} = \frac{1}{2}\ tab$$

x = 0.5 or 1/2 tab.

This is an acceptable answer (0.5 or 1/2 tab) since it states the tablets are scored. The dosage ordered is less than what's available. You would need less than one tablet to administer the required dose.

27. No conversion needed.

200 mg : 1 tab = 400 mg : x tab

$$\frac{200\,x}{200} = \frac{400}{200}$$

OR

$$\frac{400\,mg}{200\,mg} = 2\ tab$$

x = 2 tabs

The dosage ordered is more than what's available. You would need more than one tablet to administer the dose.

28. No conversion needed:

75 mg : 1 cap = 150 mg : x cap

$$\frac{75\,x}{75} = \frac{150}{75}$$

OR

$$\frac{150 \text{ mg}}{75 \text{ mg}} = 2 \text{ cap}$$

x = 2 caps.

The dose ordered is more than what's available. You would need more than one capsule to administer the dose.

29. Change 1 g to 1000 mg (1000 mg = 1 g)

500 mg : 1 tab = 1000 mg : x tab

$$\frac{500 \, x}{500} = \frac{1000}{500}$$

OR

$$\frac{1000 \text{ mg}}{500 \text{ mg}} = 2 \text{ tab}$$

x = 2 tabs

The dosage ordered is greater than what's available. You need more than one tab to administer the dose.

30. 25 mg : 1 tab = 12.5 mg : x tab

$$\frac{25 \, x}{25} = \frac{12.5}{25}$$

OR

$$\frac{12.5 \text{ mg}}{25 \text{ mg}} = \frac{1}{2} \text{ tab}$$

x = 1/2 tab

The dosage ordered is less than what's available. You would need less than one tablet to administer the dose.

31. It would be best to adminster 1 - 75 mcg tablet and 1 - 25 mcg for a total of 100 mcg. This would be the least number of tablets.
(75 mcg + 25 mcg = 100 mcg)

Answers to Pratice Problems on Oral Liquids:

Note: The set-up shown for problems that required conversions reflect converting of what the doctor ordered to what's available.

32. 20 mg : 5 mL = 100 mg : x mL

OR

$$\frac{100 \text{ mg}}{20 \text{ mg}} \times 5 \text{ mL} = x$$

Answer: 25 mL. In order to administer the dose required more than 5 mL would be necessary. The dosage ordered is 5x larger than what the available strength is.

33. Conversion required. 1g = 1000 mg.

500 mg : 10 mL = 1000 mg : x mL

OR

$$\frac{1000 \text{ mg}}{500 \text{ mg}} \times 10 \text{ mL} = x$$

Answer: 20 mL. To administer the required dose which is 2x larger than the strength it is available in, more than 10 mL is required.

34. 40 mEq : 15 mL = 40 mEq : x mL

$$\frac{40 \, x}{40} = \frac{600}{40}$$

OR

$$\frac{40 \text{ mEq}}{40 \text{ mEq}} \times 15 \text{ mL} = x \text{ mL}$$

$$\frac{40 \times 15}{40} = x$$

$$\frac{600}{40} = x$$

x = 15 mL

The dosage ordered is contained in 15 mL

of the medication.

35. $80 \text{ mg} : 15 \text{ mL} = 120 \text{ mg} : x \text{ mL}$

OR

$$\frac{120 \text{ mg}}{80 \text{ mg}} \times 15 \text{ mL} = x \text{ mL}$$

Answer: 22.5 mL, or 22 1/2 mL. To administer the dose required more than 15 mL would be necessary.

36. $200 \text{ mg} : 5 \text{ mL} = 250 \text{ mg} : x \text{ mL}$

$$\frac{200 \, x}{200} = \frac{1250}{200}$$

OR

$$\frac{250 \text{ mg}}{200 \text{ mg}} \times 5 \text{ mL} = x \text{ mL}$$

$$\frac{250 \times 5}{200} = x$$

$$\frac{1250}{200} = x$$

$x = 6.25$

$x = 6.3 \text{ mL}$

The dosage ordered is greater than what's available. The answer to the nearest tenth is 6.3 mL

37. $125 \text{ mg} : 5 \text{ mL} = 100 \text{ mg} : x \text{ mL}$

OR

$$\frac{100 \text{ mg}}{125 \text{ mg}} \times 5 \text{ mL} = x \text{ mL}$$

Answer: 4 mL. The amount ordered is less than what's available so less than 5 mL would be needed to administer the required dose.

38. Use the mcg equivalent to calculate the dosage.

$50 \text{ mcg} : 1 \text{ mL} = 125 \text{ mcg} : x \text{ mL}$

OR

$$\frac{125 \text{ mcg}}{50 \text{ mcg}} \times 1 \text{ mL} = x \text{ mL}$$

Answer: 2.5 mL, 2 1/2 mL. The dosage ordered is larger than what's available so you would need more than 1 mL to administer the dose.

39. $125 \text{ mg} : 5 \text{ mL} = 250 \text{ mg} : x \text{ mL}$

$$\frac{125 \, x}{125} = \frac{1250}{125}$$

OR

$$\frac{250 \text{ mg}}{125 \text{ mg}} \times 5 \text{ mL} = x \text{ mL}$$

$$\frac{250 \times 5}{125} = x$$

$$\frac{1250}{125} = x$$

$x = 10 \text{ mL}$

The dosage ordered is more than what's available. You would need more than 5 mL to administer the dose.

40. Conversion required. 0.5 g = 500 mg.

$125 \text{ mg} : 5 \text{ mL} = 500 \text{ mg} : x \text{ mL}$

OR

$$\frac{500 \text{ mg}}{125 \text{ mg}} \times 5 \text{ mL} = x \text{ mL}$$

Answer: 20 mL. The dosage ordered is 4 times larger than the available strength, therefore more than 5 mL would be needed to administer the dose.

41. 20 mg : 5 mL = 60 mg : x mL

$$\frac{20\,x}{20} = \frac{300}{20}$$

OR

$$\frac{60\ \text{mg}}{20\ \text{mg}} \times 5\ \text{mL} = x\ \text{mL}$$

$$\frac{60 \times 5}{20} = x$$

$$\frac{300}{20} = x$$

$$x = 15\ \text{mL}$$

The dosage ordered is more than what's available. You would need more than 5 cc to administer the dose.

42. 30 mg : 1 mL = 150 mg : x mL

OR

$$\frac{150\ \text{mg}}{30\ \text{mg}} \times 1\ \text{mL} = x\ \text{mL}$$

Answer: 5 mL. The dose ordered is 5 times larger than the available strength, you would need more than 1 mL to administer the required dose

43. 12.5 mg : 5 mL = 25 mg : x mL

OR

$$\frac{25\ \text{mg}}{12.5\ \text{mg}} \times 5\ \text{mL} = x\ \text{mL}$$

Answer: 10 mL. The dosage needed is 2 times more than the available strength, so you will need more than 5 mL to administer the required dose.

44. The label indicates that 5 mL = 300 mg of the medication.

300 mg : 5 mL = 600 mg : x mL

OR

$$\frac{600\ \text{mg}}{300\ \text{mg}} \times 5\ \text{mL} = x\ \text{mL}$$

a) 10 mL. The dosage ordered is 2 times more than the available strength. You would need more than 5 mL to administer the required dose.
b) 2 containers are needed. One container delivers 300 mg.

45. 2 mg : 1 mL = 10 mg : x mL

OR

$$\frac{10\ \text{mg}}{2\ \text{mg}} \times 1\ \text{mL} = x\ \text{mL}$$

Answer: 5 mL. The dosage ordered is 5 times greater than the available strength. More than 1 mL would be needed to administer the required dose.

46. Conversion is required. 0.5 g = 500 mg.

62.5 mg : 5 mL = 500 mg : x mL

OR

$$\frac{500\ \text{mg}}{62.5\ \text{mg}} \times 5\ \text{mL} = x\ \text{mL}$$

Answer: 40 mL. The dosage ordered is larger than the available strength. You will need more than 5 mL to adminster the required dose.

47. 200,000 U. : 5 mL = 500,000 U. : x mL

OR

$$\frac{500{,}000\ \text{U.}}{200{,}000\ \text{U.}} \times 5\ \text{mL} = x\ \text{mL}$$

Answer: 12.5 mL, or 12 1/2 mL. The amount ordered is greater than the strength available, you will need to administer more than 5 mL to administer the required dose.

48. Conversion is required. 1g = 1000 mg.

125 mg : 5 mL = 1000 mg : x mL

OR

$$\frac{1000 \text{ mg}}{125 \text{ mg}} \times 5 \text{ mL} = x \text{ mL}$$

Answer: 40 mL. The dosage ordered is more than the strength available. You would need more than 5 mL to administer the dose.

49. 16 mg : 5 mL = 24 mg : x mL

OR

$$\frac{24 \text{ mg}}{16 \text{ mg}} \times 5 \text{ mL} = x \text{ mL}$$

Answer: 7.5 mL, or 7 1/2 mL. The dosage ordered is greater than the available strength. You would need more than 5 mL to administer the required dose.

50. 325 mg : 10.15 mL = 650 mg : x mL

OR

$$\frac{650 \text{ mg}}{325 \text{ mg}} \times 10.15 \text{ mL} = x \text{ mL}$$

Answer: 20.3 mL. The dosage ordered is 2 times greater than the available strength. You will need more than 5 mL to administer the dose.

51. 300 mg : 5 mL = 400 mg : x mL

$$\frac{300\, x}{300} = \frac{2000}{300}$$

OR

$$\frac{400 \text{ mg}}{300 \text{ mg}} \times 5 \text{ mL} = x \text{ mL}$$

$$\frac{400 \times 5}{300} = x$$

$$\frac{2000}{300} = x$$

$x = 6.66$

$x = 6.7$ mL

The dosage ordered is more than what's available. You need more than 5 cc to administer the dose.

Chapter 16

Answers to Practice Problems

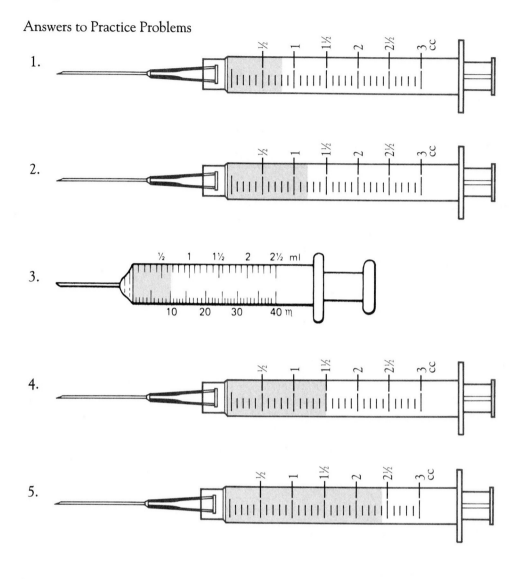

1.

2.

3.

4.

5.

6.   m 8
7.   1.4 cc
8.   1.0 cc
9.   0.9 cc
10. 0.4 cc
11. 4.4 cc
12. 7 cc
13. 3.2 cc
14. 20 mL
15. 25 mg/mL; 500 mg/20 mL is also correct
16. 10 mL
17. 20 mL
18. 2 mEq/mL

1. 0.05 mg = 50 mcg$\qquad\qquad$OR$\qquad\qquad$$\dfrac{50\text{ mcg}}{100\text{ mcg}} \times 1\text{ mL} = x$

    100 mcg : 1 mL = 50 mcg : x mL

    Answer: 0.5, or 1/2 mL. The dosage ordered is less than what is available.

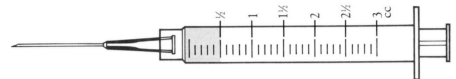

2. Demerol:

    75 mg : 1 mL = 50 mg : x mL$\qquad$OR$\qquad$$\dfrac{50\text{ mg}}{75\text{ mg}} \times 1\text{ mL} = x$

    Answer: 0.66 mL = 0.7 mL. The dosage ordered is less than what is available. Therefore less than a cc would be required to administer the dosage.

    Vistaril:

    50 mg : 1 mL = 25 mg : x mL$\qquad$OR$\qquad$$\dfrac{25\text{ mg}}{50\text{ mg}} \times 1\text{ mL} = x$

    Answer: 0.5, 1/2 mL. The dose ordered is less than what's available. Therefore less than a cc would be required to administer the dosage.

    The total number of cc you will prepare to administer is 1.2 mL. This dosage is measureable on the small hypodermics. These two medications are often administered in the same syringe.

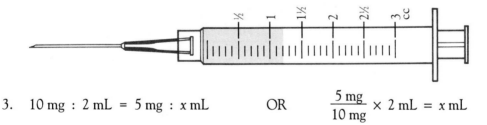

3. 10 mg : 2 mL = 5 mg : x mL$\qquad$OR$\qquad$$\dfrac{5\text{ mg}}{10\text{ mg}} \times 2\text{ mL} = x\text{ mL}$

    x = 1 mL. The dosage required is less than the dosage available, therefore less than 2 cc would be needed to administer the dosage.

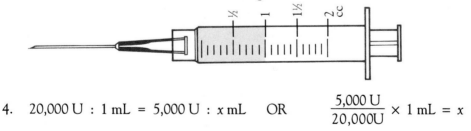

4. 20,000 U : 1 mL = 5,000 U : x mL$\quad$OR$\quad$$\dfrac{5,000\text{ U}}{20,000\text{ U}} \times 1\text{ mL} = x$

    Answer: 0.25 mL. The dosage ordered is less than what's available therefore less than a mL is required to administer the dosage. This dosage can be measured accurately on the 1 cc syringe, since it is measured in hundredths of a mL. The dosage you are administering is 25/100.

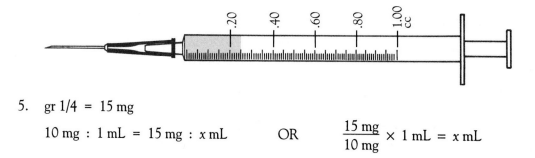

5. gr 1/4 = 15 mg

$$10 \text{ mg} : 1 \text{ mL} = 15 \text{ mg} : x \text{ mL} \qquad \text{OR} \qquad \frac{15 \text{ mg}}{10 \text{ mg}} \times 1 \text{ mL} = x \text{ mL}$$

Answer: 1.5 mL. The dosage ordered is more than what is available, therefore more than a cc is required to administer the dosage.

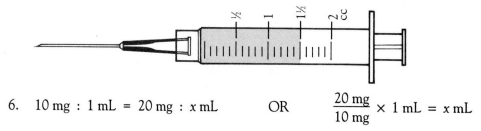

6. $10 \text{ mg} : 1 \text{ mL} = 20 \text{ mg} : x \text{ mL} \qquad \text{OR} \qquad \frac{20 \text{ mg}}{10 \text{ mg}} \times 1 \text{ mL} = x \text{ mL}$

Answer: 2 mL. The dosage ordered is more than what's available, therefore more than 1 mL is needed to administer the required dose.

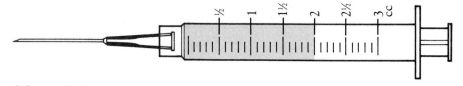

7. 0.3 g = 300 mg

$$\frac{300 \text{ mg}}{150 \text{ mg}} \times 1 \text{ mL} = x \text{ mL}$$

Answer: 2 mL. The dosage ordered is more than the dosage available, therefore more than 1 mL is required to administer the dosage.

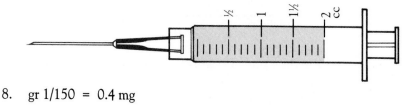

8. gr 1/150 = 0.4 mg

$$0.4 \text{ mg} : 1 \text{ mL} = 0.4 \text{ mg} : x \text{ mL} \qquad \text{OR} \qquad \frac{0.4 \text{ mg}}{0.4 \text{ mg}} \times 1 \text{ mL} = x \text{ mL}$$

Answer: 1 mL. After making the conversion you can see that although the dosage ordered was in gr, it is equivalent to the same number of mL as what's available.

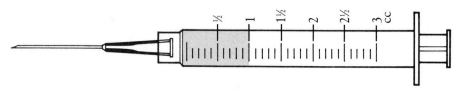

9. $0.5 \text{ g} = 500 \text{ mg}$

   $225 \text{ mg} : 1 \text{ mL} = 500 \text{ mg} : x \text{ mL}$ OR $\dfrac{500 \text{ mg}}{225 \text{ mg}} \times 1 \text{ mL} = x \text{ mL}$

   Answer: 2.2 mL. The dosage ordered is more than what's available, therefore more than 1 cc is required. The dosage here was rounded off to the nearest tenth of a mL. The small hypodermics are marked in tenths of a mL. To round to the nearest tenth the math is carried to the hundredths place.

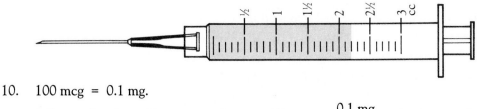

10. $100 \text{ mcg} = 0.1 \text{ mg}.$

    $0.5 \text{ mg} : 2 \text{ mL} = 0.1 \text{ mg} : x \text{ mL}$ OR $\dfrac{0.1 \text{ mg}}{0.5 \text{ mg}} \times 2 \text{ mL} = x \text{ mL}$

    Answer: 0.4 mL. The dosage ordered is less than what's available. The dosage required would be less than 2 mL.

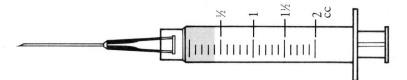

11. $\text{gr } 1/2 = 30 \text{ mg}$

    $120 \text{ mg} : 1 \text{ mL} = 30 \text{ mg} : x \text{ mL}$ OR $\dfrac{30 \text{ mg}}{120 \text{ mg}} \times 1 \text{ mL} = x \text{ mL}$

    Answer: 0.25 mL. This is rounded off to 0.3 mL in order to administer one dosage on the small hypodermic. The dosage ordered is less than what's available.

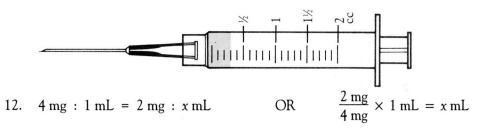

12. $4 \text{ mg} : 1 \text{ mL} = 2 \text{ mg} : x \text{ mL}$ OR $\dfrac{2 \text{ mg}}{4 \text{ mg}} \times 1 \text{ mL} = x \text{ mL}$

    Answer: 0.5 mL, or 1/2 mL. The dosage ordered is less than what's available, therefore less than a mL is required to administer the dosage.

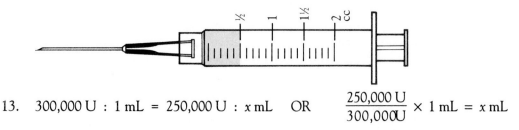

13. $300,000 \text{ U} : 1 \text{ mL} = 250,000 \text{ U} : x \text{ mL}$ OR $\dfrac{250,000 \text{ U}}{300,000 \text{ U}} \times 1 \text{ mL} = x \text{ mL}$

    Answer: 0.8 mL. The dosage ordered is less than what's available therefore you would need less than 1 mL to administer the dose.

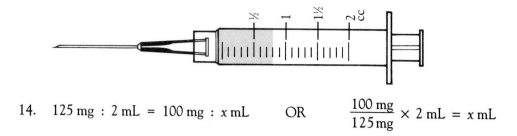

14.   125 mg : 2 mL = 100 mg : x mL   OR $\dfrac{100 \text{ mg}}{125 \text{ mg}} \times 2 \text{ mL} = x \text{ mL}$

Answer: 1.6 mL. The amount ordered is less than what is available, therefore less than 2 mL is needed to administer the required dose.

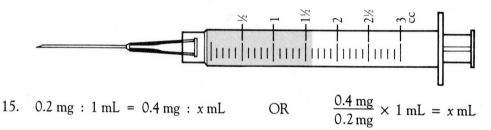

15.   0.2 mg : 1 mL = 0.4 mg : x mL   OR $\dfrac{0.4 \text{ mg}}{0.2 \text{ mg}} \times 1 \text{ mL} = x \text{ mL}$

Answer: 2cc. The dosage ordered is more than what's available, therefore you would need more than 1cc to administer the required dosage.

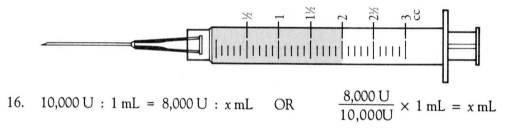

16.   10,000 U : 1 mL = 8,000 U : x mL   OR $\dfrac{8,000 \text{ U}}{10,000 \text{U}} \times 1 \text{ mL} = x \text{ mL}$

Answer: 0.8 mL. The dosage ordered is less than what's available. You would need less than a mL to administer the dose.

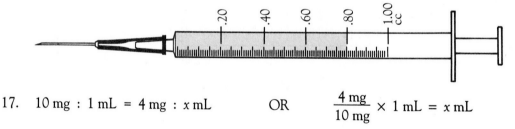

17.   10 mg : 1 mL = 4 mg : x mL   OR $\dfrac{4 \text{ mg}}{10 \text{ mg}} \times 1 \text{ mL} = x \text{ mL}$

Answer: 0.4 mL. The dosage ordered is less than what is available, therefore less than a mL would be required to administer the dose.

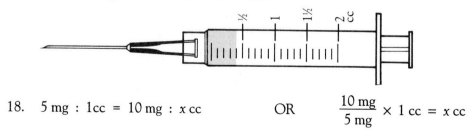

18.   5 mg : 1cc = 10 mg : x cc   OR $\dfrac{10 \text{ mg}}{5 \text{ mg}} \times 1 \text{ cc} = x \text{ cc}$

Answer: 2cc. The dosage ordered is more than what's available, therefore you would need more than 1cc to administer the dosage.

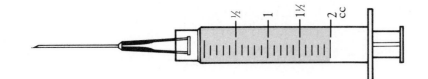

19. gr 1/4 = 15 mg

30 mg : 1 mL = 15 mg : x mL or   OR $\dfrac{15 \text{ mg}}{30 \text{ mg}} \times 1 \text{ mL} = x \text{ mL}$

gr 1/2 : 1 mL = gr 1/4 : x mL

If fractions used:

$\dfrac{\text{gr } \dfrac{1}{4}}{\text{gr } \dfrac{1}{2}} \times 1 \text{ mL} = x$

Answer: 0.5 mL or 1/2 mL. The dosage ordered is less than what's available, therefore you would need less than a mL to administer the dose.

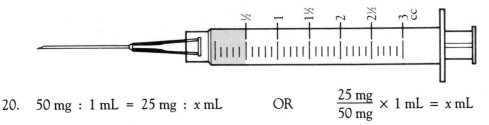

20. 50 mg : 1 mL = 25 mg : x mL   OR $\dfrac{25 \text{ mg}}{50 \text{ mg}} \times 1 \text{ mL} = x \text{ mL}$

Answer: 0.5 mL or 1/2 mL. The dosage ordered is less than what's available, therefore you would need to administer less than a mL.

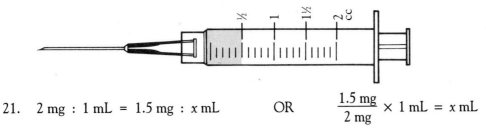

21. 2 mg : 1 mL = 1.5 mg : x mL   OR $\dfrac{1.5 \text{ mg}}{2 \text{ mg}} \times 1 \text{ mL} = x \text{ mL}$

Answer: 0.8 mL. The dose ordered is less than what's available. You would need less than 1 mL to administer the dose.

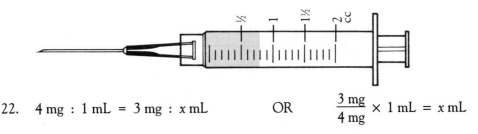

22. 4 mg : 1 mL = 3 mg : x mL   OR $\dfrac{3 \text{ mg}}{4 \text{ mg}} \times 1 \text{ mL} = x \text{ mL}$

Answer: 0.8 mL. The dose ordered is less than what's available. You would need less than 1 mL to administer the dose.

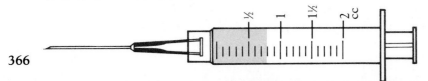

23. Conversion is needed: gr 1 = 60 mg
therefore, gr 1/300 = 0.2 mg

0.4 mg : 1 mL = 0.2 mg : x mL   OR $\dfrac{0.2 \text{ mg}}{0.4 \text{ mg}} \times 1 \text{ mL} = x \text{ mL}$

Answer: 0.5 mL.

The dosage ordered is 1/2 of what's available. You would need less than a mL to administer the dose.

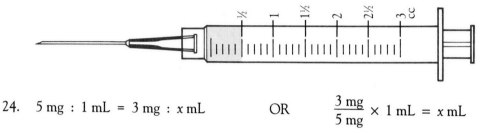

24.   5 mg : 1 mL = 3 mg : x mL   OR $\dfrac{3 \text{ mg}}{5 \text{ mg}} \times 1 \text{ mL} = x \text{ mL}$

Answer: 0.6 mL. The dosage ordered is less than what's available. You would need less than 1 mL to administer the dose.

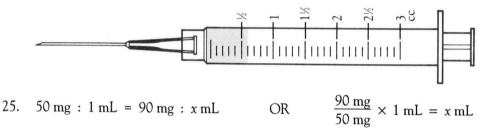

25.   50 mg : 1 mL = 90 mg : x mL   OR $\dfrac{90 \text{ mg}}{50 \text{ mg}} \times 1 \text{ mL} = x \text{ mL}$

Answer: 1.8 mL. The dosage ordered is more than what's available you would need more than 1 mL to adminster the dose.

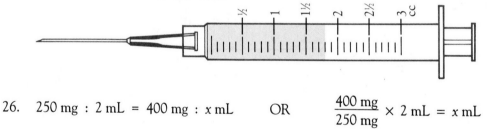

26.   250 mg : 2 mL = 400 mg : x mL   OR $\dfrac{400 \text{ mg}}{250 \text{ mg}} \times 2 \text{ mL} = x \text{ mL}$

Answer 3.2 mL. The dosage ordered is more than what's available. You would need more than 2 mL to administer the dose.

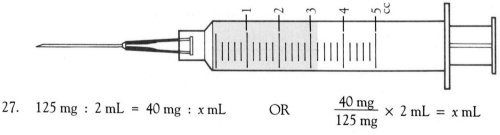

27.   125 mg : 2 mL = 40 mg : x mL   OR $\dfrac{40 \text{ mg}}{125 \text{ mg}} \times 2 \text{ mL} = x \text{ mL}$

Answer 0.6 mL. The dosage ordered is less than the available dose. You need less than a mL to administer the dose.

28. Conversion needed.
    Equivalent (1000 mcg = 1 mg)
    200 mcg = 0.2 mg

    0.2 mg : 1 mL = 0.2 mg : x mL   OR $\dfrac{0.2\ mg}{0.2\ mg} \times 1\ mL = x\ mL$

    Answer: 1 mL. Since 200 mcg = 0.2 mg. You would need 1 mL to administer the required dose.

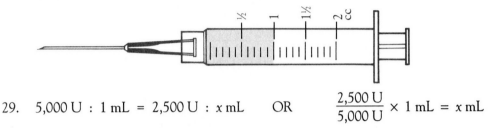

29.   5,000 U : 1 mL = 2,500 U : x mL   OR $\dfrac{2,500\ U}{5,000\ U} \times 1\ mL = x\ mL$

    Answer: 0.5 mL. The dosage ordered is less than what's available. You would need less than 1 mL to administer the dose.

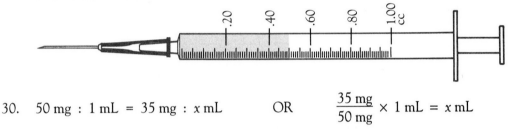

30.   50 mg : 1 mL = 35 mg : x mL   OR $\dfrac{35\ mg}{50\ mg} \times 1\ mL = x\ mL$

    Answer: 0.7 mL. The dosage ordered is less than what's available. You would need less than 1 mL to administer the required dose.

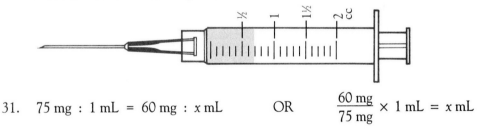

31.   75 mg : 1 mL = 60 mg : x mL   OR $\dfrac{60\ mg}{75\ mg} \times 1\ mL = x\ mL$

    Answer: 0.8 mL. The dosage ordered is less than what's available. You would need less than 1 mL to administer the required dose.

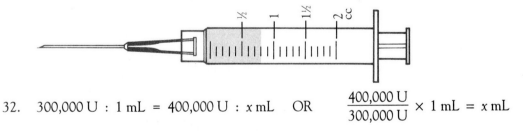

32.   300,000 U : 1 mL = 400,000 U : x mL   OR $\dfrac{400,000\ U}{300,000\ U} \times 1\ mL = x\ mL$

    Answer: 1.3 mL. The dosage ordered is more than what's available. You would need more than 1 mL to administer the required dose.

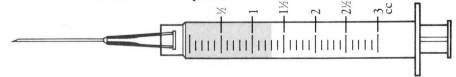

33.　0.5 mg : 2 mL = 0.4 mg : x mL

OR

$$\frac{0.4 \text{ mg}}{0.5 \text{ mg}} \times 2 \text{ mL} = x \text{ mL}$$

Answer: 1.6 mL. The dosage ordered is less than what's available. You would need less than 2 mL to administer the required dose.

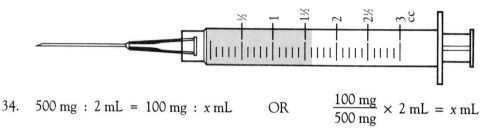

34.　500 mg : 2 mL = 100 mg : x mL　　　OR　　　$\frac{100 \text{ mg}}{500 \text{ mg}} \times 2 \text{ mL} = x \text{ mL}$

Answer: 0.4 mL. The dosage ordered is less than what's available. You would need less than 2 mL to administer the required dose.

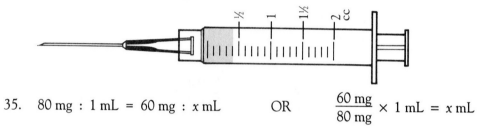

35.　80 mg : 1 mL = 60 mg : x mL　　　　OR　　　$\frac{60 \text{ mg}}{80 \text{ mg}} \times 1 \text{ mL} = x \text{ mL}$

Answer: 0.8 mL. The dosage ordered is less than what's available. You would need less than 1 mL to administer the dose.

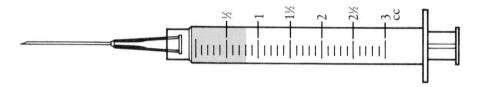

Chapter 17

Answers to Practice Problems

1. 3.5 mL
2. none stated.
3. 250 mg/mL
4. 1 hour
5. 2 mL

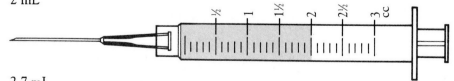

6. 2.7 mL
7. sterile water for injection
8. 250 mg per 1.5 mL.

9. 3 days
10. 7 days
11. 2.4 mL

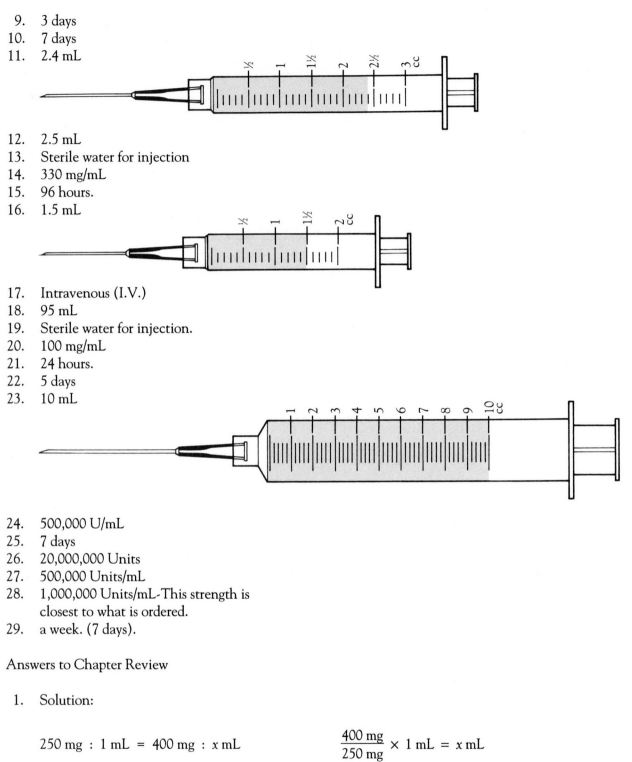

12. 2.5 mL
13. Sterile water for injection
14. 330 mg/mL
15. 96 hours.
16. 1.5 mL

17. Intravenous (I.V.)
18. 95 mL
19. Sterile water for injection.
20. 100 mg/mL
21. 24 hours.
22. 5 days
23. 10 mL

24. 500,000 U/mL
25. 7 days
26. 20,000,000 Units
27. 500,000 Units/mL
28. 1,000,000 Units/mL-This strength is closest to what is ordered.
29. a week. (7 days).

Answers to Chapter Review

1. Solution:

$$250 \text{ mg} : 1 \text{ mL} = 400 \text{ mg} : x \text{ mL}$$

$$\frac{400 \text{ mg}}{250 \text{ mg}} \times 1 \text{ mL} = x \text{ mL}$$

OR

$$\frac{250 \, x}{250} = \frac{400}{250}$$

$$\frac{400}{250} = x$$

$$x = 1.6 \text{ mL}$$

$$x = 1.6 \text{ mL}$$

The dosage ordered is more than what's available. You need more than 1 mL to administer the dose.

2. $1g : 10 \text{ mL} = 1g : x \text{ mL}$ OR $\dfrac{1 \text{ g}}{1 \text{ g}} \times 10 \text{ mL} = x \text{ mL}$

$x = 10 \text{ mL}$ $x = 10 \text{ mL}$

The dosage ordered is equal to the volume of the reconstituted solution. 10 mL I.V. is acceptable. Large volumes of I.V. solution may be administered I.V.

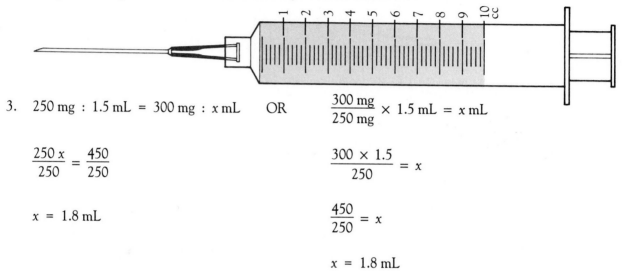

3. $250 \text{ mg} : 1.5 \text{ mL} = 300 \text{ mg} : x \text{ mL}$ OR $\dfrac{300 \text{ mg}}{250 \text{ mg}} \times 1.5 \text{ mL} = x \text{ mL}$

$\dfrac{250 \, x}{250} = \dfrac{450}{250}$ $\dfrac{300 \times 1.5}{250} = x$

$x = 1.8 \text{ mL}$ $\dfrac{450}{250} = x$

$x = 1.8 \text{ mL}$

The dosage ordered is greater than what's available; you would need more than 1.5 mL to administer the dose.

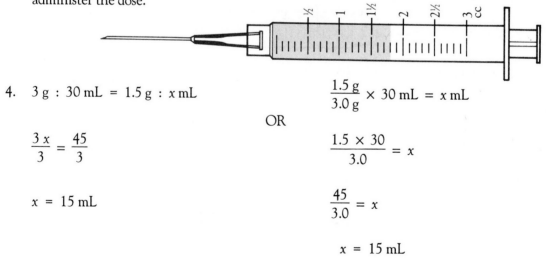

4. $3 \text{ g} : 30 \text{ mL} = 1.5 \text{ g} : x \text{ mL}$ $\dfrac{1.5 \text{ g}}{3.0 \text{ g}} \times 30 \text{ mL} = x \text{ mL}$

OR

$\dfrac{3 \, x}{3} = \dfrac{45}{3}$ $\dfrac{1.5 \times 30}{3.0} = x$

$x = 15 \text{ mL}$ $\dfrac{45}{3.0} = x$

$x = 15 \text{ mL}$

The dosage ordered is less than the available dosage less than 30 mL would be needed to administer the dosage 15 mL I.V. can be administered.

5. a) 2 mL
    b) sterile water or Lidocaine 1% HCl.
    c) 1 g/2.6 mL
    d) 2.6 mL.

Solution:

$$1g : 2.6 \text{ mL} = 1g : x \text{ mL}$$ OR $$\frac{1 g}{1 g} \times 2.6 \text{ mL} = x \text{ mL}$$

$$x = 2.6 \text{ mL}$$ $$\frac{1 \times 2.6}{1} = x$$

$$x = 2.6 \text{ mL}$$

When mixed according to directions the solution gives 1 g/2.6 mL. Therefore you would administer 2.6 mL to give 1g.

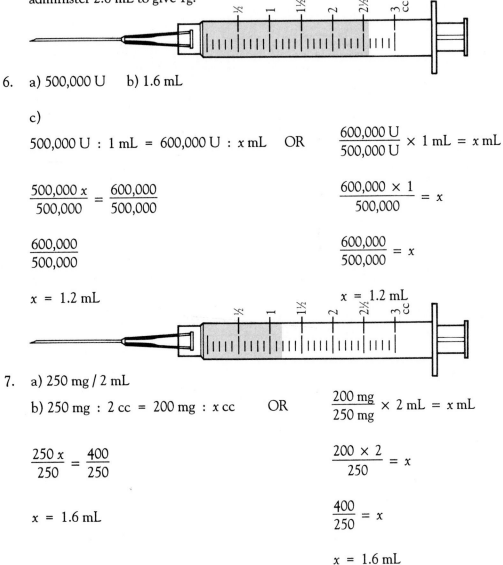

6. a) 500,000 U   b) 1.6 mL

c)

$$500,000 \text{ U} : 1 \text{ mL} = 600,000 \text{ U} : x \text{ mL} \quad \text{OR} \quad \frac{600,000 \text{ U}}{500,000 \text{ U}} \times 1 \text{ mL} = x \text{ mL}$$

$$\frac{500,000 \, x}{500,000} = \frac{600,000}{500,000}$$ $$\frac{600,000 \times 1}{500,000} = x$$

$$\frac{600,000}{500,000}$$ $$\frac{600,000}{500,000} = x$$

$$x = 1.2 \text{ mL}$$ $$x = 1.2 \text{ mL}$$

7. a) 250 mg / 2 mL

b) 250 mg : 2 cc = 200 mg : x cc   OR $$\frac{200 \text{ mg}}{250 \text{ mg}} \times 2 \text{ mL} = x \text{ mL}$$

$$\frac{250 \, x}{250} = \frac{400}{250}$$ $$\frac{200 \times 2}{250} = x$$

$$x = 1.6 \text{ mL}$$ $$\frac{400}{250} = x$$

$$x = 1.6 \text{ mL}$$

The dosage ordered is less than what's available. Less than 2 cc would be required to administer the dose.

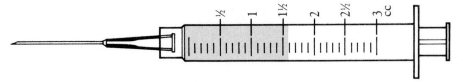

8. a) Sterile water for injection.

b) $1\text{g} : 2.5 \text{ mL} = 1\text{g} : x \text{ mL}$ 　　　OR　　　 $\dfrac{1\text{ g}}{1\text{ g}} \times 2.5 \text{ mL} = x \text{ mL}$

$x = 2.5 \text{ mL}$ 　　　　　　　　　　　　　　　 $\dfrac{1 \times 2.5}{1} = x$

$\dfrac{2.5}{1} = x$

$x = 2.5 \text{ mL}$

When mixed according to directions 1g will be contained in 2.5 mL. Administer 2.5 mL.

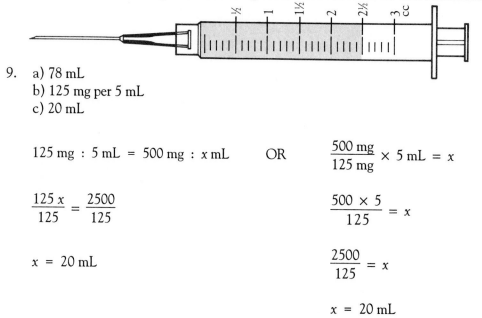

9. a) 78 mL
   b) 125 mg per 5 mL
   c) 20 mL

$125 \text{ mg} : 5 \text{ mL} = 500 \text{ mg} : x \text{ mL}$ 　　OR　　 $\dfrac{500 \text{ mg}}{125 \text{ mg}} \times 5 \text{ mL} = x$

$\dfrac{125\,x}{125} = \dfrac{2500}{125}$ 　　　　　　　　　　 $\dfrac{500 \times 5}{125} = x$

$x = 20 \text{ mL}$ 　　　　　　　　　　　　　　 $\dfrac{2500}{125} = x$

$x = 20 \text{ mL}$

The dosage ordered is more than what's available. More than 5 mL would be required to give the dosage. 20 mL p.o. can be administered since its a p.o. liquid and sometimes large volumes are administered.

10. a) 5.7 mL of sterile water or Sodium Chloride for injection

b) $1\text{g} : 2 \text{ mL} = 1\text{g} : x \text{ mL}$ 　　　OR　　　 $\dfrac{1\text{ g}}{1\text{ g}} \times 2 \text{ mL} = x$

$x = 2 \text{ mL}$ 　　　　　　　　　　　　　　　 $\dfrac{1 \times 2}{1} = x$

$\dfrac{2}{1} = x$

$x = 2 \text{ mL}$

If mixed according to directions 2 mL would contain 1g of the medication.

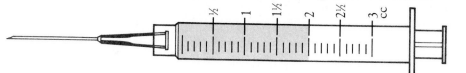

11. a) 2.5 mL of sterile water
    b) 330 mg/mL

    c) 330 mg : 1 mL = 500 mg : x mL   OR $\dfrac{500 \text{ mg}}{330 \text{ mg}} \times 1 \text{ mL} = x \text{ mL}$

    Answer: 1.5 mL. The dosage ordered is more than what's available. You will need more than 1 mL to administer the dose.

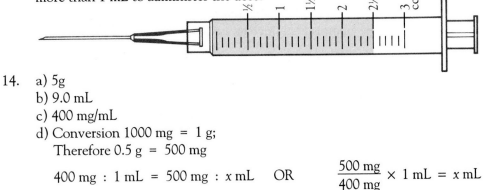

12. a) 250 mg/mL
    b) A conversion is necessary.
        1000 mg = 1g

        250 mg : 1 mL = 1000 mg : x mL   OR $\dfrac{1000 \text{ mg}}{250 \text{mg}} \times 1 \text{ mL} = x \text{ mL}$

    Answer: 4 mL. The dosage ordered is more than what's available. You would need more than 1 mL to administer the dose.

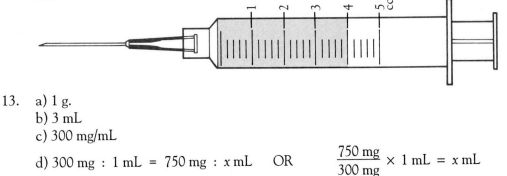

13. a) 1 g.
    b) 3 mL
    c) 300 mg/mL

    d) 300 mg : 1 mL = 750 mg : x mL   OR $\dfrac{750 \text{ mg}}{300 \text{ mg}} \times 1 \text{ mL} = x \text{ mL}$

    Answer: 2.5 mL. The dosage ordered is more than what's available therefore you will need more than 1 mL to administer the dose.

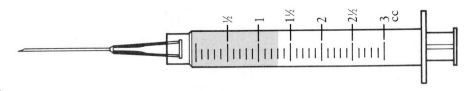

14. a) 5g
    b) 9.0 mL
    c) 400 mg/mL
    d) Conversion 1000 mg = 1 g;
        Therefore 0.5 g = 500 mg

        400 mg : 1 mL = 500 mg : x mL   OR $\dfrac{500 \text{ mg}}{400 \text{ mg}} \times 1 \text{ mL} = x \text{ mL}$

    Answer: 1.25 mL rounded up to 1.3 mL. The dosage ordered is more than what's available per mL; therefore, more than 1 cc is required. The dosage here (1.25) was rounded off to the nearest tenth of a mL (1.3). The small hypodermics are marked in tenths of a mL. To round to the nearest tenth, the math is carried to the hundredths place.

15. a) 10 mL

b) 100 mg/mL

c) Conversion 1000 mg=1 g, therefore 0.5 g = 500 mg

$$100 \text{ mg} : 1 \text{ mL} = 500 \text{ mg} : x \text{ mL} \quad \text{OR} \quad \frac{500 \text{ mg}}{100 \text{ mg}} \times 1 \text{ mL} = x \text{ mL}$$

Answer: 5 mL. The dosage ordered is more than what's available therefore you need more than 1 mL to administer the dose.

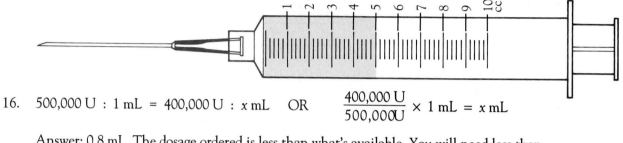

16. $500,000 \text{ U} : 1 \text{ mL} = 400,000 \text{ U} : x \text{ mL} \quad \text{OR} \quad \frac{400,000 \text{ U}}{500,000 \text{ U}} \times 1 \text{ mL} = x \text{ mL}$

Answer: 0.8 mL. The dosage ordered is less than what's available. You will need less than 1 mL to administer the dose.

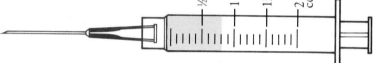

17. a) 500,000 U/mL - closer to doctor's order, client will receive less volume.

b) 1.6 mL

c) $500,000 \text{ U} : 1 \text{ mL} = 600,000 \text{ U} : x \text{ mL} \quad \text{OR} \quad \frac{600,000 \text{ U}}{500,000 \text{ U}} \times 1 \text{ mL} = x \text{ mL}$

Answer: 1.2 mL. The dosage ordered is greater than what's available. More than 1 mL would be needed to administer the dose.

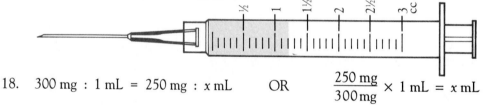

18. $300 \text{ mg} : 1 \text{ mL} = 250 \text{ mg} : x \text{ mL} \quad \text{OR} \quad \frac{250 \text{ mg}}{300 \text{ mg}} \times 1 \text{ mL} = x \text{ mL}$

Answer: 0.8 mL. The dosage ordered is less than what's available, therefore less than 1 mL would be needed to administer the dose.

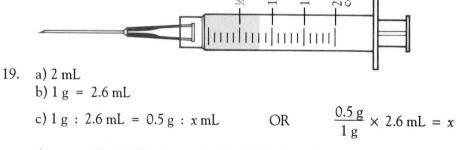

19. a) 2 mL

b) 1 g = 2.6 mL

c) $1 \text{ g} : 2.6 \text{ mL} = 0.5 \text{ g} : x \text{ mL} \quad \text{OR} \quad \frac{0.5 \text{ g}}{1 \text{ g}} \times 2.6 \text{ mL} = x$

Answer: 1.3 mL. The dose ordered is half of the dose available. Less than 2.6 mL would be necessary to administer the dose.

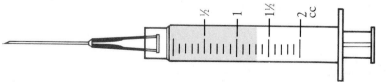

20. a) 5.7 mL
    b) 1g = 2 mL

    c) 1g : 2 mL = 1g : x mL   OR $\dfrac{1\,g}{1\,g} \times 2\,mL = x\,mL$

    Answer: 2 mL. The dose ordered is equivalent to 2 mL therefore 2 mL would be needed to administer the dose.

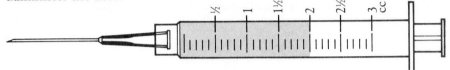

Chapter 18

Answers to Practice Problems

1. Lente; human
2. Protamine Zinc; beef and pork.
3. NPH; beef and pork
4. Ultralente; human.
5. 22 U.
6. 41 U.
7.

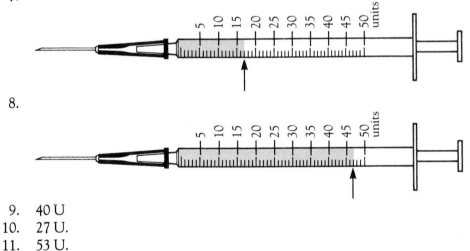

8.

9. 40 U
10. 27 U.
11. 53 U.
12. 14 U.

13.   14.   15.

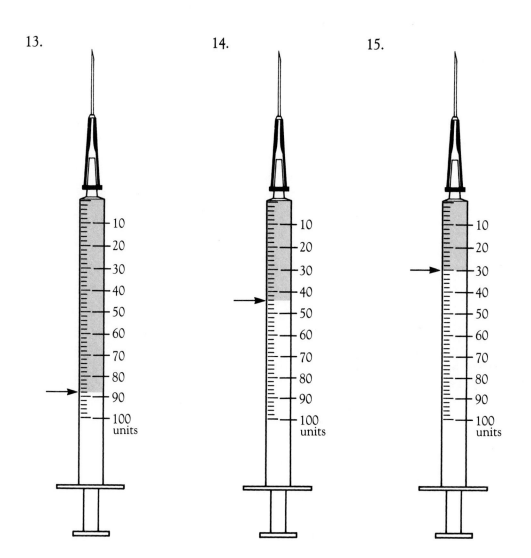

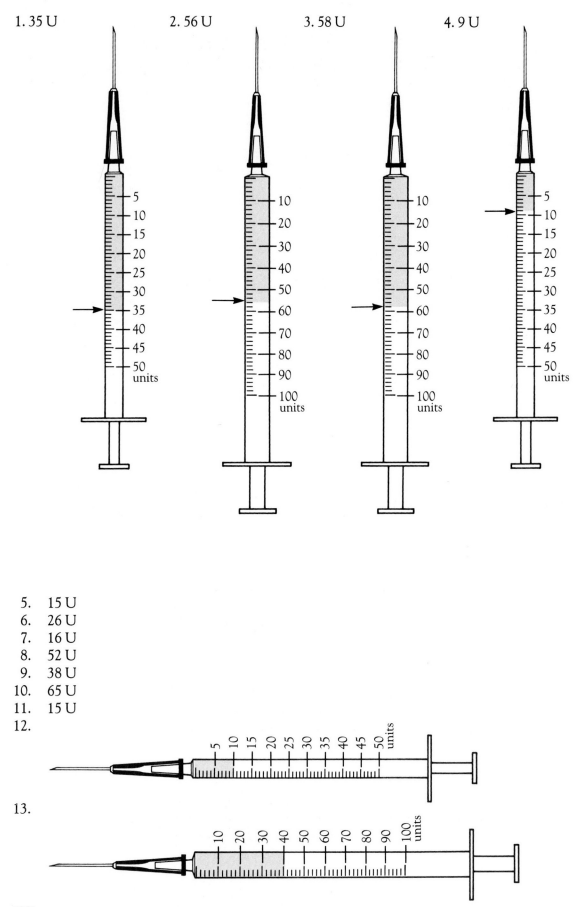

1. 35 U
2. 56 U
3. 58 U
4. 9 U

5.   15 U
6.   26 U
7.   16 U
8.   52 U
9.   38 U
10. 65 U
11. 15 U
12.

13.

14.

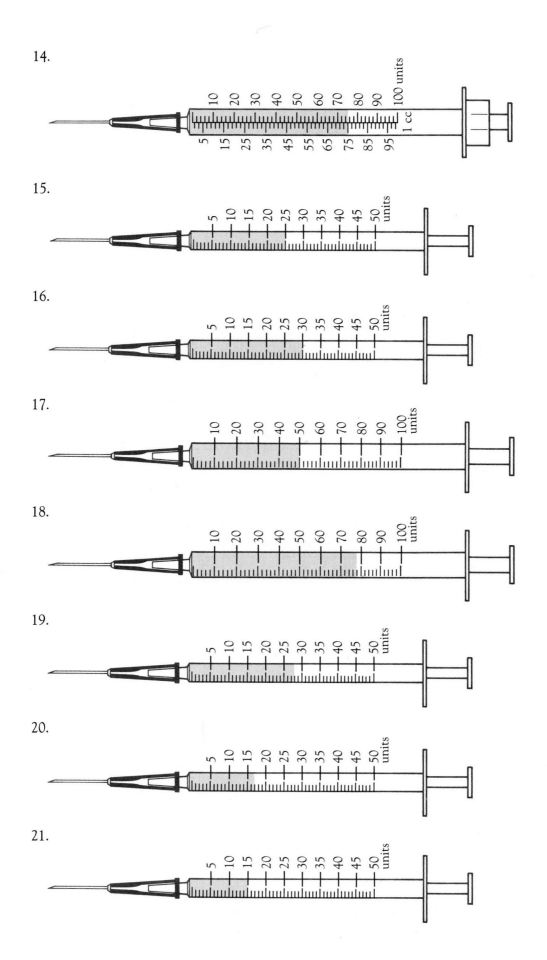

15.

16.

17.

18.

19.

20.

21.

22.

23.

24.

25.

26.

27.

28. 6 Units for blood sugar 364

29.

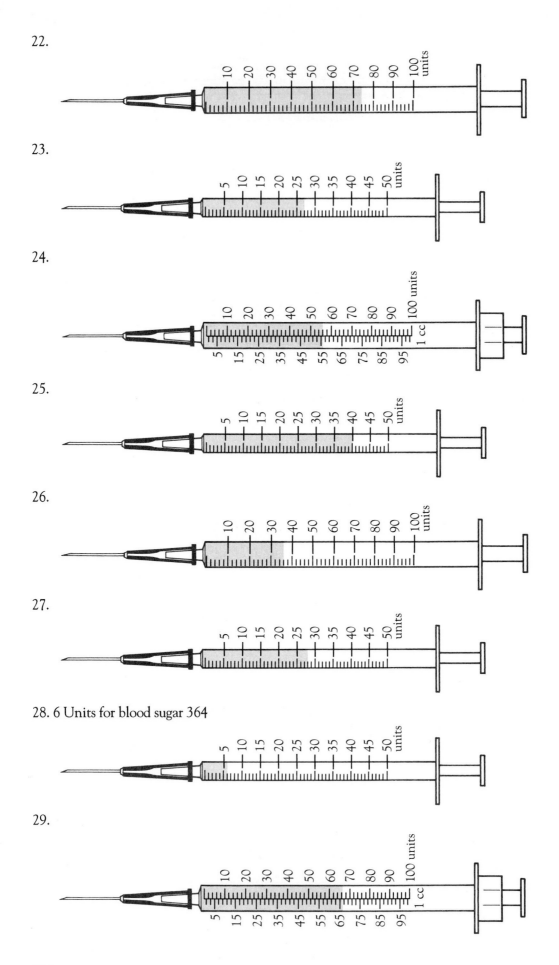

30.

31. 38 U = 0.38 mL

32. 12 U = 0.12 mL

33. 60 U = 0.60 mL

34. 64 U = 0.64 mL

35. 35 U = 0.35 mL

36. 9 U = 0.9 mL

37. 24 U = 0.24 mL

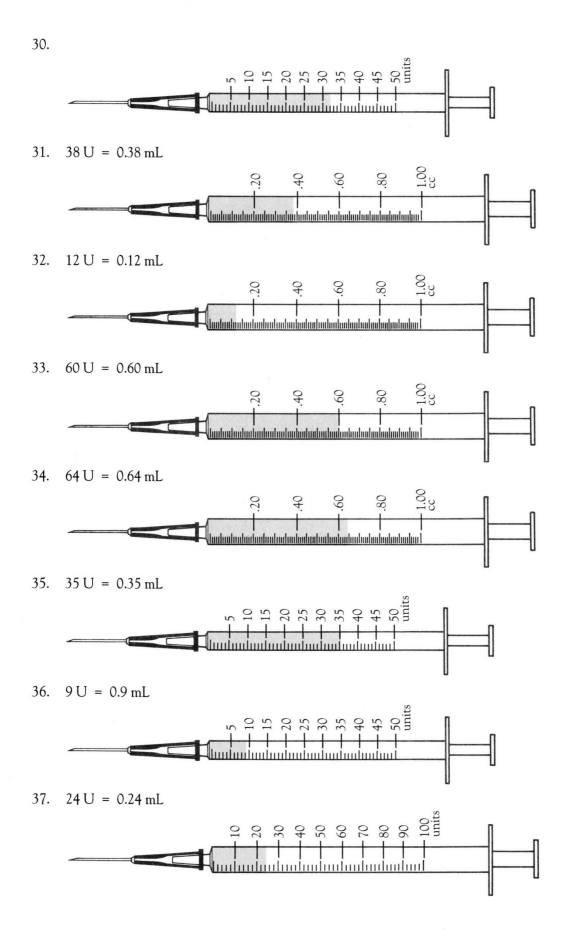

Chapter 19

Answers to Practice Problems

1. 9.1 kg
2. 29.1 kg
3. 10 kg
4. 23.6 kg
5. 32.3 kg
6. 44 lb
7. 101.2 lb
8. 48.4 lb
9. 33 lb
10. 74 .8 lb

Answers to Practice Problems

11. a) 25-50 mg/kg/day.
    b) Convert weight first (2.2 lbs = 1 kg)
       $35 \div 2.2 = 15.90$ kg

    $$\frac{25 \text{ mg}}{x \text{ mg}} = \frac{1 \text{ kg}}{15.90 \text{ kg}} =$$

    $25 \text{ mg} \times 15.90 = 397.5 \text{ mg}$

    $$\frac{50 \text{ mg}}{x \text{ mg}} = \frac{1 \text{ kg}}{15.90 \text{ kg}} =$$

    $50 \text{ mg} \times 15.90 = 795 \text{ mg}$

    Range of dosage is 397.5 mg – 795 mg

    c) The dosage ordered falls within the range that is safe.
       (150 mg × 4 = 600 mg).

    d) 125 mg : 5 mL = 150 mg : x

       OR

       $$\frac{150}{125} \times 5$$

       $x = 6 \text{ mL}$

12. a) $\dfrac{15 \text{ mg}}{x \text{ mg}} = \dfrac{1 \text{ kg}}{35 \text{ kg}}$

    $x = 35 \times 15$

x = 525 mg - maximum dose for 24 hours.

b) $\dfrac{525 \text{ mg}}{3} = 175 \text{ mg}$

c) No. 200 × 3 = 600 mg. This is greater than the maximum dose. Check order with doctor.

13. a) $\dfrac{8 \text{ mg}}{x \text{ mg}} = \dfrac{1 \text{ kg}}{40 \text{ kg}} = 320 \text{mg}$

    $$\frac{25 \text{ mg}}{x} = \frac{1 \text{ kg}}{40 \text{ kg}} = 1{,}000 \text{mg}$$

    Answer: 1000 mg.

    b) Four divided doses.

    320 mg ÷ 4 = 80 mg

    1000 mg ÷ 4 = 250 mg

    Answer: 80 – 250 mg

14. a) 4.1 kg.

    b) $\dfrac{3 \text{ mg}}{x \text{ mg}} = \dfrac{1 \text{ kg}}{4.1 \text{ kg}} = 12.3 \text{ mg}$

    $$\frac{5 \text{ mg}}{x \text{ mg}} = \frac{1 \text{ kg}}{4.1 \text{ kg}} = 20.5 \text{ mg}$$

    Safety range for the child for a day is 12.3 mg – 20.5 mg. The divided dose is 6.2 mg – 10.3 mg.

    c) The dosage ordered is safe.
       10 mg × 2 = 20 mg. The maximum dose per day is 20.5 mg.

    d) 20 mg : 5 mL = 10 mg : x

       OR

       $$\frac{10 \text{ mg}}{20 \text{ mg}} \times 5 \text{ ml}$$

       $x = 2.5$

You need to give 2.5 mL to administer

the ordered dose of 10 mg.

15. Convert weight to kg.
84 lbs = 38.2 kg

a) 38.2 × 0.1 mg = 3.82 mg = 3.8 mg
38.2 × 0.2 mg = 7.64 mg = 7.6 mg

The dose ordered is safe.
You would administer 0.5 mL.

15 mg : 1 mL = 7.5 mg : x mL

OR

$$\frac{7.5 \text{ mg}}{15 \text{ mg}} \times 1 \text{ ml}$$

x = 0.5 mL

16. Convert weight.
11 lbs = 5 kg

$$\frac{4 \text{ mg}}{x \text{ mg}} = \frac{1 \text{ kg}}{5 \text{ kg}} = 20 \text{ mg}$$

$$\frac{8 \text{ mg}}{x \text{ mg}} = \frac{1 \text{ kg}}{5 \text{ kg}} = 40 \text{ mg}$$

The dose that is ordered is safe.
It falls within the safe range
15 mg × 2 = 30 mg.

You would give 0.6 mL.

17. Convert the child's weight to kg.
44 lbs = 20 kg

$$\frac{2.5 \text{ mg}}{x \text{ mg}} = \frac{1 \text{ kg}}{20 \text{ kg}}$$

x = 50 mg

18. a) 17.3 kg

b) $$\frac{40 \text{ mg}}{x \text{ mg}} = \frac{1 \text{ kg}}{17.3 \text{ kg}}$$

x = 692 mg/day

c) $$\frac{692 \text{ mg}}{4} = 173 \text{ mg}$$

d) The dose ordered is not safe.

19. 0.60
20. 0.27
21. 0.90
22. 0.8
23. 0.28
24. 0.52
25. 0.45
26. a) 0.52

b) $$\frac{0.52}{1.7} \times 25 = \frac{0.52 \times 25}{1.7} =$$

$$\frac{13}{1.7} = 7.64$$

Answer: 7.6 mg.

27. a) 0.52

b) $$\frac{0.52}{1.7} \times 200 = \frac{0.52 \times 200}{1.7} =$$

$$\frac{104}{1.7} = 61.17$$

61.17 mg = 61.2 mg

$$\frac{0.52}{1.7} \times 400 = \frac{208}{1.7} =$$

122.35 mg = 122.4 mg

Answer: 61.2 mg – 122.4 mg

28. $$\frac{1.5}{1.7} \times 5 \text{ mg} = \frac{1.5 \times 5}{1.7} =$$

$$\frac{7.5}{1.7} = 4.41 = 4.4 \text{ mg}$$

$$\frac{1.5}{1.7} \times 15 \text{ mg} = \frac{22.5}{1.7} =$$

13.23 mg = 13.2 mg

Answer: 4.4 mg – 13.2 mg.

29. $\dfrac{0.8}{1.7} \times 20 \text{ mg} = \dfrac{0.8 \times 20}{1.7} =$

$\dfrac{16}{1.7} = 9.41 \text{ mg} = 9.4 \text{ mg}$

No; the correct dose is 9.4 mg.

30. $\dfrac{0.92}{1.7} \times 25 \text{ mg} = \dfrac{0.92 \times 25}{1.7} =$

$\dfrac{23}{1.7} = 13.52 \text{ mg} = 13.5 \text{ mg}$

The dose is incorrect. The correct dose is 13.5 mg.

31. $\dfrac{1.5}{1.7} \times 250 \text{ mg} = \dfrac{1.5 \times 250}{1.7} =$

$\dfrac{375}{1.7} = 220.58 \text{ mg}$

Answer: 220.6 mg

32. $0.74 \times 20 = 14.8 \text{ mg}$
$0.74 \times 30 = 22.2 \text{ mg}$
Answer: 14.8 mg – 22.2 mg

33. $\dfrac{0.67}{1.7} \times 20 \text{ mg} = \dfrac{13.4}{1.7} =$

7.88 mg = 7.9 mg. The dosage is correct.

34. $\dfrac{.94}{1.7} \times 10 = 5.5 \text{ mg}$

$\dfrac{.94}{1.7} \times 20 = 11.1 \text{ mg}$

Range: 5.5 – 11.1 mg

35. a) 0.45
   b) $\dfrac{0.45}{1.7} \times 500 \text{ mg} = \dfrac{225}{1.7} = 132.35$

Answer: 132.4 mg

Answers to Chapter Review

1. Convert weight (2.2 lb = 1 kg).
   22 lb = 22 ÷ 2.2 = 10 kg
   1 mg × 10 kg = 10 mg
   The dose ordered for this child is safe.

2. Convert weight (2.2 lb = 1 kg).
   a) 23 lb = 23 ÷ 2.2 = 10.5 kg
   b) 20 mg × 10.5 kg = 210 mg/day
      40 mg × 10.5 kg = 420 mg/day
      The safety range for this 10.5 kg child is 210 – 420 mg/day.
   c) The drug is given in divided doses q8h.
      q8h = 24 ÷ 8 = 3 doses per day.
      210 mg ÷ 3 = 70 mg per dose
      420 mg ÷ 3 = 140 mg per dose
      The dosage range is 70 – 140 mg per dose q8h.
   d) The dose ordered is not safe since
      10 mg q8h 150 mg × 3 = 450 mg.
      Notify the doctor and question the order.

3. a) Convert child's weight in kg to lb. The recommended dose is stated in lb.
      2.2 lb = 1 kg
      17 kg = 17 × 2.2 = 37.4 lb.
      The dosage range is stated as
      2.2 – 3.2 mg/lb/day
      2.2 mg × 37.4 = 82.28 mg = 82.3 mg
      3.2 mg × 37.4 = 119.68 mg = 119.7 mg
      The dosage range is 82.3 – 119.7 mg
      q6h = 4 doses
      82.3 mg ÷ 4 = 20.57 mg = 20.6 mg
      119.7 mg ÷ 4 = 29.92 mg = 29.9 mg
      The dosage range is 20.6 – 29.9 mg per dose.
      The dosage ordered 25 mg q6h.
      This dose is safe.
   b) 5 mg : 1 mL = 25 mg : x mL

      OR

      $\dfrac{25 \text{ mg}}{5 \text{ mg}} \times 1 \text{ mL} = 5 \text{ ml}$

      $x = 5$ mL
      Give 5 mL per dose.

4. No conversion of weight is required. The child's weight is in kg, and the recommended dose is expressed in kg. (12.5 mg/kg)
   12.5 mg × 35 = 437.5 mg/day
   q6h = 4 doses.
   437.5 mg ÷ 4 = 109.37 =

109.4 mg per dose.
The dose ordered is safe.
100 mg × 4=400 mg.

5. No conversion of weight is required. The child's weight is in lb, and the recommended dose is expressed in lb (2 mg/lb)
2 mg × 30 lbs = 60 mg/day
60 mg ÷ 2 = 30 mg per dose
75 mg × 2 = 150 mg. This dose is too high, notify the doctor.

6. Convert the child's weight in lb to kg. The recommended dose is expressed in kg (60 mg/kg)
2.2 lbs = 1 kg.
42 lb = 42 ÷ 2.2 = 19.1 kg
60 mg × 19.1 = 1,146 mg/day
1,146 mg ÷ 4 = 286.5 mg per dose
The dose ordered is safe
250 mg × 4 = 1000 mg

7. Convert the child's weight in lbs to kg. The recommended dose is stated in kg.
(10 to 25 mg/kg)
36 lb = 36 ÷ 2.2 = 16.4 kg
10 mg × 16.4 = 164 mg/day
25 mg × 16.4 = 410 mg/day
The safety range is 164 mg – 410 mg/day.
The drug is given q6-8h. The dose in this problem is ordered q8h.
24 ÷ 8 = 3 doses
164 mg ÷ 3 = 54.7 mg/dose
410 mg ÷ 3 = 136.7 mg/dose
The dose ordered is 150 mg q8h.
150 mg × 3 = 450 mg.
Notify the doctor, the dose is high.

8. Convert the child's weight in lb to kg. The recommended dose is expressed in kg.
(25 – 50 mg/kg)
66 lbs = 66 ÷ 2.2 = 30 kg
25 mg × 30 = 750 mg/day
50 mg × 30 = 1500 mg/day
The safety range is 750 – 1500 mg/day.
The drug is given in divided doses (4).
The dosage ordered is q6h.
24 ÷ 6 = 4 doses.
750 mg ÷ 4 = 187.5 mg/per dose
1500 mg ÷ 4 = 375 mg/per dose

The dosage range is 187.5 – 375 mg per dose q6h. 250 mg × 4 = 1000 mg. This is a safe dose since the total dose falls within the safety range for 24h, and the divided dose also falls within the safe range. You would give 10 mL for one dose.
125 mg : 5 mL = 250 mg : x mL

OR

$$\frac{250 \text{ mg}}{125 \text{ mg}} \times 5 \text{ mL}$$

x = 10 mL.

9. a) No conversion of weight is required. The child's weight is stated in kg and the recommended dosage is (20 – 40 mg/kg).
20 mg × 35 = 700 mg
40 mg × 35 = 1400 mg
The safety range is 700 – 1400 mg/day.
The drug is given in divided doses q12h.
24 ÷ 12 = 2 doses.
700 mg ÷ 2 = 350 mg
1400 mg ÷ 2 = 700 mg
350 – 700 mg per dose is safe.
The doctor ordered 400 mg I.M. q12h.
This dose is safe.
400 mg × 2 = 800 mg.
    b) Administer 1 mL
400 mg : 1 mL = 400 mg : x mL

OR

$$\frac{400 \text{ mg}}{400 \text{ mg}} \times 1 \text{ mL}$$

x = 1 mL

10. Convert the child's weight in lb to kg. The recommended dose is expressed in kg. (120 mg/kg)
46 lb = 46 ÷ 2.2 = 20.9 kg
120 mg × 20.9 = 2,508 mg/day
The drug is given in four equally divided doses.
The dose for this child is ordered q6h.
24 ÷ 6 = 4 doses.
2508 mg ÷ 4 = 627 mg per dose
250 mg × 4 = 1000 mg

The dosage ordered is low. Notify the doctor. 250 mg each dose is less than 627 mg.

11. a) $0.45 \, M^2$
    b) $\dfrac{0.45}{1.7} \times 500 \, mg = 132.4 \, mg$

12. a) $0.54 \, M^2$
    b) $\dfrac{0.54}{1.7} \times 25 \, mg = 7.9 \, mg$

13 a) $1.2 \, M^2$
    b) $\dfrac{1.2}{1.7} \times 250 \, mg = 176.5 \, mg$

14. a) $1.1 \, M^2$
    b) $\dfrac{1.1}{1.7} \times 30 \, mg = 19.4 \, mg$

15. a) $1.05 \, M^2$
    b) $\dfrac{1.05}{1.7} \times 150 \, mg = 92.6 \, mg$

16. $\dfrac{0.70}{1.7} \times 50 \, mg = 20.6 \, mg$

17. $\dfrac{0.66}{1.7} \times 10 \, mg = 3.9 \, mg$

$\dfrac{0.66}{1.7} \times 20 \, mg = 7.8 \, mg$

The dosage range is 3.9 – 7.8 mg

18. $\dfrac{0.55}{1.7} \times 2000U = 647.1 \, U$

19. $\dfrac{0.55}{1.7} \times 200 \, mg = 64.7 \, mg$

$\dfrac{0.55}{1.7} \times 250 \, mg = 80.9 \, mg$

The dosage range is 64.7 – 80.9 mg.

20. $\dfrac{0.22}{1.7} \times 150 \, mg = 19.4 \, mg$

21. Dosage incorrect, the child's dosage is 17.3 mg

$\dfrac{0.49}{1.7} \times 60 \, mg = 17.3 \, mg$

The dosage of 25 mg is too high.

22. $\dfrac{0.32}{1.7} \times 10 \, mg = 1.9 \, mg$

The dosage of 4 mg is too high.

23. Dosage correct.

$\dfrac{0.68}{1.7} \times 125 \, mg = 50 \, mg$

$\dfrac{0.68}{1.7} \times 150 \, mg = 60 \, mg$

The dosage of 50 mg falls within the range of 50 – 60 mg.

24. Dosage incorrect.

$\dfrac{0.55}{1.7} \times 25 \, mg = 8.1 \, mg$

The dosage of 5 mg is too low.

25. The dosage is correct.

$\dfrac{1.2}{1.7} \times 75 \, mg = 52.9 \, mg$

$\dfrac{1.2}{1.7} \times 100 \, mg = 70.6 \, mg$

The dosage ordered is 60 mg and falls within the dosage range of 52.9 – 70.6 mg.

Chapter 20

Answers to Practice Problems

1. $75 \, mL \times \dfrac{10 \, gtts/cc}{60} = 75 \times \dfrac{1}{6} =$

$\dfrac{75}{6} = 12.5 = 13 \, gtts/minute$

2. $\dfrac{30 \, mL}{1 \, hr} \times \dfrac{60 \, gtts/cc}{60} = \dfrac{30}{1} =$

$$\frac{30}{1} = 30 \text{ gtts/minute}$$

3. $\dfrac{125 \text{ mL}}{1 \text{ hr}} \times \dfrac{15 \text{ gtts/cc}}{60} = \dfrac{125}{1} \times \dfrac{1}{4} =$

$$\frac{125}{4} = 31.25$$

Answer: 31 gtts/minute

4. $\dfrac{1000 \text{ mL}}{6 \text{ hrs}} \times \dfrac{15 \text{ gtts/mL}}{60} = \dfrac{1000}{6} \times \dfrac{1}{4} =$

$$\frac{1000}{24} = 41.66$$

Answer: 42 gtts/minute

5. $60 \text{ mL} \times \dfrac{60 \text{ gtts/mL}}{45 \text{ minutes}} = 60 \times \dfrac{4}{3} =$

$$\frac{240}{3} = 80 \text{ gtts/minute}$$

6. $\dfrac{1000 \text{ mL}}{16 \text{ hrs}} \times \dfrac{15 \text{ gtts/mL}}{60 \text{ minutes}} = \dfrac{1000}{16} \times \dfrac{1}{4} =$

$$\frac{1000}{64} = 15.62$$

Answer: 16 gtts/minute

7. $\dfrac{150 \text{ mL}}{2 \text{ hrs}} \times \dfrac{20 \text{ gtts/mL}}{60 \text{ minutes}} = \dfrac{150}{2} \times \dfrac{1}{3} =$

$$\frac{150}{6} = 25 \text{ gtts/minute}$$

8. $\dfrac{3000 \text{ mL}}{24 \text{ hrs}} \times \dfrac{10 \text{ gtts/mL}}{60 \text{ minutes}} = \dfrac{3000}{24} \times \dfrac{1}{6} =$

$$\frac{3000}{144} = 20.83$$

Answer: 21 gtts/minute

9. $\dfrac{2000 \text{ mL}}{12 \text{ hrs}} \times \dfrac{15 \text{ gtts/mL}}{60 \text{ minutes}} = \dfrac{2000}{12} \times \dfrac{1}{4} =$

$$\frac{2000}{48} = 41.66$$

Answer: 42 gtts/minute

10. $60 \text{ cc} \times \dfrac{60 \text{ gtts/mL}}{30 \text{ minutes}} = 60 \times 2 =$

120 gtts/minute

11. $\dfrac{125 \text{ cc}}{1 \text{ hr}} \times \dfrac{15 \text{ gtts/mL}}{60 \text{ minutes}} = \dfrac{125}{1} \times \dfrac{1}{4} =$

$$\frac{125}{4} = 31.25$$

Answer: 31 gtts/minute

12. $\dfrac{2500 \text{ cc}}{16 \text{ hrs}} \times \dfrac{10 \text{ gtts/mL}}{60 \text{ minutes}} = \dfrac{2500}{16} \times \dfrac{1}{6} =$

$$\frac{2500}{96} = 26.04$$

Answer: 26 gtts/minute

13. $\dfrac{100 \text{ mL}}{1 \text{ hr}} \times \dfrac{60 \text{ gtts/mL}}{60 \text{ minutes}} = \dfrac{100}{1} \times \dfrac{1}{1} =$

$$\frac{100}{1} = 100 \text{ gtts/minute}$$

Answer: 100 gtts/minute

14. $\dfrac{2000 \text{ mL}}{10 \text{ hrs}} \times \dfrac{15 \text{ gtts/mL}}{60 \text{ minutes}} = \dfrac{2000}{10} \times \dfrac{1}{4} =$

$$\frac{2000}{40} = 50 \text{ gtts/minute}$$

Answer 50 gtts/minute

15. $\dfrac{130 \text{ mL}}{1 \text{ hr}} \times \dfrac{15 \text{ gtts/mL}}{60 \text{ minutes}} = \dfrac{130}{1} \times \dfrac{1}{4} =$

$$\frac{130}{4} = 32.5$$

Answer: 33 gtts/minute

16. $\dfrac{100 \text{ mL}}{1 \text{ hour}} \times \dfrac{20 \text{ gtts/cc}}{60 \text{ minutes}} = \dfrac{100}{1} \times \dfrac{1}{3} =$

$\dfrac{100}{3} = 33.33$

Answer: 33 gtts/minute

17. $50 \text{ cc} \times \dfrac{10 \text{ gtts/mL}}{45 \text{ minutes}} = 50 \times \dfrac{10}{45} =$

$\dfrac{500}{45} = 11.11$

Answer: 11 gtts/minute

18. $75 \text{ mL} \times \dfrac{10 \text{ gtts/cc}}{30 \text{ minutes}} = 75 \times \dfrac{1}{3} =$

$\dfrac{75}{3} = 25 \text{ gtts/minute}$

19 a) $15 \text{ mEq} : 1000 \text{ mL} = 4 \text{ mEq} : x \text{ mL}$

$\dfrac{15\,x}{15} = \dfrac{4000}{15} = 266.66$

$x = 267 \text{ mL/hr to deliver 4 mEq of}$
Potassium Chloride

b) $\dfrac{267 \text{ mL}}{1 \text{ hr}} \times \dfrac{10 \text{ gtt/mL}}{60 \text{ m}} = 45 \text{ gtts/min}$

45 gtts/min would deliver 4 mEq of
Potassium Chloride each hour.

20 a) $50 \text{ U} : 250 \text{ mL} = 10 \text{ U} : x \text{ mL}$

$\dfrac{50\,x}{50} = \dfrac{2500}{50} = 50 \text{ mL/h}$

50 mL/hr must be administered for client
to receive 10 U/h.

b) $\dfrac{50 \text{ ml}}{1 \text{ h}} \times \dfrac{15 \text{ gtt/mL}}{60 \text{ min}} = 13 \text{ gtt/min}$

13 gtt/min of this solution would deliver
10 U/h.

21.   a) $40\text{U} : 250 \text{ mL} = 15 \text{ U} : x \text{ mL}$

$\dfrac{40\,x}{40} = \dfrac{3750}{40} = 93.75 = 94 \text{ mL/hr}$

b) $\dfrac{94 \text{ ml}}{1 \text{ hr}} \times \dfrac{60}{60} = 94 \text{ gtt/min}$

94 gtt/min of this solution would deliver
15 U/h.

22. $\dfrac{150 \text{ cc}}{x} \times \dfrac{60}{60} = 60$

$\dfrac{150}{x} \times \dfrac{1}{1} = 60$

$\dfrac{150}{x} = \dfrac{60}{1}$

$\dfrac{60\,x}{60} = \dfrac{150}{60} = 2.5 \text{ hours}$

23. $\dfrac{x \text{ cc}}{5} \times \dfrac{15 \text{ gtts/cc}}{60} = 35 \text{ gtts/min}$

$\dfrac{x}{5} \times \dfrac{1}{4} = 35$

$\dfrac{x}{20} = \dfrac{35}{1}$

$x = 35 \times 20$

$x = 700 \text{ mL/cc}$

24. $\dfrac{180 \text{ cc}}{x} \times \dfrac{15 \text{ gtts/mL}}{60} = 45 \text{ gtts/min}$

$\dfrac{180}{x} \times \dfrac{1}{4} = 45$

$\dfrac{180}{4\,x} = \dfrac{45}{1}$

$\dfrac{180\,x}{180} = \dfrac{180}{180}$

Answer: 1 hour

25. $\dfrac{x \text{ cc}}{8 \text{ hrs}} \times \dfrac{15 \text{ gtts/mL}}{60} = 45 \text{ gtts/minute}$

$$\frac{x}{8} \times \frac{1}{4} = 45$$

$$\frac{x}{32} = \frac{45}{1}$$

$$x = 45 \times 32$$

Answer: 1,440 cc

26. $$\frac{90 \text{ cc}}{x} \times \frac{60 \text{ gtts/mL}}{60} = 60 \text{ gtts/min}$$

$$\frac{90}{x} \times \frac{60}{60} = 60$$

$$\frac{90}{x} = \frac{60}{1}$$

$$\frac{60\,x}{60} = \frac{90}{60}$$

Answer: 1.5 or 1 1/2 hours

27. $$\frac{250 \text{ mL}}{3 \text{ hr}} \times \frac{15}{60} = \frac{83}{1} \times \frac{1}{4} =$$

$$\frac{83}{4} = 20.75$$

Answer: 21 gtts/minute

28. $$\frac{200 \text{ mL}}{1.5 \text{ hr}} \times \frac{15}{60} = \frac{133}{1} \times \frac{1}{4} =$$

$$\frac{133}{4} = 33.25$$

Answwer: 33 gtts/min

Answers to Chapter Review

1. $$\frac{1000 \text{ mL}}{8 \text{ h}} \times \frac{20 \text{ gtt/mL}}{60 \text{ min}} = 42 \text{ gtt/min}$$

2. $$\frac{2500 \text{ mL}}{24 \text{ h}} \times \frac{10 \text{ gtt/mL}}{60 \text{ min}} = 17 \text{ gtt/min}$$

3. $$\frac{500 \text{ mL}}{4 \text{ h}} \times \frac{15 \text{ gtt/mL}}{60 \text{ min}} = 31 \text{ gtt/min}$$

4. $$\frac{300 \text{ mL}}{6 \text{ h}} \times \frac{60 \text{ gtt/mL}}{60 \text{ min}} = 50 \text{ gtt/min}$$

5. $$\frac{1000 \text{ mL}}{24 \text{ h}} \times \frac{60 \text{ gtt/mL}}{60 \text{ min}} = 42 \text{ gtt/min}$$

6. $$\frac{1000 \text{ mL}}{12 \text{ h}} \times \frac{10 \text{ gtt/mL}}{60 \text{ min}} = 14 \text{ gtt/min}$$

7. $$\frac{1000 \text{ mL}}{10 \text{ h}} \times \frac{20 \text{ gtt/mL}}{60 \text{ min}} = 33 \text{ gtt/min}$$

8. $$\frac{1500 \text{ mL}}{12 \text{ h}} \times \frac{10 \text{ gtt/mL}}{60 \text{ min}} = 21 \text{ gtt/min}$$

9. $$\frac{500 \text{ mL}}{4 \text{ h}} \times \frac{10 \text{ gtt/mL}}{60 \text{ min}} = 21 \text{ gtt/min}$$

10. $$\frac{250 \text{ mL}}{3 \text{ h}} \times \frac{10 \text{ gtt/mL}}{60 \text{ min}} = 14 \text{ gtt/min}$$

11. $$\frac{1500 \text{ mL}}{8 \text{ h}} \times \frac{20 \text{ gtt/mL}}{60 \text{ min}} = 63 \text{ gtt/min}$$

12. $$\frac{3000 \text{ mL}}{24 \text{ h}} \times \frac{15 \text{ gtt/mL}}{60 \text{ min}} = 31 \text{ gtt/min}$$

13. $$\frac{2000 \text{ mL}}{24 \text{ h}} \times \frac{15 \text{ gtt/mL}}{60 \text{ min}} = 21 \text{ gtt/min}$$

*Note: 1L = 1000 mL; therefore 2L = 2000 mL

14. $$\frac{1000 \text{ mL}}{7 \text{ h}} \times \frac{10 \text{ gtt/mL}}{60 \text{ min}} = 24 \text{ gtt/min}$$

15. $$\frac{500 \text{ mL}}{4 \text{ h}} \times \frac{60 \text{ gtt/mL}}{60 \text{ min}} = 125 \text{ gtt/min}$$

16. $$\frac{1000 \text{ mL}}{6 \text{ h}} \times \frac{20 \text{ gtt/mL}}{60 \text{ min}} = 56 \text{ gtt/min}$$

17. $$\frac{250 \text{ mL}}{8 \text{ h}} \times \frac{60 \text{ gtt/mL}}{60 \text{ min}} = 31 \text{ gtt/min}$$

18. $$\frac{50 \text{ mL}}{1 \text{ h}} \times \frac{60 \text{ gtt/mL}}{60 \text{ min}} = 50 \text{ gtt/min}$$

19. $$\frac{150 \text{ mL}}{1 \text{ h}} \times \frac{15 \text{ gtt/mL}}{60 \text{ min}} = 38 \text{ gtt/min}$$

20. $\dfrac{500 \text{ mL}}{6 \text{ h}} \times \dfrac{12 \text{ gtt/mL}}{60 \text{ min}} = 17 \text{ gtt/min}$

21. $\dfrac{1500 \text{ mL}}{12 \text{ h}} \times \dfrac{10 \text{ gtt/mL}}{60 \text{ min}} = 21 \text{ gtt/min}$

22. $\dfrac{1500 \text{ mL}}{24 \text{ h}} \times \dfrac{12 \text{ gtt/mL}}{60 \text{ min}} = 13 \text{ gtt/min}$

23. $\dfrac{2000 \text{ mL}}{16 \text{ h}} \times \dfrac{20 \text{ gtt/mL}}{60 \text{ min}} = 42 \text{ gtt/min}$

24. $\dfrac{500 \text{ mL}}{8 \text{ h}} \times \dfrac{15 \text{ gtt/mL}}{60 \text{ min}} = 16 \text{ gtt/min}$

25. $\dfrac{250 \text{ mL}}{10 \text{ h}} \times \dfrac{60 \text{ gtt/mL}}{60 \text{ min}} = 25 \text{ gtt/min}$

26. $\dfrac{75 \text{ mL}}{1 \text{ h}} \times \dfrac{60 \text{ gtt/mL}}{60 \text{ min}} = 75 \text{ gtt/min}$

27. $\dfrac{125 \text{ mL}}{1 \text{ h}} \times \dfrac{20 \text{ gtt/mL}}{60 \text{ min}} = 42 \text{ gtt/min}$

28. $\dfrac{40 \text{ mL}}{1 \text{ h}} \times \dfrac{60 \text{ gtt/mL}}{60 \text{ min}} = 40 \text{ gtt/min}$

29. $50 \text{ mL} \times \dfrac{60 \text{ gtt/mL}}{45 \text{ min}} = 67 \text{ gtt/min}$

30. $\dfrac{90 \text{ mL}}{1 \text{ h}} \times \dfrac{15 \text{ gtt/mL}}{60 \text{ min}} = 23 \text{ gtt/min}$

31. $\dfrac{150 \text{ mL}}{1 \text{ h}} \times \dfrac{10 \text{ gtt/mL}}{60 \text{ min}} = 25 \text{ gtt/min}$

32. $\dfrac{3000 \text{ mL}}{24 \text{ h}} \times \dfrac{15 \text{ gtt/mL}}{60 \text{ min}} = 31 \text{ gtt/min}$

33. $50 \text{ mL} \times \dfrac{10 \text{ gtt/mL}}{40 \text{ min}} = 13 \text{ gtt/min}$

34. $100 \text{ mL} \times \dfrac{20 \text{ gtt/mL}}{30 \text{ min}} = 67 \text{ gtt/min}$

35. $\dfrac{250 \text{ mL}}{5 \text{ h}} \times \dfrac{20 \text{ gtt/mL}}{60 \text{ min}} = 17 \text{ gtt/min}$

36. $\dfrac{80 \text{ mL}}{1 \text{ h}} \times \dfrac{20 \text{ gtt/mL}}{60 \text{ min}} = 27 \text{ gtt/min}$

37. $150 \text{ mL} \times \dfrac{12 \text{ gtt/mL}}{30 \text{ min}} = 60 \text{ gtt/min}$

38. $50 \text{ mL} \times \dfrac{60 \text{ gtt/mL}}{30 \text{ min}} = 100 \text{ gtt/min}$

39. $\dfrac{500 \text{ mL}}{3 \text{ h}} \times \dfrac{10 \text{ gtt/mL}}{60 \text{ min}} = 28 \text{ gtt/min}$

40. $\dfrac{250 \text{ mL}}{2 \text{ h}} \times \dfrac{15 \text{ gtt/mL}}{60 \text{ min}} = 31 \text{ gtt/min}$

41. $\dfrac{1750 \text{ mL}}{24 \text{ h}} \times \dfrac{10 \text{ gtt/mL}}{60 \text{ min}} = 12 \text{ gtt/min}$

42. $\dfrac{150 \text{ mL}}{1.5 \text{ h}} \times \dfrac{60 \text{ gtt/mL}}{60 \text{ min}} = 100 \text{ gtt/min}$

43. Note: 1 L = 1000 mL; Therefore,
    2 mL = 2000 mL

    $\dfrac{2000 \text{ mL}}{16 \text{ h}} = 125 \text{ mL/h}$

44. $\dfrac{500 \text{ mL}}{4 \text{ h}} = 125 \text{ mL/h}$

45. $\dfrac{200 \text{ mL}}{2 \text{ h}} = 100 \text{ mL/h}$

46. $\dfrac{500 \text{ mL}}{8 \text{h}} = 63 \text{ mL/h}$

47. $\dfrac{500 \text{ mL}}{6 \text{ h}} \times \dfrac{10 \text{ gtt/mL}}{60 \text{ min}} = 14 \text{ gtt/min}$

48. $\dfrac{1100 \text{ mL}}{12 \text{ h}} \times \dfrac{20 \text{ gtt/mL}}{60 \text{ min}} = 31 \text{ gtt/min}$

49. $\dfrac{3000 \text{ mL}}{20 \text{ h}} \times \dfrac{20 \text{ gtt/mL}}{60 \text{ min}} = 50 \text{ gtt/min}$

50. $\dfrac{500 \text{ mL}}{6 \text{ h}} \times \dfrac{10 \text{ gtt/mL}}{60 \text{ min}} = 14 \text{ gtt/min}$

51. Time remaining = 7 hours
    Volume remaining = 300 mL

    $\dfrac{300 \text{ mL}}{7 \text{ h}} \times \dfrac{15 \text{ gtt/mL}}{60 \text{ min}} = 11 \text{ gtt/min}$

Slow the IV rate from 13 gtt/min to 11 gtt/min

52. Time remaining = 4 hours.
Volume remaining = 600 mL

$$\frac{600 \text{ mL}}{4 \text{ h}} \times \frac{20 \text{ gtt/mL}}{60 \text{ min}} = 50 \text{ gtt/min}$$

53. Time remaining = 4 hours.
Volume remaining = 400 mL

a) $\frac{400 \text{ mL}}{4 \text{ h}} = 100 \text{ mL/hr}$

The hourly rate must be adjusted first; then gtt/min recalculated.

b) $\frac{100 \text{ mL}}{1 \text{ h}} \times \frac{15 \text{ gtt/mL}}{60 \text{ min}} = 25 \text{ gtt/min}$

The IV was ahead. Slow the IV from 31 gtts/min to 25 gtt/minn. The original IV order of 125 mL/hr = 31 gtt/min.

54. Time remaining = 5 hours.
Volume remaining = 250 mL

$$\frac{250 \text{ mL}}{5 \text{ h}} \times \frac{10 \text{ gtt/mL}}{60 \text{ min}} = 8 \text{ gtt/min}$$

The IV is ahead of time. The rate must be slowed to 8 gtt/min.

55. Time remaining = 4 hours.
Volume remaning = 600 mL

a) The IV is behind time.

$$\frac{600 \text{ mL}}{4 \text{ h}} \times \frac{15 \text{ gtt/mL}}{60 \text{ min}} = 38 \text{ gtt/min}$$

The IV would have to be increased from 25 gtt/min which it was originally to infuse at

$$\frac{1000 \text{ mL}}{10 \text{ h}} \times \frac{15 \text{gtt/mL}}{60 \text{ min}} = 25 \text{ gtt/min}$$

to 38 gtt/min.

56. $\frac{900 \text{ mL}}{x \text{ hours}} \times \frac{15 \text{ gtt/mL}}{60 \text{ min}} = 80 \text{ gtt/min}$

Time: 2.81 hours. Since .81 represents a fraction of an additional hour, convert it to minutes multiply by 60 minutes.

Answer: 2 hours and 49 minutes.

57. $\frac{1000 \text{ mL}}{100 \text{ cc/hr}} = 10 \text{ hours}$

58. $\frac{1000 \text{ mL}}{x \text{ hours}} \times \frac{10 \text{ gtt/mL}}{60 \text{ min}} = 20 \text{ gtt/min}$

Time: 8.33 hours. .33 × 60 = 19.8 = 20 minutes

Answer: 8 hours and 20 minutes.

59. $\frac{450 \text{ mL}}{x \text{ hours}} \times \frac{20 \text{ gtt/mL}}{60 \text{ min}} = 25 \text{ gtt/min}$

Answer: 6 hours.

60. $\frac{100 \text{ mL}}{x \text{ hours}} \times \frac{15 \text{ gtt/mL}}{60 \text{ min}} = 10 \text{ gtt/min}$

Answer: 2.5 hours = 2 1/2 hours

61. $\frac{x \text{ mL}}{8 \text{ hours}} \times \frac{15 \text{ gtt/mL}}{60 \text{ min}} = 25 \text{ gtt/min}$

800 mL

62. $\frac{x \text{ mL}}{10 \text{ hours}} \times \frac{60 \text{ gtt/mL}}{60 \text{ min}} = 40 \text{ gtt/min}$

400 mL

63. $\frac{x \text{ mL}}{5 \text{ hours}} \times \frac{15 \text{ gtt/mL}}{60 \text{ min}} = 30 \text{ gtt/min}$

600 mL

64 a) 10 mEq : 500 mL = 2 mEq : x mL

10 x = 500 × 2

$$\frac{10 x}{10} = \frac{1000}{10}$$

$x = 100$ mL. Therefore 100 mL of fluid would be needed to adminnister 2 mEq of Potassium Chloride.

b) $\dfrac{100 \text{ mL}}{1 \text{ hour}} \times \dfrac{20 \text{ gtt/mL}}{60 \text{ min}} = 33 \text{ gtt/min}$

33 gtt/min would deliver 2 mEq of Potassium Chloride each hour.

65. a) 30 mEq : 1000 mL = 4 mEq : x mL

$\dfrac{30\,x}{30} = \dfrac{4000}{30} = 133.33$

Answer: 133 mL would deliver 4 mEq of Potassium Chloride

b) $\dfrac{133 \text{ mL}}{1 \text{ hour}} \times \dfrac{15 \text{ gtt/mL}}{60 \text{ min}} = 33 \text{ gtt/min}$

33 gtt/min would deliver 4 mEq of Potassium Chloride each hour.

66. 50 U : 250 mL = 7U : x mL

$\dfrac{50\,x}{50} = \dfrac{1750}{50} = 35 \text{ mL/hr}$

Answer: 35 mL/hr

67. 100U : 250 mL = 18U : x mL

$\dfrac{100\,x}{100} = \dfrac{4500}{100} = 45 \text{ mL/hr}$

Answer: 45 mL/hr

68. 100U : 100 mL = 11U : x mL

$\dfrac{100\,x}{100} = \dfrac{1100}{100} = 11 \text{ mL/hr}$

Answer: 11 mL/hr

69. $\dfrac{150 \text{ mL}}{1 \text{ h}} \times \dfrac{10 \text{ gtt/mL}}{60 \text{ min}} = 25 \text{ gtt/min}$

70. $40 \text{ mL} \times \dfrac{60 \text{ gtt/mL}}{40 \text{ min}} = 60 \text{ gtt/min}$

71. $35 \text{ mL} \times \dfrac{60 \text{ gtt/mL}}{30 \text{ min}} = 70 \text{ gtt/min}$

72. $80 \text{ mL} \times \dfrac{15 \text{ gtt/mL}}{40 \text{ min}} = 30 \text{ gtt/min}$

73. $50 \text{ mL} \times \dfrac{10 \text{ gtt/mL}}{25 \text{ min}} = 20 \text{ gtt/min}$

74. $\dfrac{65 \text{ mL}}{1 \text{ h}} \times \dfrac{15 \text{ gtt/mL}}{60 \text{ min}} = 16 \text{ gtt/min}$

Chapter 21

Answers to Chapter Review

1. $10{,}000 \, U : 1 \, mL = 3500 \, U : x \, mL$ OR $\dfrac{3{,}500 \, U}{10{,}000 \, U} \times 1 \, mL = x \, mL$

   $x = 0.35 \, mL$. The dosage ordered is less than what's available. Therefore, less than 1 mL would be needed to administer the dose.

   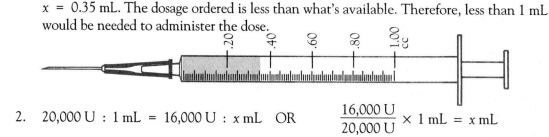

2. $20{,}000 \, U : 1 \, mL = 16{,}000 \, U : x \, mL$ OR $\dfrac{16{,}000 \, U}{20{,}000 \, U} \times 1 \, mL = x \, mL$

   Answer: 0.8 mL. The dosage ordered is less than what's available, therefore less than 1 mL would be needed to administer the dose.

   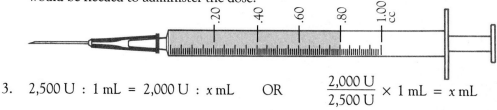

3. $2{,}500 \, U : 1 \, mL = 2{,}000 \, U : x \, mL$ OR $\dfrac{2{,}000 \, U}{2{,}500 \, U} \times 1 \, mL = x \, mL$

   Answer: 0.8 mL. The dosage ordered is less than what's available, therefore less than 1 mL would be needed to administer the dose.

   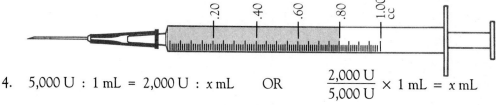

4. $5{,}000 \, U : 1 \, mL = 2{,}000 \, U : x \, mL$ OR $\dfrac{2{,}000 \, U}{5{,}000 \, U} \times 1 \, mL = x \, mL$

   Answer: 0.4 mL. The dosage ordered is less than what's available, therefore less than 1 mL is needed to administer the dose.

   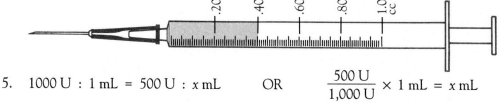

5. $1000 \, U : 1 \, mL = 500 \, U : x \, mL$ OR $\dfrac{500 \, U}{1{,}000 \, U} \times 1 \, mL = x \, mL$

   Answer: 0.5 mL. The dosage ordered is less than what's available, therefore you would need less than a mL to administer the dose.

   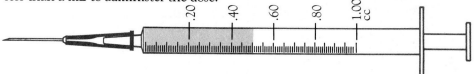

6. $10\,U : 1\,mL = 10\,U : x\,mL$ OR $\dfrac{10\,U}{10\,U} \times 1\,mL = x\,mL$

1 mL contains 10 U, so 1 mL would be needed to administer the dose.

7. $10{,}000\,U : 1\,mL = 50{,}000\,U : x\,mL$ $\dfrac{50{,}000\,U}{10{,}000\,U} \times 1\,mL = x\,mL$

Answer: 5 mL would be needed to administer the dose. The dosage ordered is greater than what's available. Therefore more than a mL would be required to administer the dose.

8. $20{,}000\,U : 1\,mL = 15{,}000\,U : x\,mL$ OR $\dfrac{15{,}000\,U}{20{,}000\,U} \times 1\,mL = x\,mL$

Answer: 0.75 mL. The dosage ordered is less than what's available. Therefore less than a mL would be required to administer the dose.

9. $2{,}500\,U : 1\,mL = 3000\,U : x\,mL$ OR $\dfrac{3{,}000\,U}{2{,}500\,U} \times 1\,mL = x\,mL$

Answer: 1.2 mL. The dosage ordered is more than what's available. Therefore you would need more than 1 mL to administer the dose.

10. $20{,}000\,U : 1\,mL = 17{,}000\,U : x\,mL$ OR $\dfrac{17{,}000\,U}{20{,}000\,U} \times 1\,mL = x\,mL$

Answer: 0.85 mL. The dose ordered is less than what's available. You would need less than 1 mL to administer the dose.

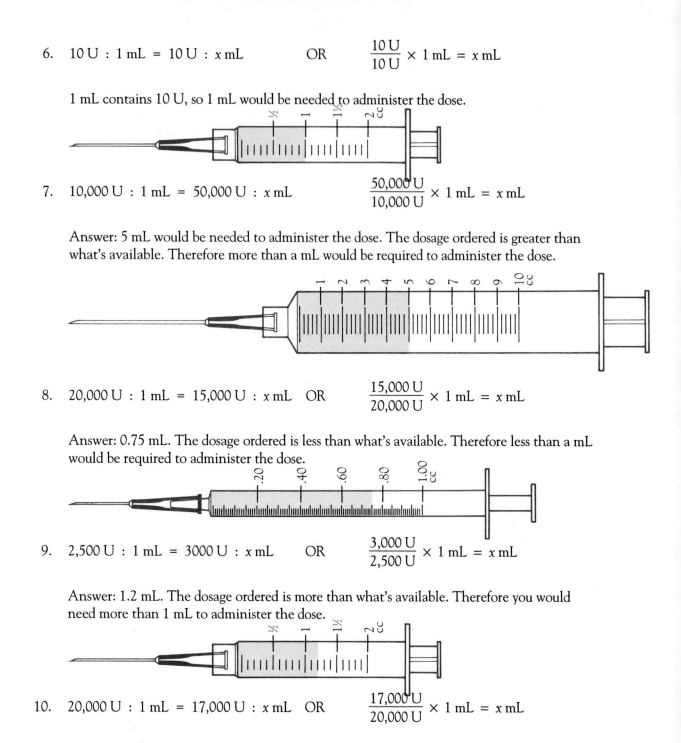

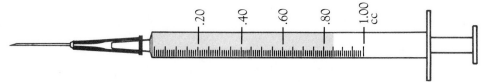

11. $10,000 \text{ U} : 1 \text{ mL} = 8,500 \text{ U} : x \text{ mL}$ OR $\dfrac{8,500 \text{ U}}{10,000 \text{ U}} \times 1 \text{ mL} = x \text{ mL}$

Answer: 0.85 mL. The dosage ordered is less than what's available. You will need less than 1 mL to administer the dose.

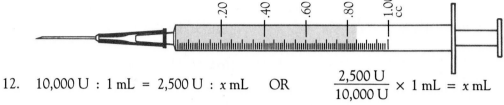

12. $10,000 \text{ U} : 1 \text{ mL} = 2,500 \text{ U} : x \text{ mL}$ OR $\dfrac{2,500 \text{ U}}{10,000 \text{ U}} \times 1 \text{ mL} = x \text{ mL}$

Answer: 0.25 mL. The dose ordered is less than what's available. Less than 1 mL would be required to administer the dose.

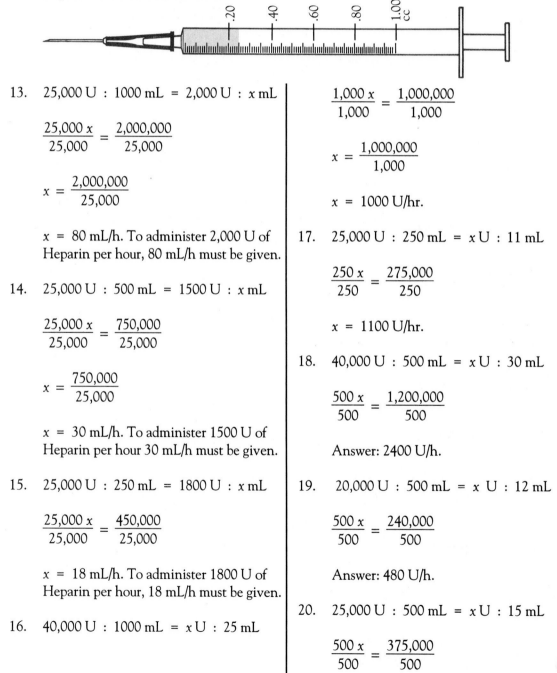

13. $25,000 \text{ U} : 1000 \text{ mL} = 2,000 \text{ U} : x \text{ mL}$

$\dfrac{25,000\, x}{25,000} = \dfrac{2,000,000}{25,000}$

$x = \dfrac{2,000,000}{25,000}$

$x = 80$ mL/h. To administer 2,000 U of Heparin per hour, 80 mL/h must be given.

14. $25,000 \text{ U} : 500 \text{ mL} = 1500 \text{ U} : x \text{ mL}$

$\dfrac{25,000\, x}{25,000} = \dfrac{750,000}{25,000}$

$x = \dfrac{750,000}{25,000}$

$x = 30$ mL/h. To administer 1500 U of Heparin per hour 30 mL/h must be given.

15. $25,000 \text{ U} : 250 \text{ mL} = 1800 \text{ U} : x \text{ mL}$

$\dfrac{25,000\, x}{25,000} = \dfrac{450,000}{25,000}$

$x = 18$ mL/h. To administer 1800 U of Heparin per hour, 18 mL/h must be given.

16. $40,000 \text{ U} : 1000 \text{ mL} = x \text{ U} : 25 \text{ mL}$

$\dfrac{1,000\, x}{1,000} = \dfrac{1,000,000}{1,000}$

$x = \dfrac{1,000,000}{1,000}$

$x = 1000$ U/hr.

17. $25,000 \text{ U} : 250 \text{ mL} = x \text{ U} : 11 \text{ mL}$

$\dfrac{250\, x}{250} = \dfrac{275,000}{250}$

$x = 1100$ U/hr.

18. $40,000 \text{ U} : 500 \text{ mL} = x \text{ U} : 30 \text{ mL}$

$\dfrac{500\, x}{500} = \dfrac{1,200,000}{500}$

Answer: 2400 U/h.

19. $20,000 \text{ U} : 500 \text{ mL} = x \text{ U} : 12 \text{ mL}$

$\dfrac{500\, x}{500} = \dfrac{240,000}{500}$

Answer: 480 U/h.

20. $25,000 \text{ U} : 500 \text{ mL} = x \text{ U} : 15 \text{ mL}$

$\dfrac{500\, x}{500} = \dfrac{375,000}{500}$

Answer: 750 U/hr.

21. a) $\dfrac{1000 \text{ mL}}{24 \text{ h}} = 41.66 = 42 \text{ mL/h}$

$40,000 \text{ U} : 1000 \text{ mL} = x \text{ U} : 42 \text{ mL}$

$\dfrac{1,000\,x}{1,000} = \dfrac{1,680,000}{1,000}$

$x = \dfrac{1,680,000}{1,000}$

$x = 1,680 \text{ U/hr}$

b) $\dfrac{42 \text{ mL}}{1 \text{ hr}} \times \dfrac{15 \text{ gtt/mL}}{60} = 11 \text{ gtt/min}$

22. a) Calculate mL/hr

$\dfrac{1000 \text{ mL}}{10 \text{ h}} = 100 \text{ mL/hr}$

b) Calculate U/hr

$15,000 \text{ U} : 1000 \text{ mL} = x \text{ U} : 100 \text{ mL}$

$\dfrac{1,000\,x}{1,000} = \dfrac{1,500,000}{1,000}$

$x = \dfrac{1,500,000}{1,000}$

$x = 1,500 \text{ U/hr.}$

23. a) $35,000 \text{ U} : 1000 \text{ mL} = x \text{ U} : 20 \text{ mL}$

$\dfrac{1,000\,x}{1,000} = \dfrac{700,000}{1,000}$

$x = \dfrac{700,000}{1,000}$

$x = 700 \text{ U/hr.}$

b) $\dfrac{20 \text{ mL}}{1 \text{ hr}} \times \dfrac{60 \text{ gtt/mL}}{60} = 20 \text{ gtt/min}$

24. a) Convert gtt/min to mL/min
$10 \text{ gtt} : 1 \text{ mL} = 20 \text{ gtt} : x \text{ mL}$

$\dfrac{10\,x}{10} = \dfrac{20}{10}$

$x = 2 \text{ mL/min}$

b) Convert mL/min to mL/hr.
$2 \text{ mL} \times 60 \text{ min} = 120 \text{ mL/hr}$

c) $10,000 \text{ U} : 500 \text{ mL} = x \text{ U} : 120 \text{ mL}$

$\dfrac{500\,x}{500} = \dfrac{1,200,000}{500}$

$x = \dfrac{1,200,000}{500}$

$x = 2,400 \text{ U/hr}$

25. $25,000 \text{ U} : 500 \text{ mL} = x \text{ U} : 25 \text{ mL}$

$\dfrac{500\,x}{500} = \dfrac{625,000}{500}$

Answer: 1250 U/hr

26. $20,000 \text{ U} : 500 \text{ mL} = x \text{ U} : 40 \text{ mL}$

$\dfrac{500\,x}{500} = \dfrac{800,000}{500}$

Answer: 1600 U/hr

27. a) Calculate mL/hr to be administered

$40,000 \text{ U} : 1000 \text{ mL} = 1400 \text{ U} : x \text{ mL}$

$\dfrac{40,000\,x}{40,000} = \dfrac{1,400,000}{40,000}$

$x = 35 \text{ mL/hr}$

b) Calculate gtts/min.

$\dfrac{35 \text{ mL}}{1 \text{ hr}} \times \dfrac{15 \text{ gtt/mL}}{60 \text{ min}} = 8.75 =$

9 gtt/min

28. a) $40,000 \text{ U} : 1000 \text{ mL} = 1000 \text{ U} : x \text{ mL}$

$$\frac{40{,}000\,x}{40{,}000} = \frac{1{,}000{,}000}{40{,}000}$$

$$x = \frac{1{,}000{,}000}{40{,}000}$$

$$x = 25 \text{ mL/hr.}$$

b) $\dfrac{25 \text{ mL}}{1 \text{ hr}} \times \dfrac{15 \text{ gtt/mL}}{60 \text{ min}} = 6.25 =$

6 gtt/min

29. a) 25,000 U : 500 mL = 1000 U : x mL

$$\frac{25{,}000\,x}{25{,}000} = \frac{500{,}000}{25{,}000}$$

$$x = \frac{500{,}000}{25{,}000}$$

$$x = 20 \text{ mL/hr}$$

b) $\dfrac{20 \text{ mL}}{1 \text{ hr}} \times \dfrac{60 \text{ gtt/mL}}{60 \text{ min}} = 20 \text{ gtt/min}$

30. a) 25,000 U : 1000 mL = 2000 U : x mL

$$\frac{25{,}000\,x}{25{,}000} = \frac{2{,}000{,}000}{25{,}000}$$

$$x = \frac{2{,}000{,}000}{25{,}000}$$

$$x = 80 \text{ mL/hr}$$

b) $\dfrac{80 \text{ mL}}{1 \text{ hr}} \times \dfrac{15 \text{ gtt/mL}}{60 \text{ min}} = 20 \text{ gtt/min}$

31. a) Convert gtt/min to mL/min

15 gtt : 1 mL = 15 gtt : x mL

$$\frac{15\,x}{15} = \frac{15}{15}$$

$$x = 1 \text{ mL/min}$$

b) Convert mL/min to mL/hr.

1 mL/min × 60 min = 60 mL/hr

c) Calculate units per hour

50,000 U : 1000 mL = x U : 60 mL

$$\frac{1{,}000\,x}{1{,}000} = \frac{3{,}000{,}000}{1{,}000}$$

$$x = \frac{3{,}000{,}000}{1{,}000}$$

$$x = 3{,}000 \text{ U/hr}$$

32. a) Convert gtt/min to mL/min
10 gtt : 1 mL = 20 gtt : x mL

$$\frac{10\,x}{10} = \frac{20}{10}$$

$$x = 2 \text{ mL/min}$$

b) Convert mL/min to mL/hr
2 mL/min × 60 min = 120 mL/hr.

c) Calculate units per hour
25,000 U : 250 mL = x U : 120 mL

$$\frac{250\,x}{250} = \frac{3{,}000{,}000}{250}$$

$$x = \frac{3{,}000{,}000}{250}$$

$$x = 12{,}000 \text{ U/hr}$$

33. a) Convert gtt/min to mL/min
60 gtt : 1 mL = 20 gtt : x mL

$$\frac{60\,x}{60} = \frac{20}{60}$$

$$x = 0.33 \text{ mL/min}$$

b) convert mL/min to mL/hr
0.33 mL/min × 60 min =
19.8 mL/hr = 20 mL/hr

c) Calculate units per hour
20,000 U : 500 mL = x U : 20 mL

$$\frac{500\,x}{500} = \frac{400{,}000}{500}$$

$$x = \frac{400,000}{500}$$

$$x = 800 \text{ units/hr}$$

34. a) Convert gtt/min to mL/min
    15 gtt : 1 mL = 14 gtt : x mL

$$\frac{15\,x}{15} = \frac{14}{15}$$

$$x = 0.93 \text{ mL/min}$$

b) Convert mL/min to mL/hr
   0.93 mL/min × 60 min = 55.8 = 56 mL/hr.

c) Calculate units per hour.
   25,000 U : 1000 mL = x U : 56 mL

$$\frac{1,000\,x}{1,000} = \frac{1,400,000}{1,000}$$

$$x = \frac{1,400,000}{1000}$$

$$x = 1400 \text{ U/hr}$$

35. a) Convert gtt/min to mL/min
    10 gtt : 1 mL = 24 gtt : x mL

$$\frac{10\,x}{10} = \frac{24}{10}$$

$$x = 2.4 \text{ mL/min}$$

b) Convert mL/min to mL/hr
   2.4 mL/min × 60 min = 144 mL/hr

c) Calculate units per hour.
   20,000 U : 1000 mL = x U : 144 mL

$$\frac{1,000\,x}{1,000} = \frac{2,880,000}{1,000}$$

$$x = \frac{2,880,000}{1000}$$

$$x = 2,880 \text{ U/hr}$$

36. 30,000 U : 500 mL = x U : 25 mL

$$\frac{500\,x}{500} = \frac{750,000}{500}$$

$$x = \frac{750,000}{500}$$

$$x = 1500 \text{ U of Heparin per hour}$$

37. 20,000 U : 1000 mL = x U : 40 mL

$$\frac{1,000\,x}{1,000} = \frac{800,000}{1,000}$$

$$x = \frac{800,000}{1000}$$

$$x = 800 \text{ units of Heparin per hour}$$

38. 40,000 U : 500 mL = x U : 25 mL

$$\frac{500\,x}{500} = \frac{1,000,000}{500}$$

$$x = \frac{1,000,000}{500}$$

$$x = 2000 \text{ U/hr.}$$

39. 35,000 U : 1000 mL = x U : 20 mL

$$\frac{1000\,x}{1000} = \frac{700,000}{1000}$$

$$x = \frac{700,000}{1000}$$

$$x = 700 \text{ U/hr}$$

40. 25,000 U : 1,000 mL = x U : 30 mL

$$\frac{1000\,x}{1000} = \frac{750,000}{1000}$$

$$x = \frac{750,000}{1000}$$

$$x = 750 \text{ U/hr.}$$

Chapter 22

Answers to Practice Problems:

1. 2 mg : 250 mL = x mg : 30 mL

    $$\frac{250\,x}{250} = \frac{60}{250}$$

    x = 0.24 mg/hr.

    Convert mg to mcg (1000 mcg = 1 mg)
    0.24 mg = 240 mcg/hr

    Convert mcg/hr to mcg/min
    240 mcg/hr ÷ 60 minutes = 4 mcg/min

2. Change g to mg. (Note you
    were asked mg/min and mg/hr)
    0.25 g = 250 mg
    Calculate mg to hr.
    250 mg : 8 hr = x mg : 1 hour

    $$\frac{8\,x}{8} = \frac{250}{8}$$

    x = 31.25 = 31.3 mg/hr

    Answer: 31.3 mg/hr

    Convert mg/hr to mg/min
    31.3 mg/hr ÷ 60 = 0.52 mg/minute

3. Note: Calculate units per hour only.

    a) 60 gtt : 1 mL : 15 gtt : x mL

    $$\frac{60\,x}{60} = \frac{15}{60}$$

    x = 0.25 mL/min

    b) 0.25 mL/min × 60 = 15 mL/hr

    c) 10 U : 1000 cc = x U : 15 mL

    $$\frac{1000\,x}{1000} = \frac{150}{1000}$$

    x = 0.15 U/hr.

4. a) Determine the dosage per minute
       60 kg × 3 mcg/kg = 180 mcg/min.

    b) Convert to dosage per hour
       180 mcg/min × 60 = 10,800 mcg/hr

    c) Convert to like units
       10800 mcg = 10.8 mg

       Calculate flow rate mL/hr.
       50 mg : 250 mL = 10.8 mg : x mL
       50x = 250 × 10.8

       $$\frac{50\,x}{50} = \frac{2700}{50}$$

       x = 54 mL/hr.

5. Solution:
    50 mg : 250 mL = x mg : 3 mL/hr

    $$\frac{250\,x}{250} = \frac{150}{250}$$

    x = 0.6 mg/hr

    Convert to mcg (1000 mcg = 1 mg)
    0.6 mg = 600 mcg/hr.

    Convert mcg/hr to mcg/min.
    600 mcg/hr ÷ 60 minutes = 10 mcg/min

    Answer:
    a) 600 mcg/hr
    b) 10 mcg/min

Answers to Chapter Review

1. a) Calculate the dosage per hr.
       2 mg : 250 mL = x mg : 30 mL

       $$\frac{250\,x}{250} = \frac{60}{250}$$

       $$x = \frac{60}{250}$$

       x = .24 mg/hr

    b) Convert mg to mcg (1000 mcg = 1 mg)
       1000 × .24 = 240 mcg/hr

c) Convert mcg/hr to mcg/min
   240 mcg/hr ÷ 60 min = 4 mcg/min.

2. a) Calculate dosage per hr
    4 mg : 500 mL = x mg : 40 mL

    $$\frac{500\,x}{500} = \frac{160}{500}$$

    $$x = \frac{160}{500}$$

    x = .32 mg/hr.

    b) Convert to mcg. (1000 mcg = 1 mg)
       1000 × .32 = 320 mcg/hr.

    c) Convert mcg/hr to mcg/min
       320 mcg/hr ÷ 60 min = 5.33 =
       5.3 mcg/min

3. a) Determine dosage per hour
    800 mg : 500 mL = x mg : 30 mL

    $$\frac{24000}{500} = \frac{500\,x}{500}$$

    $$x = \frac{24000}{500} = 48 \text{ mg/hr}$$

    b) Convert mg to mcg (1000 mcg = 1 mg)
       48 mg × 1000 = 48,000 mcg/hr

    c) Convert mcg/hr to mcg/min
       48,000 mcg/hr ÷ 60 min = 800 mcg/min

    200 mg : 5 mL = 800 mg : x mL

    OR

    $$\frac{800 \text{ mg}}{200 \text{ mg}} \times 5 \text{ mL} = x \text{ mL}$$

    Answer: 20 mL. The dose ordered is
    greater than what's available.

4. a) Determine dosage per hour
    50 mg : 250 mL = x mg : 30 mL

    $$\frac{1500}{250} = \frac{250\,x}{250}$$

    $$x = \frac{1500}{250}$$

    x = 6 mg/hr

    b) Convert mg to mcg (1000 mcg = 1 mg)
       6 mg × 1000 = 6,000 mcg/hr.

    c) Convert mcg/hr to mcg/min
       6,000 mcg hr ÷ 60 min = 100 mcg/min

5. a) Calculate mg/hr.
       100 mg : 250 mL = x mg : 25 mL

    $$\frac{250\,x}{250} = \frac{2500}{250}$$

    $$x = \frac{2500}{250}$$

    x = 10 mg/hr.

    b) Convert milligrams to mcg.
       (1000 mcg = 1 mg)
       10 mg = 10,000 mcg/hr

    c) Convert mcg/hr to mcg/min
       10,000 mcg/hr ÷ 60 min = 166.66 =
       166.7 mcg/min

6. a) Convert metric weights to the same as
       answer request.
       1g = 1000 mg
       2000 mg : 250 mL = x mg : 60 mL

    $$\frac{250\,x}{250} = \frac{120,000\ x}{250}$$

    $$x = \frac{120,000}{250}$$

    x = 480 mg/hr.

    b) Convert mg/hr to mg/min
       480 ÷ 60 = 8 mg/min

7 a) Convert g to mg. (1000 mg = 1g)
     0.25 g = 250 mg

  b) Calculate mg/hr
     250 mg : 6 hr = x mg : 1 hr

$$\frac{250}{6} = \frac{6\,x}{6}$$

$$x = \frac{250}{6}$$

$x = 41.66 = 41.7$ mg/hr.

8. a) Convert g to mg. (1000 mg = 1 g)
   2g = 2000 mg.

   b) Calculate mg/hr.
   2000 mg : 250 mL = x mg : 30 mL

   $$\frac{250\,x}{250} = \frac{60,000}{250}$$

   $$x = \frac{60,000}{250}$$

   $x = 240$ mg/hr.

   c) Convert mg/hr to mg/min
   240 mg ÷ 60 = 4 mg/min

9. a) Calculate gtt/min to mL/min
   60 gtt : 1 mL = 45 gtt : x mL

   $$\frac{60\,x}{60} = \frac{45}{60}$$

   $$x = \frac{45}{60}$$

   $x = 0.75$ mL/min

   b) Calculate units/minute
   20 U : 1000 mL = x units : 0.75 mL

   $$\frac{15}{1000} = \frac{1000\,x}{1000}$$

   $$x = \frac{15}{1000}$$

   $x = .015$ U/minute

   c) Calculate units/hr.

   .015 U/minute × 60 min = 0.9 U/hr

10. 30U : 1000 mL = x U : 40 mL

    $$\frac{1200}{1000} = \frac{1000\,x}{1000}$$

    $$x = \frac{1200}{1000}$$

    $x = 1.2$ U/hr

11. 30 U : 500 mL = x U : 45 mL

    $$\frac{1350}{500} = \frac{500\,x}{500}$$

    $$x = \frac{1350}{500}$$

    $x = 2.7$ U/hr.

12. a) Change metric measures to same as
       question. 1g = 1000 mg; therefore
       2 g = 2000 mg

    b) Calculate mg/hr.
       2000 mg : 500 mL : x mg : 30 mL

       $$\frac{60,000}{500} = \frac{500\,x}{500}$$

       $$x = \frac{60,000}{500}$$

       $x = 120$ mg/hr.

    c) mg/hr change to mg/min
       120 mg/hr ÷ 60 min = 2 mg/min

13. a) Calculate mg/hr. Change metric
       measures to same s question.
       2g = 2000 mg.

    b) Calculate mg/hr
       2000 mg : 500 mL = x mg : 45 mL

       $$\frac{90,000}{500} = \frac{500\,x}{500}$$

       $$x = \frac{90,000}{500}$$

$x = 180$ mg/hr

c) Change mg/hr to mg/min
180 mg/hr ÷ 60 min = 3 mg/min

14. a) Determine dosage per hour
400 mcg/min × 60 = 24000 mcg/hr

b) Convert mcg to mg
1000 mcg = 1 mg
24000 mcg/hr = 24 mg/hr

c) Calculate flow rate in mL/hr
50 mg : 250 mL = 24 mg : x mL

$$\frac{50\,x}{50} = \frac{6000}{50}$$

$x = 120$ mL/hr
Set at 120 mL/hr to deliver 24 mg/hr

15. 400 mg : 500 mL = x mg : 35 mL

$$\frac{500\,x}{500} = \frac{14{,}000\,x}{500}$$

$x = 28$ mg/hr

16. a) Calculate mg/hr.
2 mg : 250 mL = x mg : 30 mL

$$\frac{60}{250} = \frac{250\,x}{250}$$

$$x = \frac{60}{250}$$

$x = .24$ mg/hr.

b) Convert mg to mcg.
(1000 mcg = 1 mg)
.24 mg × 1000 = 240 mcg/hr

c) Convert mcg/hr to mcg/min
240 mcg ÷ 60 = 4 mcg/min

17. a) Convert metric weights to same as
answer. 1000 mg = 1 g

b) Calculate mg/hr
1000 mg : 10 hrs = x mg : 1 hr

$$\frac{10\,x}{10} = \frac{1000}{10}$$

$x = 100$ mg/hr

18. 150 mg : 500 mL = x mg : 30 mL

$$\frac{500\,x}{500} = \frac{4500}{500}$$

$$x = \frac{4500}{500}$$

$x = 9$ mg/hr.

19. a) Convert metric weights g to mg.
2 g = 2000 mg (1000 mg = 1g)

b) 2000 mg : 250 mL = x mg : 22 mL

$$\frac{250\,x}{250} = \frac{44{,}000\,x}{250}$$

$$x = \frac{44{,}000}{250}$$

$x = 176$ mg/hr

c) Change mg/hr to mg/min
176 mg/hr ÷ 60 min = 2.93 =
2.9 mg/min

20. a) Calculate dosage per hour
4 mg : 250 mL = x mg : 8 mL

$$\frac{250\,x}{250} = \frac{32}{250}$$

$$x = \frac{32}{250}$$

$x = .128$ mg/hr

b) Convert mg to mcg.
.128 mg × 1000 = 128 mcg/hr

c) Convert mcg/hr to mcg/min.
128 mcg/hr ÷ 60 min =
2.13 mcg/min or 2.1 mcg/min

21. a) 500 mg : 250 mL = x mg : 30 mL

$$\frac{250\,x}{250} = \frac{15{,}000}{250}$$

$$x = \frac{15{,}000}{250}$$

$$x = 60\ \text{mg/hr}$$

b) Convert mg/hr to mg/min
60 mg/hr ÷ 60 min = 1 mg/min

22. a) Calculate mg/hr.
500 mg : 500 mL = x mg : 30 mL

$$\frac{500\,x}{500} = \frac{15{,}000}{500}$$

$$x = \frac{15{,}000}{500}$$

$$x = 30\ \text{mg/hr}$$

b) Convert mg to mcg.
30 mg = 30,000 mcg/hr

c) Convert mcg/hr to mcg/min.
30,000 mcg/hr ÷ 60 min =
500 mcg/min

23. 25 g : 300 mL = 2 g : x mL

$$\frac{25\,x}{25} = \frac{600}{25}$$

$$x = \frac{600}{25}$$

$$x = 24\ \text{mL/hr to administer 2 g.}$$

24. a) Determine dosage per hour.
200 mcg/min × 60 min =
12,000 mcg/hr

b) Convert mcg to mg
(1000 mcg = 1 mg)
12,000 mcg ÷ 1000 = 12 mg/hr

c) Calculate the mL/hr.
400 mg : 500 mL = 12 mg : x mL

$$\frac{400\,x}{400} = \frac{6000}{400}$$

$$x = 15\ \text{mL/hr}$$

25. 25 g : 300 mL = 3 g : x mL

$$\frac{25\,x}{25} = \frac{900}{25}$$

$$x = \frac{900}{25}$$

$$x = 36\ \text{mL/hr to administer 3 g}$$

26. a) Convert dosage per min to dosage
per hour.
10 mcg/min × 60 = 600 mcg/hr.

b) Convert measures to like units
(mcg to mg). 1000 mcg = 1 mg
600 mcg = 600 ÷ 1000 = 0.6 mg

c) Calculate mL/hr.
50 mg : 250 mL = 0.6 mg : x mL

$$\frac{50\,x}{50} = \frac{150}{50}$$

$$x = 3\ \text{mL/hr}$$

d) Calculate the flow rate in gtt/min

To deliver 10 mcg/min the IV is to infuse
at 3 gtt/min.

27. a) Convert weight in lb to kg.
120 lb = 54.54 = 55 kg

b) Calculate dosage per minute.
55 kg × 2 mcg = 110 mcg/min

28. a) No conversion of weight is required.
80 kg × 3 mcg = 240 mcg/minute

29. a) No conversion of weight is required
73.5 kg × 0.7 mg = 51.45 mg/hr

30. a) Convert weight in lbs to kg.
110 lb ÷ 2.2 = 50 kg

b) Calculate dose per hour.
   50 kg × 0.7 mg = 35 mg/hr

c) Calculate the dose per minute
   35 mg/hr ÷ 60 minutes =
      0.58 mg/min = 0.6 mg/min

   The dose is safe; it falls within safe range.

Index